OKANAGAN COLLEGE LIBRARY

03501863

D1571600

OKANAGAN COLLEGE
LIBRARY
BRITISH COLUMBIA

# A Multilevel Approach to the Study of Motor Control and Learning

## Second Edition

**Debra J. Rose**

*California State University, Fullerton*

**Robert W. Christina**

*University of North Carolina, Greensboro*

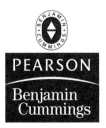

PEARSON

Benjamin
Cummings

San Francisco  Boston  New York
Cape Town  Hong Kong  London  Madrid  Mexico City
Montreal  Munich  Paris  Singapore  Sydney  Tokyo  Toronto

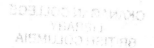

Publisher: Daryl Fox
Senior Acquisitions Editor: Deirdre Espinoza
Development Manager: Claire Alexander
Assistant Editors: Christina Pierson and Alison Rodal
Production Supervisor: Beth Masse
Manufacturing Buyer: Stacey Weinberger
Senior Marketing Manager: Sandra Lindelof
Production and Composition: The Left Coast Group
Cover Designer: Yvo Riezebos Design
Photo Researcher: Diane Austin
Copyeditor: Carla Breidenbach
Cover photo: Getty Images/Zac Macauley

Photo and art credits are found on page 421, which should be considered an extension of the copyright page.

ISBN 0-8053-6031-X

Copyright © 2006 Pearson Education, Inc., publishing as Benjamin Cummings, 1301 Sansome St., San Francisco, CA 94111. All rights reserved. Manufactured in the United States of America. This publication is protected by Copyright and permission should be obtained from the publisher prior to any prohibited reproduction, storage in a retrieval system, or transmission in any form or by any means, electronic, mechanical, photocopying, recording, or likewise. To obtain permission(s) to use material from this work, please submit a written request to Pearson Education, Inc., Permissions Department, 1900 E. Lake Ave., Glenview, IL 60025. For information regarding permissions, call (847) 486-2635.

Many of the designations used by manufacturers and sellers to distinguish their products are claimed as trademarks. Where those designations appear in this book, and the publisher was aware of a trademark claim, the designations have been printed in initial caps or all caps.

Library of Congress Cataloging-in-Publication Data

Rose, Debra J.
    A multilevel approach to the study of motor control and learning/Debra J. Rose, Robert W. Christina.—2nd ed.
        p.; cm.
    Includes bibliographical references and index.
    ISBN 0-8053-6031-X
  1. Motor learning. 2. Afferent pathways.
    [DNLM: 1. Motor Activity. 2. Learning. 3. Psychomotor Performance. WE 103 R795m 2006] I. Christina, Robert W. II. Title.
    QP301.R65 2006
    612.8'11—dc22
                                                                        2005006531

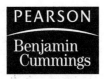

10 9 8 7 6 5 4 3 2 1 DOC 08 07 06 05
www.aw-bc.com

# CONTENTS

# PREFACE

The second edition of a *Multilevel Approach to Motor Control and Learning* expands upon the goal of the first edition: to provide a textbook for upper division undergraduate and entry-level graduate students in kinesiology that addresses motor control and motor learning concepts in the same text. What continues to differentiate this text from others that address one or both of these important subject areas is its multilevel approach. The content contained in this text is not only presented at a behavioral level of analysis but at a neurological level of analysis also. The significantly expanded content at both levels of analysis in the second edition will be particularly appropriate for students interested in pursuing postgraduate studies in health care professions such as physical therapy and/or professional careers in rehabilitation settings.

The book continues to be divided into two sections: Motor Control and Motor Learning. The first section—Chapters 1 through 5—presents an in-depth discussion of the prominent motor control theories and the scientific evidence in support of each theory and/or theoretical perspective. The underlying mechanisms that contribute to motor control are explored at both a behavioral and neurological level of analysis. At the completion of this section, the reader should have acquired a strong understanding of the behavioral and neurological processes that are involved in the planning and executing of many different movement skills.

The second section—Chapters 6 through 12—focuses on the theoretical concepts that underlie the acquisition, retention, and, in some cases, forgetting of learned movement skills. The multilevel theoretical approach is followed in this section also, as the behavioral changes associated with the learning of movement skills are once again linked to the underlying neurological mechanisms. This section of the book also emphasizes practical application as issues related to how motor skills should be introduced and practiced for optimal retention and transfer are discussed.

## New to This Edition

1. A coauthor. It is a privilege and honor to be writing this second edition with my mentor, Dr. Robert Christina. Dr. Christina brings a wealth of knowledge and history of the field of motor control and learning that adds a richness and depth to the content presented in a number of chapters, but most notably the motor learning section of the book.

2. A new chapter that addresses the issue of the transfer of learning.

3. Major restructuring and reordering of chapters. The reordering of chapters provides a more cohesive discussion of the subject matter and was based on reviewer feedback and our own critical review of the first edition.

4. Expanded and updated content in all chapters. There is a more comprehensive discussion of the major theoretical approaches that have guided the research conducted in the areas of motor control and learning.

5. Addition of practical activities at the end of selected chapters. These provide the instructor with opportunities to engage the students in classroom activities that add a practical dimension to the theoretical content presented in the book.

6. Addition of more highlight boxes. Each addresses an important theoretical concept or controversy, a classic experiment, or examples of how motor control and learning theory has been applied to practice.

## Pedagogical Features

The pedagogical features in the second edition have been expanded to include practical activities at the end of selected chapters, additional summary boxes that emphasize important points presented in the text, and new highlights in every chapter that address pivotal research findings from sport and clinical settings, important theoretical concepts, or practical applications of research.

## Acknowledgements

This second edition would not have come to fruition without the significant contributions and support of my coauthor, Bob Christina, and the encouragement of so many of my colleagues in motor control and learning who adopted the first edition of this textbook over six years ago and kept asking when the second edition was going to be published. Of course, our book editors at Benjamin-Cummings kept asking us the same question, as we missed our submission deadlines on multiple occasions. Fortunately for us, Christina Pierson and Deirdre Espinoza both recognized that writing a textbook, even a second edition, is a serious undertaking and one that cannot be rushed if it is to be a product of which everyone can be proud. I would also personally like to thank my faculty colleagues in motor control and learning at Cal State-Fullerton, David Chen and Michelle Barr, who provided me with excellent feedback on the first edition based on their own personal teaching experiences using the book. Finally, I wish to thank each and every undergraduate and graduate student who I have taught in the six years since this book was first published. They have been my very best critics as the target audience for whom this book is intended. I hope that this second edition addresses many of their criticisms of the first edition.

## Reviewers

Laurie Lundy-Ekman, Pacific University; Jeffrey M. Haddad, University of Massachusetts–Amherst; Rachel D. Seidler, University of Michigan; Amy Haufler, University of Maryland; Shane Frehlich, California State University–Northridge; Richard Stratton, Virginia Tech; Steven J. Radlo, Western Illinois University; Ann Gentile, Teachers College, Columbia University; Daniel Corcos, University of Illinois at Chicago; Qin Lai, Wayne State Univeristy; Lori Ploutz-Snyder, Syracuse University; Gabriele Wulf, University of Nevada–Las Vegas.

# INTRODUCTION TO MOTOR CONTROL

*In order to understand the nature of motor control, it is necessary to discover what is actually being controlled and how the various processes governing that control are organized.*

## CHAPTER OBJECTIVES

After studying this chapter, you should be able to:

- Explain why it is important to adopt a multilevel approach to the study of motor control and learning.

- Understand and be able to explain the importance of scientific theory to practice.

- Compare and contrast the underlying assumptions associated with the major theories of

motor control that have guided research over the past century.

- Describe the strengths and weaknesses of each theory of motor control in describing various characteristics of human action.

- Understand and be able to describe how the available degrees of freedom within the human system are organized to produce skilled action.

The book you are about to begin reading is quite unlike most of the textbooks currently available to students interested in learning more about human motor behavior. How is it different? It is different in two important ways. First, it attempts to explore the principles governing both the control *and* the learning of movements in a single textbook, and second, it adopts a multilevel approach to the study of motor control and learning. Not only does it seek to explore the learning and control of human actions at a behavioral, or psychological, level of analysis, but where possible, it also conducts a similar exploration at the neuromotor level of analysis.

By adopting a multilevel approach, we acknowledge the two most important bodies of knowledge that have shaped the field of study known as motor control and learning: neurophysiology and psychology. And we also reveal the many levels of complexity that characterize the learning and control of movement. Historically, writers of motor control and/or motor learning textbooks have tended to describe human motor behavior by drawing from only one of the two bodies of knowledge (Brooks, 1986; Latash, 1998; Magill, 2004;

Schmidt & Lee, 1999). As a result, students acquire a good understanding of such behavioral processes as those believed to be involved in the control and learning of movement skills (e.g., stimulus identification, response selection, response programming) but learn little if anything about where these processes actually occur within the nervous and/or musculoskeletal systems. The students we have introduced to the multilevel approach to motor control and learning believe they have a better understanding of why a particular behavior is occurring because of the knowledge they have acquired about the inner workings of the nervous and musculoskeletal systems with which it interfaces. In short, we feel that more pieces of the puzzle known as motor control and learning fall into place for students when a multilevel approach is used.

## Defining Motor Control

*Motor control:* The study of postures and movements and the mechanisms that underlie them.

What exactly *is* the nature of motor control, and how broadly should the term be applied when describing movement? For example, should the term be reserved for describing the quality of movement expressed by accomplished athletes such as the diver pictured on the cover of this textbook? Or can it also be used to describe the movements of an infant attempting to stand for the first time, a child swinging and missing a pitched baseball, and a frail adult attempting to negotiate a corridor with the assistance of a walker? Perhaps the best way to begin to address this question is by defining the term. Simply stated, **motor control** is the study of postures and movements and the mechanisms that underlie them. This definition suggests that all movements and postures, irrespective of quality, are expressions of motor control.

Theories of motor control must address the "what" and "how" of human control.

In order to understand the nature of motor control, it is necessary to discover *what* is actually being controlled and *how* the various processes governing that control are organized. Although it is clear that muscles and joints are the final targets of motor control, the process by which these agents of movement are recruited remains a subject of considerable interest and controversy among researchers. Throughout the years, systematic research efforts have led to the development of a number of theories and related models of motor control, each of which has contributed significantly to our understanding of human motor control.

We have found over the years that presenting the different theories of motor control in our undergraduate classes, in particular, is not always greeted enthusiastically. In fact, many students have asked us why it is so important to study the different theories of motor control in order to be good teachers, coaches, or clinicians. Our answer is that "theory guides practice." As researchers it influences the types of research questions we ask and the types of experiments we conduct, and as practitioners it influences how we teach new movement skills or apply different treatment strategies with a patient. Certainly a good deal of evidence exists to support this statement as you will learn during the reading of this textbook. Not only have a number of therapeutic techniques and strategies been developed on the basis of different theories of motor control, but many different strategies and methods used by practitioners to assist learners to acquire new motor skills can be directly traced back to a particular theory of motor control. A number of examples of how motor control theories have influenced practice will be provided in the section of this chapter describing the major motor control theories that have been developed over the course of many decades.

What exactly is a theory, and how can it help us better understand how movements are controlled? According to Kerlinger (1973), a **theory** is a set of concepts, propositions, or definitions that are interrelated in some way. They are used to specify relationships among different variables so that we can obtain a systematic view of specific types of phenomena. In the motor control section of this book you will be introduced to a number of different theoretical concepts used to explain different aspects of the planning and control process. For example, you will be introduced to concepts such as reflex chaining, generalized motor programs, and self-organization in the sections describing the different motor control theories that have been developed to explain how movements are planned and executed at a behavioral level of analysis.

*Theory:* A general principle used to account for certain observable phenomena.

In science, theories become powerful tools for not only explaining a specific set of observations cohesively, but for testing certain predictions or **hypotheses** about what might occur in other similar situations. For example, in the study of human motor control, certain behavioral theories have been developed over the years that have attempted to explain the sequence of cognitive processes that are involved in the planning and control of different movements. Certain predictions or hypotheses have been subsequently formulated to explain how the observed processes are adapted or modified in the face of changing task demands and/or environmental constraints. If more than one hypothesis is formulated to explain how the sequencing of the various cognitive processes is altered as a function of different task demands, for example, then a series of tests will be conducted to systematically test each hypothesis. The hypotheses being tested will either be supported or rejected based on whether they match the predicted behavioral outcomes.

*Hypothesis:* A tentative statement or explanation for observed events, which can then be tested by conducting a scientific experiment.

In science, theories are modified to account for new observations or discoveries or are discarded in favor of a new theory with greater explanatory power. As you will learn when you read the section on different motor control theories, some motor control theories have been discarded in favor of others that are better able to account for the myriad of movement patterns we can produce over the course of our lives.

Becoming familiar with the basic assumptions of the different motor control theories will also influence how you practice, whether it is in a physical education, sport, or rehabilitation setting. Embracing the assumptions associated with one or more of the motor control theories may change how you look at control of movements. You are also likely to think more about how you can better identify errors in performance and then develop strategies that will assist the performer to correct them. Once you have been introduced to each of the theories of motor control you will find yourself beginning to re-evaluate certain teaching or treatment strategies you currently use, modifying some, and perhaps discarding others. Most importantly, each of the motor control theories presented in this chapter will provide you with the knowledge and tools needed to develop and implement evidence-based programs and then systematically evaluate the effectiveness of your teaching or treatment methods.

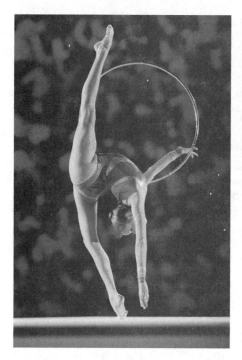
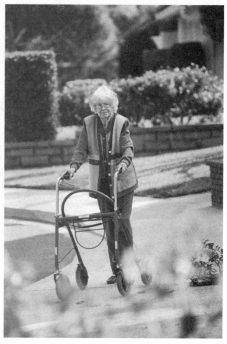

Whether the movements and postures are those of a skilled gymnast or frail older adult, both are expressions of motor control.

## Open- and Closed-Loop Motor Control

One important and defining feature of human motor control is the ability to initiate and control movements differently, based on the availability of sensory feedback. Two types of motor control have been described in the literature to address this ability and are central to at least two of the theories of motor control we will describe in the next section of this chapter. These different types are referred to as **open-loop control** or **closed-loop control.** Although these terms were originally used to describe different models of control in the field of mechanical engineering, they have also proved useful to motor control theorists in their development of different models of human motor control at both a behavioral and neurological level of analysis. As you can see in Figures 1.1a and b, the existence of a hypothetical movement control center and a set of effectors are central to both types of control. What constitutes the primary difference between the two models of motor control is whether feedback is involved in the planning and execution of the movement.

## Open-Loop Motor Control

The open-loop control system depicted in Figure 1.1a does not require that sensory feedback be available and or used to control movements. For movements governed by open-loop control, the central movement executive sends

Movements of short duration and many well-learned skills are performed using an open-loop system of control.

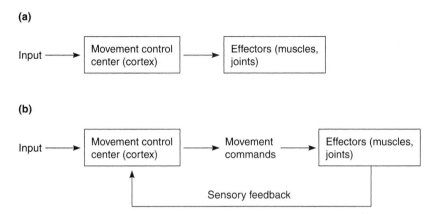

**Figure 1.1** **(a)** Open-loop systems of motor control do not require that sensory feedback be available and/or used to control movements. **(b)** In a closed-loop system of motor control, feedback is involved in the planning and execution of movement.

a movement plan to the effectors (e.g., muscles, joints) that contains all the details necessary to perform the movement. The most convincing evidence in support of an open-loop model of motor control has come from animal studies. Using a surgical technique that deprives the animal of sensory information from one or more limbs, researchers have demonstrated that animals can still perform quite complex movements (Wilson, 1961; Taub & Berman, 1968). These **deafferentation** studies will be referred to again when we discuss motor–program-based theories of motor control in the next section of this chapter.

In the case of closed-loop motor control, feedback derived from the effectors (muscles, joints) directly involved in the movement and from other sensory systems (e.g., vision, audition) is used to inform the movement control center about the movement currently in progress or just completed. This **afferent (sensory) information** is then used by the movement control center to determine whether the intended movement is being executed as planned. If there is a match between the intended plan and the movement in progress, then the movement will proceed without modification. In the case of an already completed movement, a match between the intended plan of action and the movement outcome would result in the individual repeating the movement pattern in the same way on the next attempt.

In the case of a mismatch occurring between the intended movement plan and the actual movement performed, however, the role of the afferent feedback would be to signal a need for the movement control center to modify or change the plan of action. If the movement is still in progress, the movement control center will determine if small changes are needed to correct the errors or a new plan of action is needed because the demands of the task or the environment have changed so much that the original plan is no longer workable.

A closed-loop system of control is used to perform slow and precise movements.

Evidence for closed-loop motor control has largely come from studies using relatively slow aiming movements. In order to determine the extent to which feedback might be used to control these types of movements, researchers eliminate or degrade the sensory information that is normally available in these situations. Not surprisingly, the results of these studies show that performance accuracy declines as one or more sources of feedback (vision, audition, proprioception, etc.) are removed or degraded. This type of motor control is fundamental to the reflex theories of motor control (described on page 7), as well as the closed-loop theory of motor learning (Adams, 1971; see Chapter 6).

## Use of Open- versus Closed-Loop Motor Control

When are we most likely to use one type of motor control in preference to the other? At least part of the decision appears to depend on what type of movement skill is to be accomplished. For example, when performing slow movements that require precision, it would be preferable to use a closed-loop type of motor control so we can use sensory feedback to guide the action by making numerous small corrections as the movement unfolds over time.

Hammering a nail into a piece of wood, performing a balance beam sequence, and threading a needle are all movements to which closed-loop motor control is well suited. That is because in each of these movement scenarios, the movement control center need only send a movement plan to the effectors that contains sufficient information to get the movement started. Thereafter, the available sensory feedback can be used to provide the additional details needed to ensure that the movement plan is carried out as it was originally intended. For the simple skill of hammering a nail into a piece of wood, for example, the movement control center will send out a plan that is sufficiently detailed to get the hammering movement started but will then rely on the afferent information provided by the cutaneous (skin) receptors and proprioceptors (position sensors) of the hammering arm, in addition to vision, to guide the control of the movement until the nail is flush with the wood. Try hammering a nail with your eyes closed and you will soon learn how integral feedback is to the successful performance of this particular movement.

Conversely, movement skills that must be executed in much shorter periods of time will be better suited to an open-loop system of control because it is unlikely that there will be sufficient time available to use the sensory feedback to make changes in the movement plan during its execution. Consider the sport skills of pitching, throwing, or pistol shooting. Each of these skills is performed in a very short period of time, providing insufficient time for feedback to be used to correct errors in the movement plan. In these movement skill scenarios, the movement control center will need to send out a more complete plan of action that contains all the details necessary to perform the skill.

One additional factor that influences which type of motor control is used or the *degree* to which a closed- or open-loop system of control is used is the skill level of the performer. Novice performers need to rely more on sensory feedback to guide their performance, while more skilled performers are capable of performing most, if not all, aspects of a chosen movement without resorting to feedback. Contrast the slow and frequently interrupted playing of novice piano players, who must carefully follow the notes displayed on a music sheet in front of them, with the rapid finger movements of experienced pianists who often do not use sheet music to play musical pieces.

# Theories of Motor Control

Three general categories of theories have dominated the literature related to motor control during the past century. These include reflex theories, hierarchical theories, and (more recently) dynamical and ecological theories. The predictions associated with each of these theoretical approaches to motor control have been tested using a variety of measurement techniques and levels of analysis. Whereas some researchers have worked primarily at a behavioral, or psychological, level of analysis, others have employed animal models in an attempt to identify the actual neurological mechanisms underlying action. Complex mathematical analyses have also been used to quantify the physical dynamics of motion. Let us begin by discussing the defining characteristics of each theory and their respective contributions to our present understanding of human motor control.

## Reflex Theories

One of the earliest neurologically based **reflex theories** developed to explain how movements are controlled was based on the work of Charles Sherrington (1857–1952), a prominent neurophysiologist who considered the reflex to be the fundamental unit of motor control. A basic assumption of this theory was that physical events occurring in the environment served as the **stimulus** for action, triggering a chain of individual reflex circuits that were responsible for producing a movement **response.** According to Sherrington (1906), "the outcome of the normal reflex action of the organism is an orderly coadjustment and sequence of reactions" (p. 8). Consistent with this theory is the idea that the individual is a passive recipient of externally produced sensory input. Sensory receptors in the skin, muscles, and joints are stimulated, triggering other sensory systems that, in turn, excite motor systems responsible for producing motor output in the muscles and joints that were originally stimulated.

Sherrington considered the reflex to be the fundamental unit of motor control.

To test his ideas, Sherrington conducted a series of experiments that involved severing the spinal cord of animals immediately below the brain. This procedure greatly simplified the circuitry of the nervous system and made it possible to study the mechanisms of the spinal cord in isolation from the higher cortical centers. In this way, Sherrington could focus his attention on what he believed to be the elementary unit of behavior: the reflex.

During the 1920s and 1930s, various forms of **reflex chaining models** of motor control were also being studied at a psychological level of analysis by a group of psychologists who came to be known as the behaviorists (Skinner, 1938; Thorndike, 1927). This group of researchers viewed the acquisition of movement patterns and motor skills as the linking of individual movements into a chain of behavior. A chain of action was thought to be triggered by some external stimulus that resulted in an observable movement response.

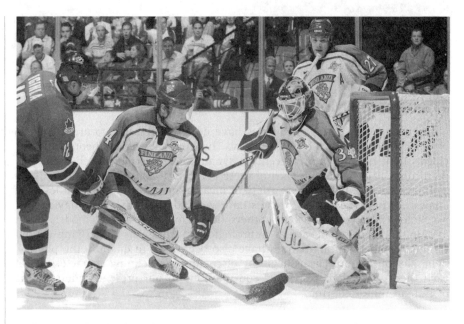

In the game of ice hockey, players must often anticipate the actions of other players rather than waiting for them to occur.

Behaviorists were more interested in studying the observable outcomes than underlying processes of motor control.

This response would then generate a second stimulus for subsequent action. Behaviorists were primarily interested in studying observable movement outcomes, as opposed to the underlying processes responsible for producing the outcomes. Thus the theories developed during this period offered little insight into how the motor system was being organized to produce movement.

Although the reflex theories of motor control provided straightforward explanations of how movements are controlled, they were much too simple to account for a person's ability to perform a wide variety of goal-directed actions. The inadequacies of these theories are particularly evident when we begin to consider the vast array of voluntary movements that require us to anticipate changes in the environment, rather than wait for them to occur. As we are well aware from our sports activities and daily living experiences, many of our actions must be proactive—as opposed to reactive—in order for us to avoid undesirable consequences.

A player tending goal during a game of soccer or ice hockey, for example, has no time to wait for the ball or puck to be contacted before deciding on his or her own plan of action. Instead, by carefully watching the movements of a number of key offensive players for important clues, the goalie must attempt to *predict* which player will attempt the shot on goal. In this way the goalie can begin to plan his or her movements before the ball or puck is actually struck. Similarly, drivers who have previously experienced winter road conditions drive at significantly lower speeds, decelerating as they approach curves in the road where ice is known to accumulate. In situations such as these, the performer must draw on existing knowledge about the situation and anticipate changes in the environment in order to be successful.

A second weakness of reflex theories of motor control is their inability to account for movements performed in the absence of sensory feedback. This open-loop control of movement has been demonstrated not only in studies using animals subjected to deafferentation, the surgical cutting of sensory pathways between peripheral receptors and spinal cord/brain (Grillner, 1975; Taub & Berman, 1968a and b), but also in human sensory block studies (Kelso, 1977; Smith, 1969) and in clinical observations of patients who have sustained damage to sensory pathways (Lashley, 1917). The collective findings of these studies have demonstrated that sensory feedback is not essential for the execution of all movements, an argument that directly contradicts Sherrington's own research findings and the basic assumptions underlying reflex theories of motor control.

Although reflex theories of motor control have largely been dismissed in favor of alternative theoretical explanations, reflex theories have influenced practice in a number of ways, most notably in the field of physical therapy. These theories provided the basis for the development of at least one very well-known treatment technique called neurodevelopmental treatment (NDT). Although still used by physical therapists to treat certain types of patient populations today, the treatment technique has evolved considerably since its formulation by Karel and Berta Bobath (1965, 1978, 1984). In fact, the NDT techniques used today are believed to be more in line with the principles underlying the dynamical and ecological perspectives (Szklut & Breath, 2001), as described on page 14.

> Sensory feedback is not essential for the execution of all movements.

## Hierarchical Theories

In stark contrast to earlier reflex theories, **hierarchical theories** of motor control assume that *all* aspects of movement planning and execution are the sole responsibility of one or more cortical centers representing the highest command level within the hierarchy of the CNS. This cortical "executor" contains all the information necessary for action and directs lower centers within the nervous system to carry out the prescribed movement. Moreover, it is capable of coordinating and regulating movement with or without referring to externally generated sensory feedback.

One of the first models developed to test the predictions of these hierarchical theories of motor control was devised by Hughlings Jackson in the 1850s. Jackson argued that movements were represented in the higher levels of the brain and then were used to guide subsequent performances. Accordingly, he believed, the flow of information is unidirectional. That is, higher centers convey information for action to lower subordinate centers, and no other communication occurs. This rigid top-down view of motor control has since been modified to allow for communication between levels within the hierarchy, the lowest spinal centers conveying information to higher cortical centers in the form of feedback related to how the movement is being carried out.

According to hierarchical theories, representations of movement are stored in memory in the form of plans or programs for movement. These **motor programs** are believed to consist of prestructured sets of motor commands that are constructed at the highest cortical levels and then conveyed to the lowest

> Higher cortical centers command lower centers to carry out prescribed movements.

> Motor programs are prestructured sets of motor commands developed in the cerebral cortex.

centers in the hierarchy responsible for executing the movement. This view of motor control guided the research of notable motor control scholars such as Henry (Henry & Rogers, 1960; Henry, 1961) and Keele (1968, 1981). According to Henry and Rogers (1960), who developed the "memory drum" theory of motor control, a motor program stored in motor memory is accessed and then translated into neural commands that are sent to the muscles. This idea of a motor program was later to be more specifically defined by Keele (1968) as "a set of muscle commands that are structured before a movement sequence begins, and that allow the entire sequence to be carried out uninfluenced by peripheral feedback" (p. 387).

Three important lines of research have provided empirical support for hierarchical theories over the years. These include (a) deafferentation studies, (b) response complexity studies, and (c) limb blocking studies. The major findings derived from each of these studies are briefly described here.

### Deafferentation Studies.

A number of motor control theorists and neuroscientists have used deafferentation techniques to study how animals control their movements in the absence of sensory feedback. In these studies, a surgical technique was used to sever (deafferent) the afferent (sensory) pathways at the level of the spinal cord, thereby isolating the central nervous system from the peripheral nervous system. These surgical techniques could be used to effectively eliminate sensory information from one or more limbs.

Despite the absence of sensory feedback from one or more limbs involved in the movement, the deafferented animals were still able to perform movement skills such as climb, groom, and feed themselves (Taub, 1976; Taub & Berman, 1968). The performance of fine motor skills (e.g., manipulating or picking up small objects with the fingers) were much more difficult for the animals to perform, however. Researchers concluded that their findings provided clear evidence that sensory feedback was not essential for successful movement production due to the existence of a central representation of movement that could be used to guide movement. These central representations were believed to be in the form of motor programs that were formulated in advance of the movement and then executed using an open-loop system of control.

### Response Complexity Studies.

The time to initiate a movement increases as its complexity increases.

A second area of research that provided good evidence for the hierarchical control of movement and the existence of motor programs involved the examination of movement responses of increasing complexity. These types of studies formed the basis of Franklin Henry's research related to the memory drum concept of motor programming and involved the use of reaction time measures to examine how the number of parts comprising a movement sequence influenced the time required to initiate the movement. **Reaction time (RT)** measures are used to determine the period of time that elapses between the presentation of a stimulus or signal to "go" and the start of the actual movement. Henry hypothesized that if the time required to initiate a movement increased as the movement response became more complex then that would be strong evidence for the pre-programming of movements. In what has become an often-cited research experiment, Henry and Rogers (1960) required a group of study participants to perform three different movement sequences that differed according to the number of component parts. The first and simplest task involved the participant lifting his or her finger from a response button, the second task required the participant to lift his or her finger from the same response button and then reach forward to grasp a tennis ball suspended from a string, while the third and most complex movement response required the subject to once again lift his or her finger from the same response button, and then perform a series of movements such as hitting a ball suspended from a string, depressing a second response button, and then hitting a second ball suspended from a string. What Henry and Rogers' findings indicated was that the time required to initiate a movement response, as measured using RT, increased from an initial time of 150 milliseconds (ms) for the simplest movement to 208 ms in the case of the third and most complex movement pattern. These findings provided support for the idea that each of the three movement response sequences was planned in advance of the movement. They correctly reasoned that if only a portion of the movement response had been planned in advance and then subsequently guided by feedback (i.e., closed-loop system of motor control) then the time to initiate the response should have remained similar across the three movement sequences. In addition to the classic work of Henry and Rogers (1960), other researchers also used RT measures to demonstrate that many voluntary movements, particularly those that must be executed quickly, can be planned in advance (Christina, 1992; Rosenbaum, Inhoff, & Gordon, 1984; Sternberg, Monsell, Knoll, & Wright, 1978). Certainly the idea that movements are planned in advance of time-constrained movements better explains how it is possible for hockey goalkeepers and drivers to plan their actions before changes actually occur in the environment.

***Limb Blocking Studies.***    A third area of research that provided support for hierarchical theory came from limb blocking studies (Wadman, Denier van der Gon, Geuze, & Mol, 1979). In these studies, participants were required to move a lever as quickly as possible to a designated target by extending the elbow. On a certain random number of trials, however, the limb was prevented from completing the movement by the insertion of a mechanical block. Surface electromyography (EMG) was used to record the activity of the **agonist** (contracting muscle, in this case the triceps) and **antagonist** (muscle that opposes an agonist, in this case the biceps) during both the trials in which participants were allowed to complete the movement and those in which they were not. What the researchers found was that not only did the EMG activation patterns of the agonist and antagonist muscles look very similar through the first 100 ms of the movement in both the blocked and unblocked trials, but the antagonist muscle continued to fire during the blocked trials even though the movement of the limb was stopped during those trials. This latter finding was most surprising given that it is the role of the antagonist muscle group in this movement to slow down the moving limb prior to arriving at the end target. The authors reasoned that, since the limb was blocked from reaching the target on certain trials, the activation patterns of both the agonist and antagonist muscles must have been planned in advance and continued until blocking of the limb resulted in altered muscle activity.

Limb blocking studies demonstrated that muscle activation patterns are planned in advance for short duration movements.

***The Generalized Motor Program (GMP) Concept.***   Although the earlier conceptions of a motor program were to serve as an important catalyst for several research endeavors in the early 1970s, certain weaknesses with the definition became evident. First, the idea that motor programs were comprised of prestructured muscle commands was difficult to reconcile with the knowledge that individuals do not always perform the same movement in exactly the same way each time and are even capable of performing movements that are considered to be novel because they have not been experienced before. A second criticism that led to a broader conception of the motor program was related to storage. Critics argued that if a motor program is stored for every conceivable movement ever performed, as early definitions implied, then memory would soon run out of space unless it had an unlimited storage capacity. A third criticism related to the diminished role given to sensory feedback in the execution of movements. In contrast to the insignificant role prescribed for feedback in Keele's earlier definition of a motor program, it was subsequently acknowledged that sensory feedback is used to ensure a movement's accuracy when sufficient time is available to use it. The importance of sensory feedback in the control and learning of movements will be discussed in more detail in later chapters of this book.

By the late 1970s, a broader definition of the motor program had emerged, largely thanks to the research efforts of Schmidt and colleagues (Schmidt, 1976, 1982a and b, 1988; Shapiro, 1978; Shapiro, Zernicke, Gregor, & Diestel, 1981). Although the **generalized motor program (GMP)** described by Schmidt (1991) still consists of a stored pattern of movement, its actual structure is more abstract than the one described by Steven Keele. Because of its broader  definition, the GMP can also be applied to a wider range of movements and can be altered or modified during execution in response to changing environmental conditions.

The GMP is comprised of variant and invariant movement parameters.

Central to this more general theoretical concept is the existence of **parameters,** some variant (changeable) and others invariant (not changeable). Variant movement parameters that specify such things as the overall duration of the movement (e.g., overall speed of a tennis serve, golf swing, or time to transfer from a chair to standing) or the absolute force needed to accomplish the movement (e.g., throw a javelin as far as possible, free-throw shot in basketball) assist us in varying a class of actions in a number of different ways. As a result, we can achieve greater flexibility in the type of movements we can produce. Conversely, the existence of invariant movement parameters provides us with the ability to consistently reproduce the spatial and temporal features of a specific movement pattern once it has been learned, even though the overall speed, size, force, or trajectory of the movement pattern changes from one movement attempt to the next. At least one movement parameter that has been demonstrated to be invariant is relative timing. This particular movement parameter is believed to provide the fundamental temporal structure, spatial organization, or rhythm associated with a particular movement pattern (Schmidt & Wrisberg, 2000). Support for the idea that the relative timing of a movement pattern is invariant has been provided by studies examining the various phases of the gait cycle during walking and running (see highlight, The Same Motor Behavior with a Different Theoretical Explanation), as well as other skills such as handwriting (Terzuolo & Viviani, 1980).

# HIGHLIGHT

### The Same Motor Behavior with a Different Theoretical Explanation

Although the types of movement skills selected for study by researchers aligned with a hierarchical view of motor control are quite different from those studied by advocates of dynamical approaches to motor control, one movement pattern that has been studied by both groups is human locomotion. Specifically, both groups of researchers have studied the transition that occurs between walking and running as gait velocity increases to provide evidence in support of certain theoretical assumptions associated with their respective theories. Not surprisingly, both groups of researchers have explained the walk-to-run transition very differently.

Shapiro, Zernicke, Gregor, and Diestel (1981) studied the gait cycle at different speeds for the purpose of testing the hypothesis that relative timing between limbs constitutes an invariant parameter of a generalized motor program (GMP) used to control a class of movements. They further hypothesized that, because walking and running belong to different classes of movement, the relative timing would differ between the two movement patterns. The relative timing associated with each of the four phases of the gait cycle plotted for the right limb (i.e., heelstrike and midstance, midstance to toe-off, toe-off to midswing, and midswing to heelstrike) was invariant. That is, the duration of each phase of the step cycle expressed as a percentage of the total step cycle was similar for walking speeds that ranged between 3 and 6 mph. Once the speed of the treadmill on which the subjects were initially walking was increased to 8 mph, the relative timing characteristics of the step cycle changed as the subject transitioned to running. The relative timing of the four phases did not vary, however, for running speeds ranging

between 8 and 12 mph. On the basis of their findings the authors not only concluded that relative timing constitutes an invariant parameter of a GMP, but that a different GMP is used to produce a walking versus running pattern because the relative timing characteristics were markedly different between the two gait patterns.

Researchers aligned with the dynamical approach to motor control (Diedrich & Warren, 1995, 1998) have also studied the same walk-to-run transition sequence for the purpose of understanding why people transition from a walking to running movement pattern as the task demands or environmental constraints change. Using a very similar experimental protocol, the authors observed a similar change in behavior but interpreted it in a very different way. In contrast to the explanation advanced by hierarchical advocates, the authors of these more recent studies interpreted their findings within the framework of the dynamical approach referred to as *dynamic systems theory*. They argued that transitions between movement patterns arise from the self-organizing properties of the human system and its desire to maintain stability. In order to achieve this stability, individuals adopt preferred patterns of coordination, or attractor states. In the face of changing task and/or environmental demands (e.g., increasing speed of the treadmill) that disrupt the stability of the preferred attractor state, individuals spontaneously transition from one attractor state or preferred pattern of coordination to another attractor state that is more stable. According to dynamic systems theorists this transition does not require any conscious processing on the part of the individual or the need to switch to a different motor program.

A GMP that can be used to perform a large number of similar movements simply by adding the appropriate set of movement parameters to the abstract plan of action considerably reduces the number of programs one must store in memory. The idea that GMPs do not specify which groups of muscles will

A generalized motor program (GMP) is more abstract in structure and can be applied to a broader range of movements.

*Motor equivalence:* The ability to perform the same movement using different muscle groups.

be activated during the planning of movements also permits greater flexibility of action and can better explain how it is possible to achieve the same movement outcome using different muscle groups. This somewhat surprising ability was empirically demonstrated by Raibert (1977), who tried to complete the following palindrome, "Able was I ere I saw Elba," first with his dominant hand, then with the wrist of his dominant hand immobilized, followed by his nondominant hand, his teeth, and finally with a pen taped to his foot. What was most remarkable about this single-subject experiment was that the writing in each of the sentences looked quite similar even though parts of the body we would think are not well suited for the skill of writing were used. This ability to produce the same movement outcome with a variety of different muscle groups is called **motor equivalence.** This same ability explains how it is possible to write by using very small print on a check or much larger print. All one has to do in this situation is "scale up" the same general movement pattern, using the larger muscle groups of the arm (Merton, 1972).

## Dynamical and Ecological Approaches

Two alternative theoretical approaches to the study of human motor control that have risen to prominence over the past 15 years are ones that embrace the principles of physical biology, mathematics, and/or ecological psychology. Although many different names have been used to describe these alternative approaches in the literature (dynamical or dynamic systems theory, dynamic pattern theory, action systems theory, ecological theory, and so on) we have chosen to broadly categorize these specific theories as dynamical and ecological approaches, respectively. While both theoretical approaches share many similar features and assumptions, the ecological approach distinguishes itself from dynamical approaches by focusing more on the perceptual interface between the individual and the environment.

In addition to being applied to human motor control, many of the principles that characterize each of these approaches have been used to describe a variety of different biological (including cardiac rhythms, the development of infant stepping, diving behavior of birds) and nonbiological (such as cloud formations, transformation of water to steam or ice) phenomena for many years. While many of the basic concepts embodied in the different dynamical approaches to motor control can be traced back to synergetic theory (Haken, 1977, 1983) and the early work of Nicolai Bernstein (1967), a Russian physiologist who contributed much to our understanding of how the many degrees of freedom available within the human system are coordinated, it was the early work of a psychologist named James Gibson (1966, 1979) that largely shaped the ecological approach. Both theoretical perspectives have been further advanced over the course of the past 25 years by a number of notable motor control and motor development theorists (e.g., Scott Kelso, Peter Kugler, Michael Turvey, Alan Lee, George Schoner, and Esther Thelen) who have chosen to explain different aspects of human motor behavior using one or both of the two approaches we will describe in this section.

***Dynamical Approaches.***     There are five basic assumptions that perhaps best differentiate **dynamical approaches** from other theories of motor control. The first assumption is that new spatial and temporal patterns of coordination emerge as a result of the interaction that occurs among the subsystems or components that make up the system as a whole. This process has been defined as *self-organization* in the literature. Second, individuals adopt preferred patterns of behavior that are referred to as *attractor states*. Third, changes in behavior can occur in a **nonlinear** and abrupt fashion. The fourth assumption is that new movement patterns emerge as a result of scalar changes in one or more *control parameters*. Finally, the parameters that exhibit the nonlinear changes are identified using *order parameters*. Let's briefly consider how each of these assumptions provides an alternative explanation of how movements are controlled.

*The system is capable of self-organization.*   Unlike previous theories, theorists aligned with dynamical and ecological approaches argue that actions do not occur as a result of a **cortical executor** (a control center at the level of the cerebral cortex that specifies all the details of a movement to be performed). Instead, they argue that motor behavior emerges from a complex and dynamic interaction among the multiple subsystems that are intrinsic to the individual, extrinsic factors such as the movement itself, and the environment in which the movement is performed. The term that these theorists apply to this phenomenon is **self-organization.** This self-organizing capability of the system is fundamental to all dynamical explanations of human motor behavior and has been used to provide an alternative explanation for how the control of different skills can be constrained by the demands of the task itself and/or the environment, how different skills are acquired (such as infant stepping, juggling), and how an individual transitions from one pattern of coordination to another pattern (e.g., walk-to-run transition).

> Motor behavior is self-organized. It results from the interaction of subsystems, and no single subsystem is capable of prescribing the entire action.

> Individuals adopt preferred patterns of behavior called attractor states.

For example, Thelen and Fisher (1982) demonstrated that, by simply manipulating the task demands, the stepping reflex that is observed in newborns but then disappears could be reinstated. By having infants lie supine on the floor, thus eliminating the constraints imposed by gravity, a kicking pattern that closely resembled the kinematics of the stepping pattern was observed. Similarly, placing infants in water also resulted in the reemergence of the stepping pattern. The researchers attributed the reemergence of the stepping pattern in this second environmental context by offsetting the weight of the infants' legs with the added buoyancy of the watery environment. This landmark research not only provided evidence for the important role played by the movement environment in shaping movement behavior, but also demonstrated how properties of the musculoskeletal system alone could constrain the type of movement behavior observed. Additional evidence for this type of self-organizing behavior has been provided using other movement skills such as rhythmically bouncing a ball on a racket (Schaal, Sternad, & Atkeson, 1996), juggling (Beek, 1989), and the control of walking (Kay & Warren, 1997).

> Properties of the musculoskeletal system alone can constrain the type of movement behavior observed.

*Individuals adopt preferred patterns of coordination to enhance stability.*   A second and related assumption of dynamical approaches is that humans naturally adopt preferred patterns of behavior or coordination modes referred to as **attractor states.** The adoption of attractor states is thought to promote stability within the complex human system. How variable a particular attractor state is depends on intrinsic factors such as the individual's level of experience or amount of practice on a given skill, as well as extrinsic factors such as the environment or the nature of the task itself (Buchanan &

Ulrich, 2001). As Buchanan and Ulrich (2001) further explain, a stable attractor state or behavior can be good in some cases (a well-learned motor skill) but also problematic (maladaptive sitting or standing postures). The idea that the stable attractor states can be associated with good or problematic behaviors has important implications for practitioners working in movement skill and rehabilitation settings.

*Not all changes in movement behavior proceed in a gradual and linear manner.*

***Changes in movement behavior can occur in a nonlinear and abrupt fashion.*** A third assumption of dynamical approaches to the study of human motor control is that qualitative changes in behavior do not always proceed in a gradual and linear fashion but can also occur suddenly and abruptly (Schoner & Kelso, 1998). These often abrupt transitions from one attractor state or preferred pattern of coordination to another are not believed to be governed by a central motor program or conscious decision made in advance but rather as a function of the complex and changing interaction that exists between the various subsystems and the external environment, including the task being performed.

Evidence for nonlinear changes in behavior have been demonstrated in a series of experiments conducted by Scott Kelso and colleagues (Kelso, 1981, 1984; Kelso & Schoner, 1988; Kelso, Buchanan, & Wallace, 1991) using different single limb, multijoint movement tasks (e.g., arms, hands, fingers, and feet). More recently, researchers have begun to study nonlinear changes in behavior using whole-body tasks such as walking and running (Diedrich & Warren, 1995, 1998; Hanna, Abernethy, Neal, & Burgess-Limerick, 2000) or the lifting and lowering of loads (Burgess-Limerick, Shemmell, Barry, Carson, & Abernethy, 2001). (See highlight, The Same Motor Behavior with a Different Theoretical Explanation, on page 13.)

Collectively, the research findings have demonstrated that if the demands of the task being performed are altered systematically (e.g., speed at which limb segments are required to move in the multijoint tasks or the height of the shelf in the lifting and lowering task) or the environmental inputs are altered (e.g., speed or grade of the treadmill during a walking or running task), the preferred movement pattern becomes increasingly more variable and then abruptly transitions to a new mode of coordination (e.g., stooping to squatting at a critical shelf height; walking to running as the treadmill reaches a critical speed).

*Control Parameter: Any variable that, when altered, can lead to changes in the pattern of coordination produced by the dynamic system.*

***Changes in preferred patterns of coordination are the result of scalar changes in control parameters.*** A fourth assumption of all dynamical approaches is that transitions between preferred movement patterns are thought to be facilitated by changes in one or more control parameters. A **control parameter** is defined as any variable that, when altered, can lead to changes in the pattern of coordination produced by the dynamic system. These control parameters can be either internal (e.g., frequency of limb movement, weight of a given limb segment) or external (e.g., changes in the environment, the demands of the task, or even the type of verbal instructions provided by a coach, teacher, or physical therapist) to the dynamic system. The pattern of coordination is believed to change when the control parameter reaches a critical value (e.g., the speed of a treadmill, height of a shelf, the speed at which limbs are moving). (See highlight, Is Ankle Motion the Control Parameter in a Supine-to-Standing Task?)

# HIGHLIGHT

## Is Ankle Motion the Control Parameter in a Supine-to-Standing Task?

According to researchers aligned with the dynamical approach to motor control, qualitative changes in a person's motor behavior are believed to result from scalar changes in one or more control parameters. To help you better understand how this basic assumption is theoretically tested, let's briefly review a study conducted by King and Van Sant (1995) in which they hypothesized that ankle motion serves as a control parameter for a supine-to-standing movement task. To test this hypothesis, the movement patterns used by 39 nondisabled young adults to rise from a supine position on the floor were compared across four experimental conditions: rising while wearing a solid-ankle-foot orthosis (SAFO) on the right leg, left leg, both legs, and while not wearing the SAFO. The coordination patterns of the upper extremity, torso (trunk), and lower extremity were videotaped, combined to produce a total body action profile, and subsequently analyzed for each of the four rising conditions.

The results revealed that the study participants varied the type of whole-body movement pattern used in the rising conditions that required them to wear a SAFO on one leg only, or both legs. Twenty of the 39 participants changed the type of movement pattern used between the no SAFO and left leg SAFO condition, while 30 subjects changed at least one component of the whole body movement when the bilateral SAFO and no SAFO conditions were compared. Participants tended to use a more asymmetrical movement pattern in each of the three body components more often in the SAFO conditions, with a large majority of the participants demonstrating increased asymmetry in at least one of the three components when wearing a SAFO on each leg.

Adequate ankle motion appears to be most needed as the individual transfers weight from the buttocks to the feet when moving from a sitting to squatting position. Wearing the SAFOs acted as a constraint on ankle motion and resulted in the need to use a compensatory movement strategy to overcome this constraint.

In general, the findings supported the original hypothesis that ankle motion does indeed constitute a control parameter in a supine-to-standing movement task. The authors indicated, however, that many other variables may have contributed to the changing patterns observed. Among those listed as possible candidates were the individual's balance abilities, general flexibility, and ability to take advantage of gravity through momentum. The characteristics of the support surface, proximity of stable objects to assist the individual in completing the task, and even the instructions provided to the subject were also listed as possible additional control parameters.

The take-home message from this study is that compensatory movement strategies often provide a positive solution to a given movement problem. As such, it would follow that the environment in which a patient (and any other learner for that matter) works should include a variety of movement contexts that promote the manipulation of control variables identified so that the broadest repertoire of successful movement strategies can be acquired. The focus of the practitioner would be more on constructing (the most favorable learning environment) than instructing if this set of theoretical findings were applied to practice.

*An order parameter is used to identify the parameter that exhibited the non-linear change leading to the abrupt transition to a new pattern of coordination.* The final assumption associated with dynamical approaches is that **order parameters** (specific variables that are used to describe the observed motor behavior) are used in conjunction with control parameters to study the conditions that lead to a change in behavior or loss of system stability (via

Order parameters are used to quantify the effect of a change in behavior on a dynamic system.

control parameters) and then to quantify the effect of the change on the system (via order parameters). For example, in the highlight box on the previous page, the authors videotaped the participants rising when wearing none, one, or two ankle-foot orthoses and then quantified the changes occurring in the movement patterns used to rise from the floor. The total body movement profiles generated from the researchers' two-dimensional movement analysis constituted the order parameter used to quantify the temporal and spatial changes occurring in the behavior observed. In studies exploring the intrinsic dynamics of other movement patterns such as locomotion, researchers have also studied how selected movement parameters such as joint angle, stride length, and/or stride duration vary across multiple step cycles as a means of discriminating between variability that is (a) an essential component of a flexible coordination pattern, (b) signaling an imminent transition between coordination patterns, or (c) symptomatic of an unstable pattern of coordination associated with different neurological diseases (Heiderscheit, 2000). Of course, as Balko Perry (1998) points out, in order to measure the actual change in the system, "one must look in the right place, or measure the correct variable" (p. 7). The appropriate selection of order parameters is therefore critical if one is to capture the true nature of the change occurring in the system.

*Ecological Approaches.*    Although many of the basic tenets that are central to dynamical approaches to motor control are also embraced in the **ecological approaches** to motor control (e.g., mathematical analyses of human motion), ecological approaches distinguish themselves by focusing more on the perceptual interface between the individual and the environment. The primary goals of ecological theorists are to first discover and then explain how lawful properties, or **affordances,** of the environment permit a certain action. In fact, a central tenet of ecological approaches is that "optical properties specific to an affordance can *directly* trigger action" (Colley, 1989, p. 169). For example, seeing the height of a step is sufficient to inform us as to whether the set of stairs in front of us is climbable and what type of action should be needed to successfully negotiate the stairs. A related assumption is that there is a continuous interaction occurring between the processes of perceiving and acting. This assumption alone distinguishes the ecological approach from the dynamical approach in that individuals are able to detect, through the perceptual process, meaningful intrinsic and extrinsic information that can then be used to organize actions that are appropriate for the movement context.

The goal of the ecological approach is to discover and then explain how lawful properties, or affordances, permit action.

These environmental affordances, as they are often called, also drive the nature of the action we produce as a result of our perception of what might be possible. For example, based on our perception of what is possible, seeing a four-foot-high fence in front of us might lead us to climb over it, crawl under it, or walk along side it until a gate is reached. This theoretical assumption has been used successfully to explain not only how we determine whether a set of stairs are climbable or not, but also whether door openings of different widths can be navigated and even how quickly an object (either the body or an external object) arrives at a particular contact point in space (Lee, Lishman, & Thomson, 1982; Sidaway, McNitt-Gray, & Davis, 1989; Warren, 1984; Warren & Whang, 1987). In the case of the stair-climbing experiments, for example, the research findings provide support for the idea that an invariant perceptual variable is used that combines body-scaled information (e.g., leg length and/or distance of the toe from the base of the step) with actual stair height to first perceive which stair heights are climbable and then to guide our actions in these situations (Warren, 1984; Ulrich, Thelen, & Niles, 1990; Cesari, Formenti, & Olivato, 2003). One additional perceptual variable that has been examined over the years is an optic variable called tau that is believed to be used to predict time-to-contact with an object. This variable has been shown experimentally to guide our actions in a variety of different movement settings (e.g., catching or hitting balls, jumping from different height platforms, driving a car). This optical variable will be discussed in greater detail in Chapter 4.

## Does One Theoretical Approach Better Explain How Movements Are Controlled?

The relative strengths and weaknesses of each of the theoretical approaches described in this chapter as all-encompassing descriptions of motor control have been debated in a number of articles and books published since the late 1980s (e.g., Colley & Beech, 1988; Meijer & Roth, 1988; Heuer & Keele, 1996; Piek, 1998). One notable set of review articles published in the *Research Quarterly for Exercise and Sport* in recent years critically examined the tenability of the basic assumptions associated with motor program explanations of motor control and a specific theory known as Dynamic Systems within the dynamical approach to motor control. The intent of the sequence of articles was to identify the strengths and weaknesses of each specific theoretical approach to motor control (Lee, 1998; Sternad, 1998; Walter, 1998). In general, the authors agreed that each theoretical perspective could provide an equally compelling account of the motor behavior observed in some movement scenarios and that one theoretical perspective provided a better explanation in other movement scenarios, but neither perspective alone was capable of explaining *what* is actually being controlled or *how* the various processes governing motor control were organized in all movement scenarios.

> Motor program theories better explain a performer's actions in rule-based sport settings.

In some cases, the authors argue that motor program explanations of motor control offer a more persuasive account of our motor behavior in certain movement scenarios. For example, having a generalized representation of a class of movements stored somewhere in memory appears to better explain motor behavior in sport settings governed by rules of play. How would a player know how to interact with a soccer ball during a game, for example, unless he had some stored cognitive representation to draw upon? Similarly, motor program explanations appear better able to explain our ability to plan actions on the basis of advance cues as would be needed in sports comprised of different anticipation timing skills (e.g., returning a serve or hitting a pitched ball in baseball or softball). Being able to apply meaning to the physical gestures of dancers and mimes that are intended to convey a certain emotion or movement pattern also require the existence of some type of cognitive representation. Walter (1998) further argues that dynamical approaches appear unable to explain a number of cognitively reliant practice strategies such as contextual interference, reduced frequency of feedback schedules, mental imagery, and deliberate practice that significantly enhance the learning of many different types of motor skills. Each of these different practice methods will be discussed in much greater detail in later chapters in the motor learning section of this book.

Dynamical and ecological approaches better explain how well-learned skills are performed.

Although motor programs were favored as theoretical explanations of motor behavior in a number of movement scenarios, Walter (1998) also identified three examples of motor behavior that might be better explained using a dynamical approach. The first example related to the emergence of "bad habits" during the learning of a particular motor skill. Drawing on the basic assumption that individuals adopt a preferred pattern of coordination, it was suggested that a bias in performance, or bad habits, emerge when new and complex movement skills are being learned that require the performer to alter a very stable pattern of coordination.

A second area in which a dynamical approach to motor control is thought to provide a more useful explanation of behavior is in the performance of continuous skills such as juggling or cycling, which require a continuous interplay between perception and action. This continuous perception–action cycle provides the performer with uninterrupted environmental information that can be matched to the demands of the task without the need for a stored cognitive representation to guide the continuous action. Of course, you may recall that we attributed this particular assumption to ecological as opposed to dynamical approaches in the previous section of this chapter. As with many motor control theories that have emerged over the years, it is not unusual to find that the boundaries between one theoretical approach and another become blurred as scholars who are not aligned with a particular school of thought have adopted a more eclectic approach to the study of motor control. Rather than interpret their empirical findings within one particular theoretical framework, these researchers have looked to other theoretical approaches (e.g., dynamical and ecological) for additional insight. Unfortunately, because of this emerging hybridization of theoretical viewpoints, it has become increasingly difficult for both new and seasoned students interested in human motor control to fully understand where the boundaries of one theoretical approach end and a second one begins (e.g., Beek & Meijer, 1988; Magill, 2004; Rosenbaum, 1991; Summers, 1998; Walter, 1998).

The third area in which dynamical approaches are believed to provide a useful explanation of the observed behavior is in the control of well-learned skills. As Walter (1998) points out, the fact that previous scholars (e.g., Fitts, 1964), have already acknowledged that cognitive processes significantly decline as a result of a skill becoming well-learned makes a dynamical approach to skilled movement control very attractive. One has only to ask elite athletes to verbally describe their skilled behavior to realize that very little attention and/or cognitive processing is being allocated to the actual coordination and control of the movement.

In summary, despite the obvious limitations of motor programs and dynamical or ecological perspectives as singular accounts of human motor behavior, each approach provides a useful theoretical framework for understanding how different types of movements are controlled in different environments. Given the relatively short period of time, in scientific years, that a concentrated effort has been devoted to the development of any of the theoretical approaches to motor control discussed in this chapter, it is perhaps unrealistic to think that a unitary theory of motor control that can account for our ability to produce a dizzying array of movement patterns in response to any number of different task demands and/or environmental contexts should already be in place. Perhaps a quote made by Newell (1998, p. 410) in a commentary following a similar critique of the strengths and weaknesses of the ecological approach to action written by Summers (1998) and published in the same year as the critical review papers published by Walter (1998) and others best summarizes the current state of motor control research: ". . . One of the values of critiques such as this is that they should serve to remind us of how much work there is to be done in order to develop a theory of movement coordination and control. . . ."

## Characteristics of Human Action

Having briefly outlined the major assumptions underlying the three most prominent theories of motor control, let us now begin to explore how the defining principles associated with each approach can be used to describe certain characteristics associated with human action. To help us in this task, Sheridan (1984) has identified four important characteristics of human motor behavior that he believes any theory of motor control must address. These are flexibility of action, uniqueness of action, consistency of action, and modifiability of action.

Any theory of motor control must be able to account for multiple characteristics of human action.

### Flexibility

Flexibility of action is thought to be achieved by recruiting different muscles and joints to achieve the same action. This characteristic enables us to write legibly even when we control the pen with limbs other than our fingers (Raibert, 1977), and it helps us push open doors and turn on light switches using other body parts when our arms are laden with parcels. In this way, the many degrees of freedom available in the human motor system can be used

Flexibility of action is achieved by recruiting different muscles and joints to perform the same action.

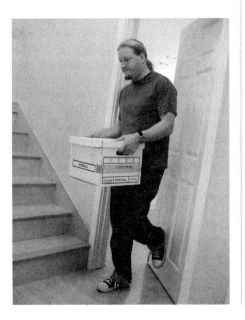

The same action, that of pushing open a door, can be achieved by recruiting different muscles and joints in the body.

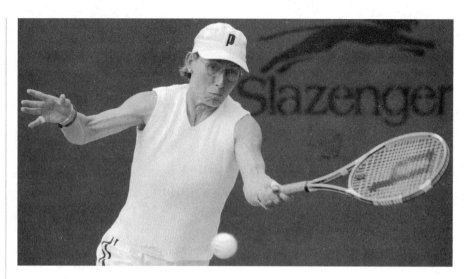

Even a tennis player as skillful as Martina Navratilova is unlikely to perform two movements in exactly the same way during a tennis match and is also capable of producing novel patterns of coordination when attempting to return a difficult shot.

to our advantage in a number of movement situations. In an earlier section of this chapter, we used the term *motor equivalence* to describe this ability. A more thorough description of this concept is provided in the degrees-of-freedom problem (page 26).

## Uniqueness

No two movements are ever performed in exactly the same way.

The uniqueness of action—the fact that no two movements are ever performed in exactly the same way—is a second characteristic of human action that any theory of motor control must account for. One has only to watch an accomplished tennis player hitting balls projected by a ball machine to see that every forehand stroke is performed differently. Slight variations are evident in how the body is positioned prior to ball contact and in how the striking limb is moved through space during each successive stroke. This suggests that the movement pattern underlying the forehand stroke is not rigidly constructed.

Related to this characteristic of human action, but not specifically identified by Sheridan, is our ability to perform movements that we may never have seen or experienced before. For example, even though many readers may never have seen or participated in the game of cricket, we are sure that a good majority could successfully hit a cricket ball that was bowled to them with the bat used in the game. Even skilled performers are capable of novel actions during the course of a game, whether it be hitting a tennis ball between the legs in an attempt to return a difficult shot or returning a volleyball back over the head as the player is running toward the baseline. These very novel patterns of coordination are not part of the player's normal repertoire of motor skills, are rarely if ever practiced, but can be produced in unusual circumstances.

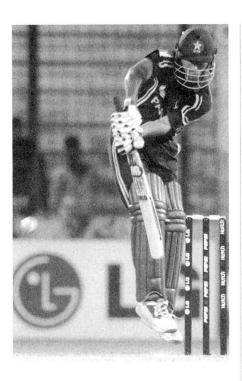

Even though the skill of batting in cricket may never have been experienced before, it is still possible to perform the skill quite successfully on the first attempt.

## Consistency and Modifiability

The third characteristic described by Sheridan involves the consistency with which actions can be reproduced. That is, the temporal and spatial characteristics of the movement remain relatively stable from one performance to the next. The fourth and final characteristic for which any theory of motor control must account is a skilled performer's ability to modify an action, even as it is being executed. How many times have you observed skilled performers change the path of their movements as a result of a change in the situation that was not apparent before the movement began? (One example is a defender jumping to obstruct a forward's view of the basketball rim.) This is a particularly important ingredient for successful performance in varied or unstable environments, whether they are associated with a sport or with conditions that arise in daily life (such as walking along a busy sidewalk). How well does each of the three theoretical approaches to the study of motor control account for these characteristics of skilled action?

The temporal and spatial characteristics of movement remain relatively stable between performances.

Skilled performers can modify actions, even as they are being performed.

## Does One Theory of Motor Control Better Explain the Characteristics of Skilled Actions?

It is clear that reflex theories of motor control are unable to provide an adequate explanation for at least three of the characteristics identified by Sheridan. Certainly they describe no mechanisms that would permit actions to be modified in any way, particularly during their execution. Recall that a

The reflex theory of motor control can only explain how actions are performed consistently.

stimulus or set of sensory inputs triggers a response, which then serves as the stimulus for the subsequent response. Nor do the rigid frameworks of these theories explain our ability to produce unique and/or novel actions on subsequent attempts. Only the characteristic of consistency can be explained in terms of reflex theories of motor control. The direct link between the stimulus and response provides a mechanism for achieving spatial and temporal consistency between movement attempts.

Hierarchical theories, on the other hand, provide one or more mechanisms that capably address each of the human characteristics identified by Sheridan. The more recently developed GMP concept is particularly helpful in explaining each of the four characteristics. For example, flexibility of action is made possible by the existence of certain movement parameters within the GMP that can be varied. By applying one or more of these variant parameters, we can apply different levels of overall force to an object we wish to throw over different distances or speed up or slow down movements by manipulating the variant parameter of overall timing. We can therefore use the same GMP but apply different parameters in order to throw a baseball from deep in the outfield to second base or a much shorter distance to another player in the outfield. Similarly, we can speed up the throw easily if a runner is trying to advance to the next base during the course of the play.

The existence of variant parameters also makes it possible for us to accomplish unique actions—at least those that belong to a class of actions for which we have a cognitive representation. Recall the example of being able to play the sport of cricket even though you may never have seen it played or experienced it before. Despite the odd-looking bat you will be required to use to hit the fast approaching ball, it is more than likely that you will be able to produce a pattern of coordination that will accomplish the goal of hitting the ball on the first attempt. Although it is unlikely that the first few attempts will resemble a well-learned batting stroke, previous striking experiences you have had with other types of implements (e.g., baseball bat, tennis racket, golf club) will help you produce that first movement attempt. Because the GMP also does not consist of a prestructured set of muscle commands, but is more abstract in nature, it is also unlikely that any two consecutive movements will be performed in exactly the same way. Recall the example in which the same movement, writing a sentence, was performed using such different parts of the body as the mouth and toes and yet the writing looked remarkably similar from one sentence to another.

Hierarchial theory can also account for our ability to modify actions in progress, at least up to a point determined by the amount of time available to produce the movement. Because it is now believed that the GMP does not provide *all* the details needed to perform a given movement, or at least those movements that are longer than 200–300 ms in duration, it is certainly possible to modify it after it has been initiated (Schmidt, Heuer, Ghodsian, & Young, 1998). As Schmidt et al. (1998) acknowledge, "current evidence shows that the centrally produced, programmed activities are blended with inputs from a variety of sources (vision, touch, and so forth) to provide the final movement output" (p. 331). Therefore, if the performer has enough time to use the sensory information that is usually available, then it is possible to modify the GMP so it better meets the performer's intended goal. Of course, in those situations where insufficient time exists to modify an action already in progress, it is assumed that the sensory information that was available during the movement can still be recalled after the movement has been completed and incorporated into the GMP used to guide the next movement attempt.

The fact that certain movement parameters applied to any general plan of action are invariant whereas others are variant ensures our ability to achieve consistency in our actions. By manipulating the parameters of overall force and time, we are able to preserve the spatial and temporal patterning of a movement even though different muscle groups are used. This ability was nicely demonstrated by Hollerbach (1978), who asked a group of subjects to write the word *hell* in both small and large print. Measurement of the two different acceleration patterns created by the moving pen revealed a surprisingly consistent temporal pattern in the application of force despite the fact that the level of overall force applied varied between the two print sizes. Hollerbach reasoned that the same underlying plan of action was being used even though the goal of the task was to write using larger print.

Finally, how do the more recently developed dynamical and ecological approaches address each of the characteristics identified by Sheridan? The self-organizing properties embodied within the dynamic approach, in particular, provide for flexibility and modifiability of action in that no single structure within the nervous system is responsible for producing the action. As a result, none of the details of the action exists before the start of the action; all simply emerge as the performance unfolds. Immediate adjustments for any sudden disturbance or obstacles encountered are therefore possible within groups of muscles that are only temporarily constrained to perform the action. This same temporary organization of muscle groups also permits uniqueness of action. Lacking the permanence of "hard-wired" reflexes, these functional muscle groups can be reorganized in an almost infinite number of ways to produce variations in action that may be considered unique. The very fact that no representations of specific movement patterns are stored also facilitates unique action.

The consistency of action characteristic identified by Sheridan is accounted for in dynamical approaches by the basic assumption that individuals adopt preferred patterns of coordination for the purpose of maintaining stability. Once acquired, these preferred patterns or attractor states ensure that a movement pattern is organized similarly from one practice attempt to another. Of course, as Buchanan and Ulrich (2001) suggested, consistency of action should not be viewed as a positive attribute in all situations. Ecological approaches to motor control are equally capable of explaining how movements can be performed consistently but are more likely to attribute this ability to the fact that the individual is able to directly perceive the environmental property or affordance that relates to the action in question.

Despite their vastly different basic assumptions, both hierarchical theories (specifically those that incorporate the GMP concept) and dynamical and ecological approaches to the study of human motor control can account for each of the characteristics of human action. On the basis of these findings and our earlier discussion in this chapter (where we first identified the primary assumptions that distinguished one theoretical perspective from another and then described the relative strengths and weaknesses of each theoretical approach), it will be our goal in the remaining chapters of this book to apply the theoretical perspective that best explains the motor behavior being studied and the context in which it is occurring.

## The Degrees-of-Freedom Problem

One very important issue that remains to be discussed in this chapter is what is often referred to as the degrees-of-freedom (df) problem in the motor control literature. A central concern for Nicolai Bernstein (1967), who was the first scholar to identify this problem, was to understand how the human performer could successfully organize a complex system of bony segments, linked by joints and layers of musculature, that was capable of moving in a variety of different ways. The term **degrees of freedom** has often been used to describe the number of ways in which any given unit of control is capable of moving. These units of control may be described in terms of the number of joints moving or the number of muscles or even motor units activated during the performance of a given movement.

For example, if we consider how many joints we need to move, it is estimated that a total of seven df must be controlled just to move the arm. That is because three df are available at the shoulder, one each at the elbow and radioulnar joint, and two at the wrist joint. If we go one step further and consider the muscle as the unit that is controlled during movement, the number of df available rises dramatically. In order to move the arm successfully, we must now regulate a minimum of 26 df: at least ten muscles at the shoulder joint, six more at the elbow joint, four at the site of the radioulnar joint, and six controlling the different movements of the wrist joint. As you might expect, the estimated number rises exponentially when the motor unit is considered the unit of control.

One solution to the degrees-of-freedom problem is to constrain muscles and joints to work together to produce the desired action.

Now that you have a better understanding of what constitutes a degree of freedom, let's consider how we might actually organize the available degrees of freedom (df) into the smallest number needed to perform a given task. According to hierarchical theory, the GMP is responsible for first determining which df will be involved in the movement to be executed and then organizing them into a single behavioral unit that is most likely to produce the most efficient movement possible. This is particularly true for the execution of ballistic movements that occur in less than 300 ms. In the case of these very short duration movements, it is believed that the GMP is responsible for controlling all aspects of the movement to be performed—specifically which muscles will be activated, when they will be activated, and how forcefully they will contract as the movement is being executed. If the movement does not need to be performed rapidly, however, sensory information that is available to the performer from intrinsic and extrinsic sources can also be used to complement the actions of the GMP by providing feedback that can be used to modify certain movement parameters in response to the changing task demands or environmental constraints or even to change the entire plan of action if sufficient time is available.

In contrast to motor programming accounts, ecological theorists such as Michael Turvey (1977) have argued that control of individual muscles by a cortical executive or motor program is not tenable. Not only does he view the individual turning on of muscles to be wasteful because of the fact that they are so closely interrelated, but he also points out that triggering the innervation of a particular muscle does not always lead to the same movement being produced every time. Rather, the end result is more likely a product of the

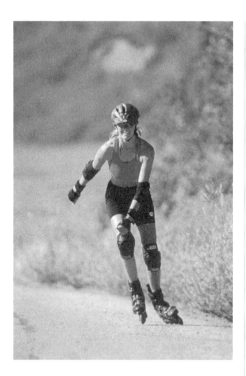

Athough some muscle response synergies are hard-wired at birth, most are developed and learned throughout life as specific ontogenetic or cultural skills, such as rollerblading.

prior condition of the muscle (e.g., length, level of tension) or how it relates to another muscle. Ecological theorists propose that we are able to solve the df problem by constraining muscles and joints to function in a manner that is appropriate for a desired action. These behavioral units are often referred to as **muscle response synergies,** or **coordinative structures.** Although some of these muscle response synergies, or coordinative structures, are believed to be functional at birth (examples include reaching, grasping, and locomotion), the majority of these synergies are developed throughout life as specific onto-genetic, or cultural, skills are learned. Examples of learned cultural skills include rollerblading, ice skating, tennis, and volleyball.

Unlike those synergies inherent in the dynamic human system, the second group of muscle response synergies are less rigidly organized and are often only temporarily constrained for the purpose of simplifying a particular motor act. For example, the muscle response synergies we recruit to lift an object to the mouth are not the same as those muscle synergies organized to assist us in lifting a chair from the floor. The size of the movement being performed, in and of itself, often determines the number and types of muscle response synergies recruited.

*Mechanical Properties of Limbs.*   A second mechanism that some theorists believe can assist us resolve the degrees-of-freedom problem is by exploiting the properties of the musculoskeletal system (Thelen, Kelso, & Fogel,

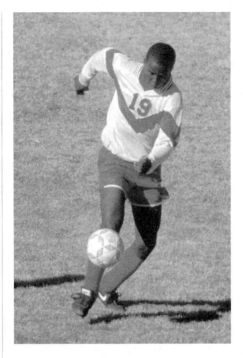

This soccer player can exploit the physical properties of his limbs and muscles to constrain the available degrees of freedom as he swings his limb forward to kick the ball.

The physical properties of the musculoskeletal system can be exploited to reduce the available degrees of freedom needed to perform an action.

1987). Simply by taking advantage of the physical properties of the different body segments and gravity, limb movements can be generated without the need for concurrent muscle activation.

This is certainly evident during the swing phase of locomotion, when passive forces generated by the mechanical properties of the muscles and their physical connections with ligaments at the various joints are sufficient to move the limb through space. Movements that are initiated at one joint invariably affect the movements of other limbs because the limb segments are linked. Swinging the hip forward, for example, naturally influences the movements of the knee and ankle joints below.

The springlike qualities of the muscle can also be exploited by the CNS to assist us in accurately positioning our limbs in space. To accomplish such goals, the stiffness of the involved musculature is manipulated, often before the movement is begun. This ability to prepare the muscles prior to movement is called **feedforward.** As we will see in later chapters, this feedforward ability serves us well in a variety of movement situations.

A coordinated movement requires the effective manipulation of multiple muscle groups and of the joints controlling each limb involved in the action. This is best achieved through a combination of resources: the assembly of various muscle response synergies into functional units of action, exploitation of the mechanical properties of limbs and muscles, and a continuous stream of sensory information triggered by performance of the movement itself.

# Summary

Despite the importance of movement as a vehicle for interacting with our immediate environment, our understanding of the mechanisms that govern such interactions remains incomplete. Over the years, a number of different motor control theories have been developed in an attempt to explain how movements are planned and executed. While each theory has provided us with important knowledge about the nature of motor control and the processes that govern its control, no single theory has been able to address how these processes are controlled in all movement situations, largely because they describe human motor control at different levels of analysis. While hierarchical theories focus primarily on the cognitive control of movement, more recently developed theories have focused on describing how movements are controlled at a physical and biological level of analysis with little attention to the cognitive processes involved.

Although it is clear that much scientific work has yet to be done to develop a theory of motor control that can explain *what* is being controlled and *how* the processes governing that control are organized, good progress has been made in the past 25 years. Practitioners can still learn much from each of the theories of motor control described in this chapter as they continue to develop and/or refine their instructional methods or treatment strategies. Becoming familiar with the basic assumptions of each theory will supplement this knowledge and provide the skills needed to develop and implement evidence-based programs of instruction or treatment, as well as enabling a more systematic evaluation of the efficacy of existing programs of instruction or treatment methods.

## IMPORTANT TERMINOLOGY

After completing this chapter, readers should be familiar with the following terms and concepts.

| | |
|---|---|
| afferent (sensory) information | hypotheses |
| affordances | motor control |
| agonist | motor equivalence |
| antagonist | motor programs |
| attractor states | muscle response synergies |
| closed-loop control | nonlinear |
| control parameter | open-loop control |
| coordinative structures | order parameters |
| cortical executor | parameters |
| deafferentation | reaction time (RT) |
| degrees of freedom | reflex chaining models |
| dynamical approaches | reflex theories |
| ecological approaches | response |
| feedforward | self-organization |
| generalized motor program (GMP) | stimulus |
| hierarchical theories | theory |

## SUGGESTED FURTHER READING

Latash, M. L. (Ed.), (1998). *Progress in motor control: Vol 1. Bernstein's traditions in movement studies.* Champaign, IL: Human Kinetics.

Walter, C., Lee, T. D., & Sternad, D. (1998). The dynamic systems approach to motor control and learning: Promises, potential limitations, and future directions. *Research Quarterly for Exercise and Sport, 69 (4),* 316–318. (Read additional papers by Sternad, D., and Lee, T. D. in same issue).

## TEST YOUR UNDERSTANDING

1. Define the term *motor control.*

2. Briefly explain why it is important, as a practitioner, to become familiar with the basic assumptions of different motor control theories.

3. How does a closed-loop system of motor control differ from an open-loop system of control?

4. Identify two factors that influence whether a closed- or open-loop system of motor control is likely to be used when performing a motor skill.

5. Briefly describe the basic assumptions underlying the hierarchical theory of motor control. Describe the research evidence in support of this theory.

6. Describe the basic assumptions underlying the dynamical approach to motor control that distinguish this approach from the hierarchical theory of motor control.

7. How does the ecological approach to motor control differ from the dynamical approach?

8. Describe the four characteristics of human action that any theory of motor control must account for.

9. Briefly discuss how each of the different theoretical approaches to motor control described in this chapter can account for each of the four characteristics of human action described in question 8.

10. Describe the degrees-of-freedom problem and how it is resolved according to each of the different theories of motor control.

# SCIENTIFIC MEASUREMENT AND MOTOR CONTROL

*The scientific method provides a cogent means of obtaining information that can be used as a solid foundation for supporting instructional decisions.*

MAGILL (1993)

## CHAPTER OBJECTIVES

After studying this chapter, you should be able to:

■ Identify and differentiate between measurement techniques used to describe the outcome of a movement and those used to describe the process by which the outcome was achieved.

■ Describe the various chronometric measures used to study the timing and duration of the cognitive operations involved in the planning and execution of actions.

■ Identify the various error scores used to determine whether a particular movement outcome was achieved and the nature of the error observed.

■ Understand and be able to differentiate between behavioral measures used to quantify the observable form of a movement and those used to quantify the various internal and external forces that influence that observable form.

■ Understand and be able to differentiate between measurement techniques used to describe the changing patterns of limb coordination and those used to describe how a particular movement is controlled.

■ Identify the different types of neurological measures used to describe and investigate the inner workings of the nervous system.

Each of the theories of motor control described in Chapter 1 is the outcome of many years of systematic research using many different and increasingly sophisticated measurement techniques. This chapter describes different types of scientific measurement techniques that are used to test the validity of various models of motor control. These measurements range from noninvasive psychological measures to considerably more invasive experimental procedures designed to monitor and/or alter CNS function directly during movement.

# Psychological Measures

The types of measures that have been used at a psychological level of analysis to test the validity of the different models of motor control can be divided into two basic categories: outcome and process measures. The measures applied to test the early reflex models of motor control were used primarily to describe the end result, or response outcome, observed as a function of manipulating one or more experimental variables. However, the assumptions underlying the more recent hierarchical and dynamic systems models have been tested using research paradigms and measurement techniques designed also to describe *how* the movement was controlled to achieve a particular outcome. We will begin this section with a discussion of two commonly used response outcome measures: chronometry and performance errors.

## Response Outcome Measures

Chronometry and performance errors are most commonly used to measure response outcomes at a psychological level of analysis.

*Chronometry.*    The **chronometry,** or timing and duration, of the cognitive operations involved in the planning of voluntary movements (as described in hierarchical models of motor control) has been extensively explored by a number of researchers using different types of **reaction time (RT)** measures (Henry & Rogers, 1960; Christina, Fischman, Vercruyssen, & Anson, 1982; Klapp, 1975). In its simplest form, RT is defined as the time interval between the presentation of a signal (such as a light or an auditory tone) and the initiation of movement. It can be used in a sports situation to determine how quickly a sprinter responds to the starter's signal and begins to leave the blocks or the time required by a quarterback to spot an open receiver and then begin the throwing action. Although both of these performance situations involve RT, they provide us with different types of information about the decision-making processes involved.

*Simple, choice, and discrimination reaction times.*    The example of the sprinter describes a **simple reaction time (SRT)** situation because the movements of the sprinter are in response to the presentation of a single stimulus, the firing of the starter's gun. Conversely, the football example describes a **choice reaction time (CRT)** situation because many possibilities for action are available to the quarterback. Depending on how the movement situation unfolds following the snap, the quarterback may choose to throw to any one of a number of possible receivers or may even decide to run with the ball. A third type of RT situation, which also involves the presentation of multiple signals, is called **discrimination reaction time (DRT).** Instead of requiring a particular movement response to a specific signal, as is the case in CRT, performers in a DRT setting are required to respond to only one of several signals presented. (The coach has instructed the quarterback to throw to a particular receiver even though several others are available.) All of these RT situations can be easily replicated using simple movement tasks in a controlled laboratory setting. Such laboratory-based RT studies have provided researchers working at a psychological level of analysis with an important means of testing certain predictions associated with hierarchical models without resorting to more invasive measurement techniques.

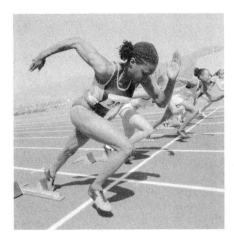 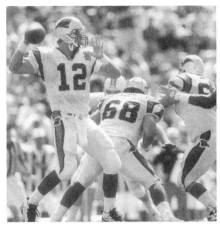

Simple reaction time and choice reaction time measures are used in the laboratory to study the speed of the decision-making processes observed in a number of different types of movement situations.

*Fractionated reaction time.*   In recent years, a more precise RT method has been used by a small number of researchers to study more closely the cognitive processes involved in the planning of action (Anson, 1982; Christina & Rose, 1985). This more precise measurement, referred to as **fractionated reaction time (FRT),** requires the use of surface electromyography (EMG) to partition RT into two parts: premotor time and motor time. **Premotor time (PRMOT)** is the time that elapses between the presentation of a reaction signal and the first change in EMG activity in the muscle that is identified as the prime mover in the action being observed (see Figure 2.1 on page 24). The prime mover might be the biceps brachialis muscle in simple flexion movements at the elbow or the middle deltoid when the movement to be performed is in a lateral direction.

Premotor time reflects the time required to receive and interpret the sensory signal presented, develop an action plan, and convey it to the appropriate musculature. **Motor time (MOT)** begins with the first change in electrical activity recorded in the prime-moving muscle and continues until the movement begins. Unlike premotor time, this second component is not directly observable and must be calculated by subtracting premotor time from the overall reaction time. This technique makes it possible to separate the more purely cognitive processes from the mechanical processes, providing researchers with more precise information about the action planning process.

The value of FRT has been demonstrated in a number of studies involving large-scale movements (Anson, 1982, 1989; Christina & Rose, 1985). It has enabled researchers to identify a number of movement characteristics (such as movement complexity, accuracy demands, and the anatomical characteristics of the responding limb) that appear to influence the speed of the decision-making process significantly. (For a detailed review of this literature, see Christina, 1992.) Moreover, the partitioning of RT into a central and a motor component has made it easier to discern whether delays in the initiation of

The fractionation of RT into premotor and motor components has made it possible to separate cognitive from mechanical processes.

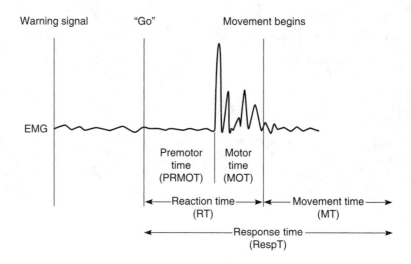

**Figure 2.1**   Surface electromyography can be used to further divide reaction time into a premotor and a motor time component. The first change in EMG activity signals the end of the premotor time and the beginning of the motor time component.

movement are due to the slowing of certain cognitive processes or are purely mechanical characteristics (such as size of limb and muscle fiber type) associated with the limb(s) performing the movement.

*Variables influencing reaction time.*   All of the RT measures have been used in more formal experimental settings in an effort to learn how certain variables affect the time needed to plan and execute movements. Proponents of hierarchical models of motor control have found RT measures particularly useful in their quest to identify the types of variables most likely to influence each of the hypothetical mental processes (stimulus identification, response selection, and response programming) involved in preparing a given action.

As a result of their experimental manipulations, researchers have identified a number of variables that significantly influence the time required to complete the mental processes believed to precede the actual movement. These include such factors as the number of response choices available to the performer, the complexity of the response to be performed, the accuracy demands associated with the movement, and the amount of practice provided on a specific task. As we will see in later chapters, the practitioner must consider the influence of each of these variables when developing and implementing strategies designed to facilitate the learning or relearning of movements.

In addition to its many applications in sports, RT methodology has also been used to investigate the impact of various types of neurological diseases and traumas on the time required to plan and initiate rapid movements. For example, both SRT and CRT measures have been used to assess the ability of patients with Parkinson's disease to prepare to execute a variety of different actions (Stelmach, Garcia-Colera, & Martin, 1989; Stelmach, Worringham, & Strand, 1987). The movement preparation abilities of individuals with cerebral

# HIGHLIGHT

### Using Fractionated Reaction Time to Study
### Developmental Coordination Disorder

Reaction time can now be fractionated into a pre-motor time (PRMOT) and a motor time (MOT) component. By doing this, researchers are better able to examine the relative contributions of the planning and execution phases of movement. The value of using FRT was also evident in a study conducted by Raynor (1998) who sought to better understand the neuromuscular processes that differentiate children with developmental coordination disorder (DCD) from children with normal coordination (NC). Although previous studies had demonstrated that children with DCD responded more slowly in simple reaction time tasks or when balance was unexpectedly disrupted, the actual locus of the delays was speculative at best.

In order to address this issue more comprehensively, Raynor studied the responses of 40 children (aged 6 and 9 years) with DCD or NC to a patellar tendon reflex (PTR) task and a simple visual reaction time (SVRT) task. In using these two different types of tasks, one reflexive and one volitional in nature, Raynor was better able to examine the respective contribution of lower and higher neural centers to the motor performance observed. In both tasks, the children responded by rapidly extending the right leg while seated on a table. In the PTR task, leg extension was triggered by the external tapping of the patellar tendon, while in the SVRT task, the child responded as soon as a visual signal was displayed.

The results of the SVRT task provided evidence that both the central (as measured using PRMOT) and peripheral (as measured using MOT) processing is adversely affected in children with DCD when compared to age-matched peers with NC. Moreover, responses in the PTR task were also significantly slower, but only for the younger children with DCD. By using FRT techniques, Raynor was able to clearly identify the locus of the differences between the DCD and NC groups. Previous studies in which researchers were limited to using SRT measures could only speculate as to the locus of the differences observed. The use of more sophisticated chronometric measures such as FRT are supported by the results of this study, particularly if the neuromuscular processes underlying motor performance are to be better understood among different clinical populations with different types and levels of motor impairments.

*Source:* Raynor 1998.

---

palsy have also been explored using the more precise FRT technique (Parks, Rose, & Dunn, 1989).

*Movement time.*   A second chronometric measure used in conjunction with RT is **movement time (MT).** This measure represents the time interval between the start of a movement and its completion. MT has proved to be a particularly useful means of demonstrating a well-known phenomenon in motor control known as the **speed–accuracy trade-off.** This phenomenon is most likely to occur in movement situations where the performer is required to move quickly *and* accurately. In a slalom kayak event, for example, the paddler strives to complete the course in the shortest period of time while also correctly negotiating several gates placed along the course. In order to be successful in this event, the paddler must delicately balance speed with accuracy because each time the paddler hits or completely misses a gate, unwanted seconds are added to the overall score. Recording MT in this type of situation therefore provides some insight into the strategy a performer uses to optimize success.

Speed–accuracy trade-offs can be demonstrated using reaction time (RT) and movement time (MT) measures of motor performance.

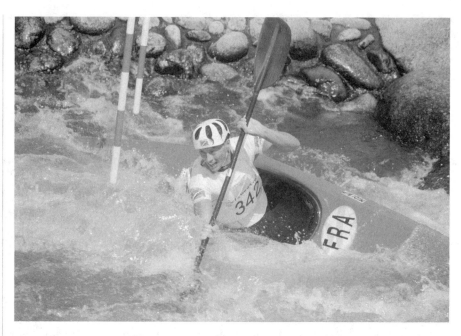

The goal of this kayaker is to paddle his boat as quickly as possible through the white-water river course but make sure that he enters the gates positioned at different points along the course in the correct direction and without hitting them with his boat, paddle, or body. This is a real-world example of a speed–accuracy trade-off.

The measurement of MT and RT can also provide important clues to whether a particular movement is being planned in advance of the movement or during its execution. Researchers have demonstrated that in certain movement situations, subjects plan only a portion of the movement in advance and then continue to plan later segments as the movement progresses (Rosenbaum, Inhoff, & Gordon, 1984; Stelmach, Worringham, & Strand, 1987). This is particularly evident in situations where movement sequences comprise multiple segments or exceed 500 ms in duration.

***Performance Errors.***   The recording of performance errors is a practice commonly used by teachers to assess performers' ability to perform a particular skill or how well they are progressing in learning a new sport skill. Similarly, a quick review of team batting averages or fielding errors provides the coach with valuable information on which to base future practice sessions. Researchers also use different types of error scores to determine whether the goal of a movement was actually achieved. For example, did the performer succeed in hitting the target or execute the movement sequence in its correct order? In addition to telling us whether a particular movement outcome was achieved, certain error scores can also help us better understand why a particular movement outcome occurred. For example, certain error scores can tell us whether performers undershot or overshot a target and how consistently they performed over multiple attempts.

A number of different performance error measures will be discussed in this section of the chapter. The type of motor skill being performed often determines which type(s) of performance error(s) will be used. Performance error measures such as absolute error, variable error, constant error, and total error are usually calculated during the performance of **one-dimensional motor tasks** (movements that require accuracy when performed in a single plane of motion or dimension). In the case of **two-dimensional movement skills** (movements that require accuracy when performed in two planes or dimensions of motion), the use of a radial error score is more useful. Finally, in order to measure the amount of error during the performance of a continuous motor skill (such as tracking objects along a predetermined pathway), root-mean-square error is used. When used appropriately, performance errors can not only assist us in identifying the type of error that is occurring during the performance of a motor skill, but also provide us with valuable information as to the possible cause of the performance error identified.

***Measuring error in one-dimensional movement skills.***   A number of error measures have been used to study the performance and learning of one-dimensional motor tasks in laboratory settings. A popular motor task that has been employed over the years involves moving a handle along a frictionless linear positioning slide. Study participants are blindfolded and then instructed to move the lever a certain distance along the track. In addition to moving the lever a certain distance, participants may also be required to reach the target in a predetermined period of time. Researchers are primarily interested in finding out whether the participants can successfully move the selected criterion distance or reach a certain position in space within a criterion time.

ABSOLUTE ERROR.   The error score that is quickest to calculate and the one most commonly used to evaluate performance on one-dimensional tasks is **absolute error (AE).** This error score simply measures the amount of error associated with a particular performance. For example, if the criterion distance selected on a linear positioning task is 20 inches and the person actually moves a distance of 25 inches, the absolute error score would be five inches. When measuring real-world skills, absolute error is used to provide a gross estimate of performance error. For example, we record how many total pins a bowler knocks down relative to the maximum number possible during each of the 10 frames played over the course of a game or count the number of times a patient recovering from knee surgery is able to achieve a criterion force level during five repetitions of a leg extension exercise. Obtaining each of these scores would be equivalent to knowing the bowler's or patient's absolute error score.

Although AE provides an overall estimate of the magnitude of the error relative to a criterion goal, it does not provide us with any information about the direction of the error. For example, it would be helpful to know how many pins, the location of the pins the bowler knocked down in each frame, in which frame the pins were knocked down, or how much force the patient performing the leg extension task applied on each trial and whether the force applied was either below the criterion level or above it. To obtain this type of information, another error score referred to as **constant error (CE)** must be calculated. This score represents the amount of response bias in a performance. Unlike AE, CE not only considers the *amount* of error, but also the *direction* of the error.

Absolute error (AE) measures the overall amount of error in performance.

Constant error (CE) is used to measure the level of bias in a performance because it considers both the amount and direction of error.

CONSTANT ERROR.   CE is the algebraic difference between a performer's response on each trial and the target of the goal response. It can be used to quantify the amount of the directional error on a single response trial or the average amount of directional error over a number of response trials. It provides a useful measure of response bias. For example, suppose our patient was asked to produce a criterion force of 40 pounds with the recovering right leg during the performance of five successive leg extension trials. If on the first trial, she generated 45 pounds, her CE score would be +5 pounds. If on trials 2 through 5, the patient generated 40, 35, 35, and 30 pounds, the patient's CE scores would be 0, −5, −5, and −10 pounds, respectively. The average CE score for all five trials would be −15 pounds, which means on average, the patient was unable to generate enough force to match the criterion level of 40 pounds per repetition. In other words, the patient's average leg extension response was negatively (−) rather than positively (+) biased. At a practical level this could mean that the criterion goal is too difficult for the patient to reach at this point in her rehabilitation and may need to be lowered until she can consistently achieve the criterion force selected.

As useful as the average CE score is when we are evaluating the performance of individuals, it offers a less accurate indication of performance bias when applied to a group of performers or patients. This is because the score of one performer negates the score of a second performer when both record the same magnitude of error in opposite directions. For example, if one performer overshoots a target by 7 inches and a second performer undershoots the same target by 7 inches, then the two scores, when summed, would be equal to zero.

To overcome this problem, Henry (1974) and Schutz (1977) suggested that the absolute values of both performers' CE scores be averaged. The overall bias of the group is then determined by comparing the number of positive and negative values associated with each individual's score. This alternative performance error score is called **absolute constant error (|CE|).** This error score is reported more often in research studies than constant error because of its greater validity.

ABSOLUTE CONSTANT ERROR.   Absolute constant error (|CE|) is the absolute value of CE over a number of trials for each learner. Each learner's average CE score is calculated over the number of response trials performed, and then the negative sign is eliminated, making it an absolute score. Using the previous CE example, the learner's average |CE| score would be 3 instead of −3. If her scores were then combined with those of four other patients who had average CE scores of −7, −10, +5, and +15, their average |CE| scores would be 7, 10, 5, and 15. The group's average CE score would be equal to zero, but the group average |CE| score would be equal to 8.

Variable error (VE) represents the degree of consistency or variability associated with a performance.

VARIABLE ERROR.   Yet another error score that provides us with useful information about the nature of performance error is **variable error (VE).** This score is equal to the standard deviation of a learner's CE scores about his or her own mean divided by the number of responses or trials. This error score is used to quantify the variability or inconsistency (or, conversely, consistency) of a performer's responses about his or her own mean. Using the previous CE example, the learner's VE score over trials 1 through 5 would be 5.09 pounds. This VE score indicates that the learner's five responses varied from trial to trial by 16.3 pounds. Often the VE score decreases with practice because the performer becomes less variable (or, conversely, more consistent) in responding from trial to trial. However, learning to become less variable in responding does not mean that the learner's responses are becoming more accurate relative to the target or goal response of 40 pounds because VE is calculated about the mean of the learner's responses and not about the target or goal response. To help you better understand the difference between these three different performance error measures and how to calculate each error score, we encourage you to complete the first problem in the Practical Activities section on page 58.

TOTAL ERROR. **Total error (E),** also referred to as root-mean-square error, is the square root of the sum of $VE^2$ and $CE^2$ (Henry, 1975).

$$E = \sqrt{VE^2 + CE^2}$$

It quantifies the total error about a target for a number of responses. In the example of the patient performing the leg extension exercise, the calculated E score would represent the total variability or the total amount of dispersion of the patient's movement responses about the 40-pound goal response. It therefore constitutes the overall measure of how successful the patient was in achieving the 40-pound criterion goal. Can you calculate the patient's E score based on the CE and VE scores presented earlier in this section? When seeking a single error score to assess how successful a person is in learning to respond to a criterion goal, E is recommended because it is a composite of CE and VE and can be analyzed in terms of response bias and variability.

*Performance errors for two-dimensional motor tasks.* **Radial error (RE)** is commonly used to assess the accuracy of performance in two-dimensional motor tasks. An example of a laboratory task that varies in two dimensions is a positioning response in which a blindfolded learner must learn to move a stylus with his or her hand and arm a criterion direction and distance on a flat surface. Thus, the stylus or hand and arm movement is free to vary horizontally (direction) and vertically (distance). Errors must therefore be assessed in these two dimensions. Examples of real-world tasks in which each response outcome can vary in two dimensions are golf putting, target archery, and target pistol or rifle shooting. Radial error is calculated on each trial by measuring the difference between the criterion response and the learner's response in both the horizontal (*x*-axis) and the vertical (*y*-axis) directions. Each value is then squared, the squared *x*- and *y*-axis values are then summed, and the square root of the total is then calculated:

> Radial error (RE) is commonly used to assess accuracy of performance in two-dimensional motor skills.

$$RE = \sqrt{(x\text{-direction error})^2 + (y\text{-direction error})^2}$$

For example, if the distance of the *x*-direction error is 3 inches and the distance of the *y*-direction error is 4 inches, the RE is 5 inches ($\sqrt{9 + 16}$) (see Figure 2.2 on page 40).

RE can also be calculated by setting the target as zero for both the *x* and *y* coordinates, which would be the criterion response. The zero target might represent the center of the hole on a putting green or bull's-eye on an archery board. Calculate RE as before. The average RE over a number of trials is calculated by summing all the RE scores and dividing by the total number of scores (trials). To see if you can successfully calculate radial error, try completing the second problem in the practical activities section on page 58.

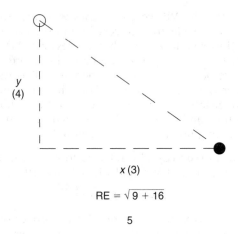

$$RE = \sqrt{9 + 16}$$

5

**Figure 2.2**   The calculation of radial error can be very useful for two-dimensional motor skills such as golf putting and target shooting. In this example, the criterion response (such as the 18th hole in golf) is marked with a closed circle and the golfer's actual response is marked with an open circle.

Often there is interest in studying *response bias* and *variability* (or, conversely, consistency) as well as accuracy (RE) in the learning of a two-dimensional task. These two measures are more difficult to determine for two-dimensional tasks when compared to one-dimensional tasks. Hancock, Butler, and Fischman (1995) provide a thorough explanation of how to calculate these two aspects of performance for two-dimensional tasks, the details of which will not be repeated here. Essentially, response bias and variability over a number of performance trials can be assessed qualitatively by examining the grouping of the performer's responses. Responses randomly scattered in all four quadrants of the target indicate little or no performance bias and considerable variability, whereas responses that are grouped together in one quadrant of the target reveal a clear performance bias and less variability. Clearly, a more complete picture of an individual's performance on a two-dimensional task over a number of practice trials is obtained when response bias, variability, and RE are all calculated.

*Performance error for continuous motor tasks.* **Root-mean-square error (RMSE)** is often used as the measure to assess performance in continuous motor tasks, which are usually tracking tasks. Tracking tasks require the learner to follow a continuous target input by matching his or her response to the target input. The difference between the target input and the learner's response is the error, which is usually in the form of timing and spatial errors but could include other errors (such as from force production). A pursuit rotor-tracking task is a traditional laboratory task in which the learner tries to keep a hand-held stylus directly over a target that is continuously moving in some pattern that can vary in difficulty or complexity.

Root-mean-square error (RMSE) is often used to assess performance error in continuous motor skills such as tracking objects or driving.

Driving a car on the correct side of a road is an example of a real-world tracking task, and driving simulators are often used to measure the amount of error in this real-world skill. In both instances, the learner attempts to keep the car on the correct side of the road by controlling the steering wheel, accelerator, and brake. As the curvature of the road becomes more irregular or unpredictable (as with more curves in the road) or as the speed of the car increases or as the distance ahead that the learner can see the road decreases, it becomes more difficult to track the road and keep the car on the correct side of the road. RMSE is calculated by determining the difference in displacement between the driver's pathway (where the car went on the road) and the criterion pathway (where the car should have gone on the road). The criterion target on the road (pathway) in this example is between the line in the middle of the road and the line marked on the right side of the road. As long as the car was between these two lines it was on the correct side of the road and not in error. However, when the car crossed over either of these two lines, it was on the wrong side of the road and was in error. RMSE is calculated by determining the amount of error between the displacement curve that represents the driver's tracking performance with the criterion displacement curve, which represents the correct performance and the pathway of the road. Typically, a computer program is used for the calculation because of the complexity involved. Essentially, it samples the car's pathway location in relation to the criterion pathway at specified points of time, and then calculates the difference between them, which is the error. All of the error scores that are sampled at the specified points in time are then averaged to produce an RMSE score for the total pathway.

## Response Process Measures

A shift in interest from simple motor skill situations involving movements of a single joint to situations characterized by complex interactions between mover and environment has prompted the use of measurement techniques designed to capture the moment-to-moment control of movement. These process-oriented measures not only have facilitated more precise descriptions of movement, but also have provided a more comprehensive means of testing the validity of hierarchical and dynamical approaches. Five of the most commonly used measurement techniques are described here. They include kinematic measures such as displacement, velocity, and acceleration; angle–angle diagrams; phase portraits; relative phasing; electromyography; and kinetic, or force production, indices. One or more of these measurement techniques are used to measure changes in movement coordination and/or movement control. Let's look at each of these measurement techniques and review their contributions to our understanding of how movements are produced.

***Kinematic Measures.***   Advances in filming equipment, coupled with the increasing availability of commercial software packages that incorporate mathematical and statistical programs (Peak Performance Systems, Qualisys, Watsmart), have given researchers an opportunity to quantify more objectively the **kinematics**—that is, the motion qualities without regard to force—that characterize the performance of a variety of motor skills. More specifically, Hall (2003) defines kinematics as "the study of the geometry, pattern, or form of

Kinematic measures are used to study the quality of motion with respect to time but not force.

motion with respect to time" (p. 318). Although our discussion in this chapter will be focused on describing quantitative forms of kinematic analysis, there are many occasions on which a teacher, coach, or clinician conducts a more qualitative kinematic analysis of a particular movement pattern. For example, a coach may visually observe the movements of an athlete over the course of several practice attempts for the purpose of identifying the quality of the movement occurring at the major joints and/or the sequencing and timing of the different body segments involved in the action. Videotape may also be used to capture the quality of the motion and to document changes in form over time.

As you will learn in this and later chapters of the book, quantitative kinematic analyses have been used to differentiate between performers at different levels of skill (elite versus novice athletes) as well as to document the changes occurring in the spatial and temporal characteristics of a movement pattern that evolve during the learning of new motor skills. Common kinematic measures used to quantify the pattern of human motion include limb and joint displacement, velocity, and acceleration. Both segmental and whole-body human motion can be analyzed in two or three dimensions and multiple planes of motion (including linear, angular). A brief description of each of these important kinematic measures follows.

*Displacement.*   This first kinematic measure provides us with quantitative information about the limb or joint's spatial position during the performance of a movement. Displacement might be quantified in a linear or angular plane of motion, depending on the movement pattern being analyzed (for example, running, somersaulting, cycling, diving). Bright, light-emitting diodes (LEDs) or electromagnetic markers are attached to the skin at predetermined anatomical reference points (such as joint centers). With the assistance of high-speed cinematography or videography and a computerized movement analysis system, the changing position of the reflective markers can be measured at a predetermined sampling rate that might range anywhere from 30 to 120 hertz (Hz), depending on the movement being studied and/or the capabilities of the movement analysis system being used.

In the case of a two-dimensional analysis, the movements of each limb segment are tracked in a horizontal and vertical direction. An $x$ coordinate is plotted and measures the distance traveled in the horizontal direction while a $y$ coordinate measures the distance traveled in a vertical direction. In a three-dimensional analysis an additional $z$ coordinate is also plotted.

*Velocity.*   How fast the pitcher's arm or individual joints move through space during the pitch can subsequently be determined using the displacement data gathered for the same movement. To quantify the speed or velocity of limb or joint movement, the change in spatial position of the limb segment measured at each time interval is divided by the time that elapses during each time interval. The velocity of the limb or joint is traditionally plotted as a function of the time it requires to complete the movement.

*Acceleration.*   The final kinematic measure to be discussed here is that of acceleration. This measure describes the rate at which velocity is changing during a given time interval. This variable can be derived from the velocity data obtained by dividing the change in velocity by the change in time. A more

---

The spatial position of a joint or limb during movement is quantified by the kinematic variable of displacement.

Speed, or velocity, of limb movement is quantified by dividing the change in spatial position of a limb segment at certain time intervals by the time that elapses during each time interval.

direct measure of acceleration can be obtained by using a device aptly called an accelerometer. One or more small transducers are directly attached to various parts of the body (forehead, spinous processes, etc.) for this purpose. The electrical output from the devices is then recorded and processed using a computer and appropriate software package. These types of devices are being more frequently used to quantify the acceleration patterns of different body segments during the performance of different types of activities (such as gait, aerial maneuvers, riding roller coasters). Both the type and/or number of accelerometers used will determine whether the body's acceleration can be tracked in multiple planes of motion.

*The acceleration of a limb segment is derived from the velocity data obtained by dividing the change in velocity by the change in time.*

### Measuring Coordination and Control.

Although it is usual to see kinematic measures used to quantify the motion of a single limb or joint plotted against time, motor researchers have begun to represent kinematic data a little differently. That is, they have begun to represent human motion by either plotting the angle between two adjacent limb segments (such as for the elbow) against the angle of one limb segment (such as the forearm) or by continuously plotting the relationship between two different kinematic measures (for example, knee angle versus knee velocity) during movement. The first of these new measurement techniques is referred to as an angle–angle diagram while the second technique of plotting two kinematic measures against each other produces a phase diagram or portrait. These two different methods of using kinematic measures to describe how movements are coordinated or controlled are described here.

### Angle–angle (A–A) diagrams.

The changing angular displacement between segments of a limb can be nicely described by plotting an **angle–angle diagram.** According to Enoka (2003), A–A diagrams are extremely useful in motor control because they can be used to describe both the quantity (range of motion about a joint) and quality (pattern of displacement) of motion as the movement pattern changes, such as occurs when we transition from a walk to running movement or as the speed of the movement increases. Although A–A diagrams are most commonly used to represent cyclical activities such as walking and running, discrete actions of short duration can also be described using the same measurement techniques (Anderson & Sidaway, 1994; McIntyre & Pfautsch, 1982; Newell, 1985).

*The nature of the intralimb coordination between segments of a limb can be described by plotting angle–angle diagrams.*

When examining an A–A diagram, the shape of the diagram and its location with respect to predetermined reference angles are considered to be the two most important features on which to focus. For example, in the A–A diagram plotted by Enoka and colleagues (1982) of an individual running (Figure 2.3a), three such reference angles are marked. The vertical line labeled $3/2\pi$ indicates when the thigh is in a vertical position during the single step cycle depicted, while the two horizontal lines indicate when the knee is extended ($\pi$) and when the knee is flexed ($\pi/2$), during the same step cycle. Seeing where the diagram is located relative to each of these reference angles and the shape of the diagram itself helps the viewer to describe the changing relationship of the included joint angles, in this case the angle of the knee relative to the thigh at each of the critical events (ipsilateral toe-off—ITO; contralateral footstrike—CFS; contralateral toe-off—CTO; ipsilateral footstrike—IFS) throughout the step cycle.

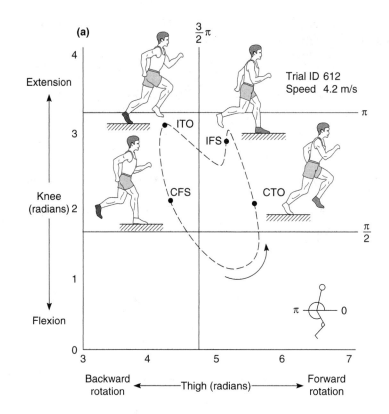

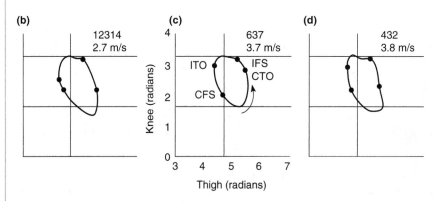

**Figure 2.3**   Knee-angle–thigh-angle diagrams comparing the running stride of a skilled runner **(a)** with those of three below-knee amputees **(b, c,** and **d)**. The labels IFS, ITO, CFS, and CTO indicate ipsilateral (left) footstrike, ipsilateral toe-off, contralateral (right) footstrike, and contralateral toe-off, respectively. These events are shown by the illustrations of the runner in **(a)**. Note that the amputee runners do not flex their knee joints at the beginning of stance.

To see the value of these types of diagrams as templates for comparing patterns of coordination across different movements and between different types of performers, let's now compare the shape and location of the A–A diagram in Figure 2.3a depicting what is considered to be a normal pattern of coordination during running with the three A–A diagrams constructed for three below-knee amputee runners (Figure 2.3b, c, and d). When we compare the topology (shape) of the curve for the skilled runner with those developed for the below-knee amputees, clear differences in the pattern of intralimb coordination are evident, particularly during the stance phase of the stride (IFS to ITO). In contrast to the characteristic knee joint flexion–extension sequence observed during the stance phase in the skilled running gait, the knee-angle–thigh-angle diagram for each of the three amputees reveals a very different pattern. This pattern indicates that the knee is not being flexed during stance, but is held rather at a constant angle. It would appear that the amputees were using the left limb as a rigid lever about which to rotate while the prosthetic foot was in contact with the ground.

Enoka (2002) suggests that these types of diagrams can be very helpful to the clinician who is interested in determining how effective a particular course of treatment was in assisting a patient achieve a more efficient movement pattern or for simply comparing the differences between different patient populations. Coaches would also find these diagrams helpful as they work with athletes to improve the quality of their performances or to correct minor problems in the movement pattern that have emerged. To illustrate how these types of diagrams could be helpful to coaches, let's consider a study that was conducted using the discrete skill of baseball batting. Although it is more common to see A–A diagrams constructed for more cyclical and continuous skills such as walking, running, and cycling, the coordination used to perform discrete skills such as hitting, kicking, and throwing can also be captured using A–A diagrams.

McIntyre and Pfautsch (1982) constructed A–A diagrams to both describe and compare the intralimb coordination of baseball batters who were considered effective opposite-field hitters with the pattern exhibited by ineffective opposite-field hitters. The relative motion of the hitter's bat and left forearm was plotted against the left elbow angle during a baseball batting swing to the same side or to the opposite side of the field. As Figure 2.4 on page 46 indicates, the A–A diagrams of the effective and the ineffective batters are quite different. Whereas the profiles for same-field and opposite-field batting swings are quite similar for the effective hitters (group 1 in Figure 2.4), this is not true for the ineffective opposite-field hitters (group 2). Significant differences are also evident when the magnitudes of the joint angles for same-field batting are compared across the two groups. With practice interpreting these types of diagrams, coaches could use this information to inform their athletes of problems with their batting form and then develop practice strategies so the athletes can correct the problems.

***Phase portraits.***   The use of topological portraits, or **phase portraits,** to describe how movements are being controlled is an important measurement technique used by researchers to explore the qualitative dynamics associated with coordinated behavior within the framework of dynamical approaches

Phase portraits are used to illustrate how a particular joint is controlled during a movement.

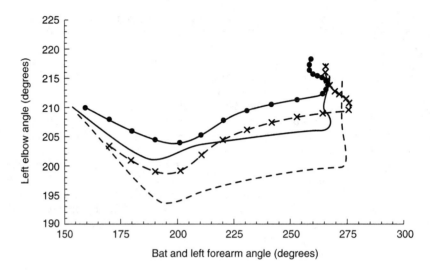

Solid = group 1, same field. Solid-dotted = group 1, opposite field.
Dashed = group 2, same field. Dashed-× = group 2, opposite field.

**Figure 2.4** Angle–angle diagram of the elbow angle and the bat-and-left-forearm angle during a baseball batting swing to either the same field or the opposite field by effective (group 1) and by ineffective (group 2) opposite-field hitters.

described in Chapter 1. Phase portraits similar to those shown in Figure 2.5a–d are geometric representations of movement that are obtained by continuously plotting the relationship between two kinematic measures of interest. According to Stergiou (2004), "a phase portrait provides a qualitative picture of the organization of the neuromuscular system" (p. 97) during the performance of a movement. The most commonly studied movement pattern using phase portraits is gait. In contrast to the A–A diagrams just described, the dynamic position of a particular joint is plotted against a movement parameter (angular velocity) rather than the position of a second limb segment. In this way, the manner in which a particular limb is coordinated *and* the way it is controlled can be measured concurrently.

Winstein and Garfinkel (1985) suggest that displaying the relationship between joint angular velocity and the position of a particular joint as a phase portrait provides a pictorial summary of the relationship between the changing velocity of a limb and its effect on joint position. Depicting the relationship between the two kinematic measures in this way also eliminates the need to review multiple graphs of single measures plotted against time (for example, limb velocity vs. time; limb position vs. time), as the more traditional approach requires. Winstein and Garfinkel used this method to compare the trajectories of movement observed in unimpaired locomotor behavior with the disordered locomotor patterns exhibited by individuals with neurological impairments. They were particularly interested in learning more about the underlying control mechanisms and how they influence the resulting action.

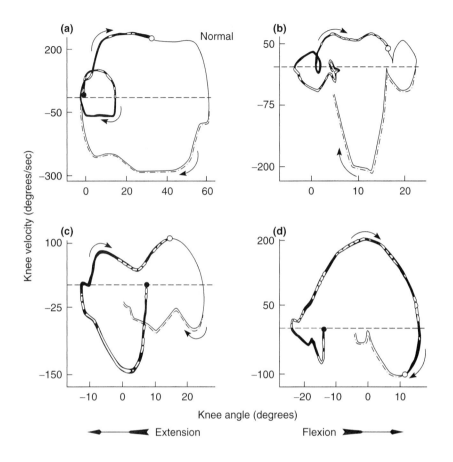

**Figure 2.5** **(a)** Normal phase trajectory of knee angle plotted against angular velocity for one gait cycle. **(b–d)** Phase trajectories plotted for each of three hemiparetic patients. These phase portraits illustrate the different levels of control exerted by the knee joint during walking.

As Figure 2.5 indicates, clear differences are evident between the phase trajectories exhibited by an unimpaired individual (a) and those exhibited by three patients with hemiparesis (b, c, and d). (An individual with **hemipare-sis** is one who has muscular weakness only on one side.) The authors identify at least four qualitative features that differentiate disordered from unimpaired locomotor patterns: (1) the absence of a square phase trajectory, indicating the loss of appropriate timing and focused control, (2) the absence of certain phase-dependent features, (3) smaller overall movement trajectories and velocities, and (4) the presence of cusps or "catches" in the movement trajectory that may indicate inappropriate activity of flexor and extensor muscle groups. Winstein and Garfinkel suggest that further development and implementation of this type of qualitative measurement technique may eventually allow researchers to identify "qualitative signatures" that characterize certain motor control pathologies.

Phase portraits have been used to examine many of the basic tenets associated with dynamical approaches, in particular (Clark & Phillips, 1993). Not only have they been used to compare the differences in neuromuscular control between healthy and abnormal gait patterns (see Figure 2.5; Winstein & Garfinkel 1985), but they have also been used to qualitatively evaluate the stability of the neuromuscular system, particularly when multiple gait cycles are plotted in the same phase portrait (Clark & Phillips, 1993). From a theoretical perspective, observable instabilities within the neuromuscular system have been associated with a pending transition from one pattern of coordination (the attractor state) to another as a result of practice or learning or with some type of underlying disease process (such as Parkinson's disease, multiple sclerosis, cerebral palsy) that renders the movement pattern unstable over time.

*Relative phasing.*  A related measure that is being used with increasing frequency by dynamical theorists to examine how limb segments are coordinated during the performance and learning of different movement skills is **relative phasing.** This measure is derived through a mathematical process that begins with the transformation of the phase portrait trajectories from $x, y$ coordinates to what are referred to as polar coordinates comprised of a radius $r$ and phase angle $\theta$. Although beyond the scope of this chapter, the reader can learn more about how to calculate this particular measure in Stergiou (2004), which describes a number of innovative methods currently being used to analyze the dynamics of human motion.

According to Kurz and Stergiou (2004), what is unique about the relative phasing measure is that it "compresses four variables (i.e., proximal and distal segments' displacement and velocities) into one measure" (p. 99). Depending on the relative phase values obtained, a researcher can determine whether two moving segments either are in-phase, or moving in the same direction (have a relative phase value of zero degrees), or are out-of-phase, or in opposite directions (have a relative phase value of 180 degrees). Whether the relative phase value is positive or negative also tells us which limb segment being studied (distal versus proximal) is ahead of the other during performance of the movement (see Figure 2.6). Relative phase analysis has been used in a number of research studies exploring the coordination and control of the neuromuscular system in both the performance and learning of many different types of movements (Barela, Whitall, Black, & Clark, 2000; Ko, Challis, & Newell, 2003; Lee, Swinnen, & Verschueren, 1995; van Emmerik & Wagenaar, 1996).

New measurement tools and statistical methods for exploring the dynamics of human motion continue to emerge in the motor control literature, providing a very different view of neuromuscular system function. Although only A–A diagrams, phase portraits, and relative phasing measures were discussed in this chapter, many other measurement tools and variations of those already discussed are currently being used to address important research questions in the area of motor control and learning. These nontraditional methods of analysis have been particularly useful for studying the physical dynamics of the human system from a nonlinear perspective as advocated by theorists aligned with both the dynamical and ecological approaches to motor control. Readers are encouraged to review Stergiou (2004) for a more in-depth discussion of a

Relative phase values can be used to describe the changing relationship between two limb segments during a movement.

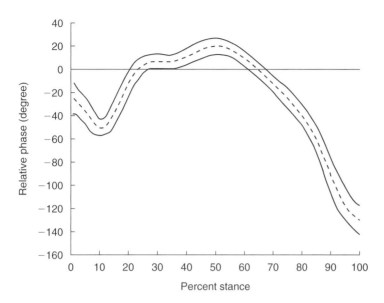

**Figure 2.6**  Relative phase–angle relationship between the thigh and shank segments of the leg during the stance phase of gait. The relative phase is represented by the dashed line, and the bold lines represent the standard deviation about the mean ensemble curve. Positive slope values indicate that the shank is leading the thigh segment, whereas negative slope values indicate the thigh segment to be ahead of the shank.

broad range of relatively new and innovative quantitative methods and analyses being applied to the study of human motor control.

*Electromyography (EMG).*  We noted earlier that **electromyography (EMG)** has enabled researchers to fractionate RT into a central and a peripheral component. It has also provided valuable information about a muscle's activity during movement. Recording electrodes are usually placed on the surface of the skin above the muscles of interest for the purpose of measuring the level of electrical activity that occurs in agonist and antagonist muscle groups during a particular movement. Once the raw EMG signal obtained from each muscle has been amplified and filtered, important spatial and temporal characteristics of the movement can be identified from the resulting output. An EMG wave form can answer questions related to the amount of force exerted by a given muscle, its amplitude and duration of contraction, and, in the case of multiple recordings, the temporal coordination between the various muscle groups.

Multiple EMG recordings have been used to describe how the various muscle groups in the leg and trunk are activated when we attempt to maintain and/or restore postural stability in a variety of environmental conditions. As Figure 2.7a and b on page 50 illustrate, when the surface below us is relatively flat and broad, balance is restored after a **perturbation** (manual disturbance of body position) by using an ankle synergy. This synergy is characterized by a muscle activation pattern that begins in the ankle joint muscles

Multiple EMG recordings have been used to describe how various muscle groups in the leg and trunk are activated when we attempt to restore balance.

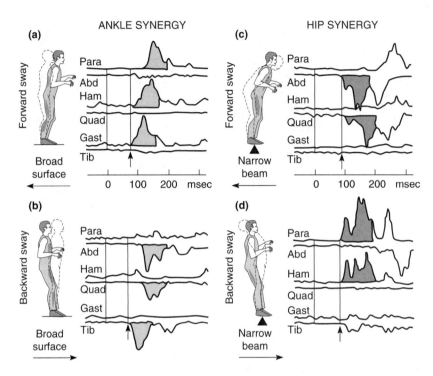

**Figure 2.7**   EMG recordings have been used to demonstrate the types of muscle response patterns to forward (**a** and **c**) and backward (**b** and **d**) sway perturbations. An ankle synergy is used on a normal, broad surface (**a** and **b**), whereas a hip synergy is used on a narrow surface (**c** and **d**).

Para = paraspinals; Abd = abdominal muscles; Ham = hamstrings;
Quad = quadricep muscles; Gast = gastrocnemius; Tib = tibialis

opposing the sway perturbation and then progresses to the proximal muscles in the thigh and lower trunk on the same dorsal or ventral aspect of the body. However, when the support surface below us (a narrow beam, for example) is shorter than the feet are long, a different postural synergy comes into play to help us maintain an upright posture. In this situation, muscles in the thigh and lower trunk muscles are activated on the opposite aspect of the body to those activated on the broader support surface. This activation pattern usually begins within 100 ms after the support surface is moved in a forward or backward direction. Figure 2.7c and d clearly indicate that a hip synergy is now being used to restore the body to an upright stance.

*Kinetic measures.*   The analysis of any movement is really not complete until all the various internal and external forces acting on the body are considered. **Kinetic measures** are used to describe the forces that produce the displacements observed in different parts of the body during the performance of a movement. Specifically, they describe the forces of individual muscles, the net movements generated by the muscles at each joint, and the associated mechanical patterns that arise from the rate at which mechanical energy is

Kinetic measures help us to understand why it is possible to achieve similar movement outcomes using different levels of force.

absorbed and generated by the muscles or transferred across limb segments as we move. Gravitational influences also contribute to the kinetics associated with a movement.

A number of different types of specialized equipment (such as electromyography and force transducers) are used to study the internal forces generated by muscle and the external forces (force plates) generated by the feet against the surface during activities such as walking, running, and jumping. While some kinetic measures can be measured directly (such as ground reaction forces and muscle force), others are calculated using algebraic equations derived from basic principles of physics or such other forms of dynamic analysis as inverse, forward, and intersegmental dynamics.

Once the amount of force applied by various limbs throughout the course of the movement has been analyzed and graphically represented, researchers can determine how it is possible to achieve a similar movement outcome using different levels of force.

*Electromyography as a kinetic measure.*   Although we have already discussed the use of EMG in the previous section related to the kinematic analysis of movement, it is also used extensively to analyze internal muscle forces during movement. Researchers have used EMG to study the neurological strategies used to control different goal-directed movements in particular. For example, by comparing the patterns of muscle activation (amplitude and duration) with the kinematics of limb movement, different control strategies used to move the limb to endpoint targets requiring different degrees of precision with or without certain time constraints imposed have been observed. On the basis of this research, a number of different theoretical hypotheses have been developed to explain how goal-directed movements are achieved in response to different task and environmental demands (Corcos, Gottlieb, & Agarwal, 1989; Gottlieb, Corcos, Agarwal, & Latash, 1990; Feldman, 1966, 1986; Latash, 1998). These different hypotheses will be discussed in greater depth in Chapter 4. The analysis of kinematic variables in conjunction with EMG activity patterns has also proven to be extremely useful in better understanding the pathophysiology associated with different movement disorders such as Parkinson's disease, cerebellar ataxia, and Huntington's disease (Berardelli, Rona, Inghilleri, & Manfredi, 1996).

# Neurological Measures

The fact that we know as much as we do about the inner workings of the nervous system is largely due to advances in recording techniques and instrumentation that have taken place over the last 100 years. These techniques have proven useful to researchers studying hierarchical theories of motor control at a neurological level of analysis. These techniques can be divided into two categories: invasive and noninvasive techniques. Two examples of invasive techniques that have been used to study CNS function in animals will be discussed in this section as well as three noninvasive brain mapping and scanning techniques that are more appropriate for use with humans. The two invasive techniques to be discussed are intracellular recordings and lesions and ablations, while the three noninvasive techniques to be discussed are positron emission tomography, functional magnetic resonance imaging, and transcranial magnetic stimulation.

## Intracellular Recordings

The development and refinement of intracellular recording techniques has provided neuroscientists with the means to explore directly the internal operations of brain cells during the execution of movement. To accomplish this goal, a micropipette with a very sharp tip is inserted directly into the brain and used to record intracellular potentials as a movement proceeds. Although the use of this invasive technique is limited to animal studies, it has provided us with a better understanding of the role of certain neurological structures in the planning and execution of movements. For example, intracellular recordings of cell activity in the basal ganglia have shown they play a much more diverse role in the planning and control of movement (Connor & Abbs, 1991; DeLong & Georgopoulos, 1981) than was previously thought. Similarly, recordings obtained from certain cells of the cerebellum have elucidated its functions in the control and learning of movements (Brooks, 1984; Gilbert & Thach, 1977).

## Lesions and Ablations

Another type of experimental method used to identify the possible role(s) played by various structures within the CNS during movement involves either the **ablation** (cutting out) of certain well-known structures in the CNS or the introduction of lesions to the same structures. The invasive nature of these two techniques restricts their use to animal applications. In these studies, the ability of animals to control and/or learn new movements is carefully studied after the removal or lesioning of the structure of interest. Evidence of the brain's ability to reorganize following the introduction of a lesion into a specific cortical area has also been demonstrated in adult monkeys that received a lesion to one side of the motor cortex during infancy (Rouiller et al., 1998). In this case, an almost complete representation of the hand had been reestablished by adulthood in a region of the motor cortex that was adjacent to the old lesion. Although the results of such animal studies have enriched our knowledge base about the functions of individual structures and the residual capabilities of other connecting structures within the CNS, one must be cautious in applying these findings to human nervous system function.

An alternative to the use of animal models to describe CNS function has been the development of pathological models of motor control based on clinically diagnosed populations. Despite the distributed processing that characterizes the human nervous system, wherein responsibility for action planning and execution is shared by a number of cortical and subcortical structures, several neurological disorders affect specific brain structures and motor behavior in clearly identifiable ways. For example, studies conducted with individuals suffering from Parkinson's disease (Della Sala, Lorenzo, Giordano, & Spinnler, 1986; Stelmach, Worringham, & Strand, 1986), known to selectively affect basal ganglia function, have yielded considerable insight into the role of the basal ganglia in the planning and coordination of movement. Clinical observations of patients with damage confined to the cerebellum (Hallett, Shahani, & Young, 1975; Nashner & Grimm, 1978), another important structure involved in the planning and coordination of movement, have also yielded valuable information about normal CNS function. In the next chapter, we will discuss in greater detail the roles of the basal ganglia and cerebellum in motor control.

# Brain Mapping and Scanning Techniques

During the course of the last decade, further advances in technology have made it possible to visualize the CNS on a grand scale. Three particularly exciting techniques that have provided considerable insight into the workings of the human brain and its capacity for reorganization following cerebral trauma will be described here. These include positron emission tomography, functional magnetic resonance imaging, and transcranial magnetic stimulation.

*Positron Emission Tomography (PET).*    A brain scanning technique that has been in use since the 1970s and has enabled scientists to study dynamic brain function is **positron emission tomography (PET).** PET scans are used for measuring the concentration of positron-emitting radioisotopes within different body tissues. Specific tracer compounds such as fluorine-18, carbon-11, or oxygen-15 are introduced into the bloodstream by injection or inhalation. Using a computerized reconstruction procedure to develop the tomographic images, scientists are able to evaluate biochemical changes occurring in different areas of the body.

Positron emission tomography (PET) has been used to study dynamic brain function.

With respect to research conducted in the area of motor control and learning, PET has been used to study, among other things, the brain mechanisms that underlie the retrieval of memories (Kapur, Craik, & Jones, 1995) and the performance of different perceptual–motor tasks (Ghatan, Hsieh, & Wirsen-Meurling, 1995). The use of PET has also contributed much to our clinical understanding of different neurological disease processes and has been used extensively in drug research and development because of its ability to monitor where a particular drug is distributed in the body once administered.

*Functional Magnetic Resonance Imaging (fMRI).*    **Functional magnetic resonance imaging (fMRI)** techniques have assisted researchers to visualize changes in brain function as a result of the chemical composition of brain areas or change in fluid flow (such as cerebrospinal fluid, blood) over a given period of recording. As with PET, fMRI can be used to find out what the brain is doing while a person responds to a range of different stimuli presented or while performing a specific motor task. Because of its better temporal and spatial resolution, however, fMRI techniques have been used in conjunction with or instead of PET scanning techniques in recent years.

Functional magnetic resonance imaging (fMRI) techniques are used to identify neural structures or brain regions involved in the learning and retention of motor skills.

The fMRI imaging technique involves taking a series of images of the brain in very quick succession and then statistically analyzing the images to see if any differences exist between them. In fact, a complete brain slice can be imaged in as little as 20 ms (Cohen & Bookheimer, 1994). These imaging techniques have been used to identify the neural structures or regions of the brain that are critical for the acquisition and retention of motor skills (Karni, 1996; Doyon & Ungerleider, 2002; Sanes & Donoghue, 2000); we will talk in more detail about these areas of the brain in the motor learning section of this book. The same techniques have also been used to document the dynamic neural changes that occur during the different phases of learning a motor skill (Karni et al., 1995; Ungerleider, Doyon, & Karni, 2002).

Using a serial reaction time task, Doyon and Ungerleider (2002) had their study participants practice pressing one of four buttons as quickly as possible as soon as a red circle corresponding to the particular button's location appeared on a screen placed in front of them. Subjects then practiced a repeating 10-item

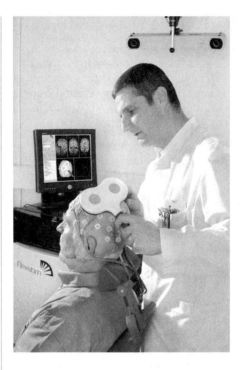

**Figure 2.8**  A study participant being prepared for transcranial magnetic stimulation (TMS). Motor evoked potentials (MEPs) are triggered using a cortical magnetic stimulator comprised of a hand-held coil device that produces a large magnetic pulse delivered by a main stimulator unit.

movement sequence taught to them for one-hour practice periods over three sessions. The results of the fMRI scans used to track the changes in brain activation patterns that occurred as the learning of the sequence progressed showed activation in certain areas of the brain early in the learning which then shifted to other regions as the skill became better learned. This study and others that have been conducted provide good evidence that functional reorganization of the cortex takes place within specific areas as a function of learning new movement skills. You will learn more about which specific areas of the brain are involved in both the control and learning of motor skills in later chapters of this book.

*Transcranial Magnetic Stimulation (TMS).*   With the development of **transcranial magnetic stimulation (TMS)** in 1985, it has become possible for researchers to not only map the exact nature of cortical motor output, but also to more clearly demonstrate the type of cortical reorganization that naturally follows injury-induced trauma to the nervous system (as with spinal cord injury or stroke) or the plastic changes that can be induced as a result of receiving a particular treatment intervention (for example, constraint-induced physical therapy following a cortical stroke). **Motor evoked potentials (MEPs)** are triggered using a cortical magnetic stimulator comprised of a hand-held coil device that produces a large magnetic pulse lasting only 150 to 200 ms. This magnetic pulse is delivered by a main stimulator unit to which the hand-held device is connected (see Figure 2.8).

In a recent study conducted by Liepert et al. (2000), for example, TMS was used to map the cortical motor output area representing a hand muscle

Transcranial magnetic stimulation (TMS) is capable of mapping the exact nature of cortical motor output in the form of motor evoked potentials (MEPs).

before and after 12 days of constraint-induced movement therapy provided to patients with chronic stroke. This type of movement therapy has become more widely used by physical therapists to assist patients who have suffered a stroke regain the use of an affected extremity. Briefly, the treatment technique requires that the patient wear some type of device (such as a hand splint and sling on the unaffected arm) that makes it extremely difficult to use the unaffected limb while performing different motor activities with the **paretic** (partially paralyzed) limb only. What the researchers were able to show using TMS was a significant increase in the level of cortical motor output in the damaged hemisphere that persisted well after the treatment had ended. This increase in cortical motor output paralleled the improvement in motor function observed in the involved limb.

In addition to being able to quantify outcomes in a number of research studies, TMS has also been used in clinical settings to assist physicians in identifying the level of dysfunction in the primary motor pathways of patients with certain neurological diseases that affect nerve conduction capabilities (including multiple sclerosis and spinal cord injury) but also as a means of predicting how much motor recovery can be expected following certain types of neurological trauma (such as stroke and spinal cord injury). We can certainly expect that the study of motor control and learning will be significantly enhanced in the years to come as these more sophisticated brain scanning and mapping techniques become more widely used by researchers. Because of their ability to provide us with a window into the inner workings of the nervous system, researchers can begin to use these different types of brain scanning and mapping techniques to more definitively identify the types of neurological mechanisms and processes that underlie the observable motor behavior that you as practitioners see after a motor skill has been practiced for a period of time or a particular method of treatment is used to assist a patient regain motor function.

## Summary

Researchers have employed a variety of measurement techniques in their attempts to understand how the human system produces an infinite number of motor actions. At a psychological level of analysis, researchers have used a combination of measurement techniques in an effort to describe what elements of the human system are being controlled and how the processes underlying performance are organized. These techniques have focused largely on the use of various kinematic, kinetic, and electromyographical measures of movement and innovative techniques for qualitatively representing the dynamic elements of action (e.g., A–A diagrams and phase portraits).

Chronometric measures (such as measures of reaction time and movement time) have been used to explore the timing and duration of cognitive operations that researchers hypothesize are involved in the planning and execution of action plans. Reaction time has been further partitioned into central (or premotor) and peripheral (or motor) components in an effort to better understand the neuromuscular processes underlying motor performance. Various types of performance error measures have also been used to learn more about the nature of the movement outcome. Typical error scores used to study movement outcomes in one-dimensional tasks have included absolute, variable, constant, and total error scores, while two-dimensional task outcomes have been explored using radial error scores. For continuous motor skills such as tracking and driving, root-mean-square error has been used to quantify the amount of error produced relative to a criterion goal. Recent technological advances have also permitted the use of neurological measurement techniques to study how a particular action is organized to achieve a given goal. While the use of more invasive neurological measures such as intracellular recordings and ablation and lesion techniques have been limited to animal studies, less invasive measures that include brain mapping and scanning techniques (such as positron emission tomography, functional magnetic resonance imaging, transcranial magnetic stimulation, and evoked potentials) have been safely used with humans. These more objective process measures have contributed many pieces to the puzzle of human motor control.

Although there are still many more questions than answers in the area of motor control, the continued development of new measurement techniques should enable researchers to test ever more effectively the predictions of present and future theories of motor control.

## IMPORTANT TERMINOLOGY

After completing this chapter, readers should be familiar with the following terms and concepts.

ablation
absolute constant error (|CE|)
absolute error (AE)
angle–angle (A–A) diagram
choice reaction time (CRT)
chronometry
constant error (CE)
discrimination reaction time (DRT)
electromyography (EMG)
fractionated reaction time (FRT)
functional magnetic resonance
    imaging (fMRI)
hemiparesis
kinematics
kinetic measures
measures
motor evoked potentials (MEPs)
motor time (MOT)

movement time (MT)
one-dimensional motor tasks
paretic
perturbation
phase portraits
positron emission topography (PET)
premotor time (PRMOT)
radial error (RE)
reaction time (RT)
relative phasing
root-mean-square error (RMSE)
simple reaction time (SRT)
speed–accuracy trade-off
total error (E)
transcranial magnetic stimulation
    (TMS)
two-dimensional movement skills
variable error (VE)

## SUGGESTED FURTHER READING

Christina, R. W. (1992). The 1991 C. H. McCloy Research Lecture: Unraveling the mystery of the response complexity effect in skilled movements. *Research Quarterly for Exercise and Sport, 63,* 218–230.

Hamill, J., Haddad, J. M., & McDermott, W. J. (2000). Issues in quantifying variability from a dynamical systems perspective. *Journal of Applied Biomechanics, 16,* 407–418.

Stergiou, N. (ed.). 2004. *Innovative analyses of human movement.* Champaign, IL: Human Kinetics.

## TEST YOUR UNDERSTANDING

1. Describe the various types of measurement that have been categorized as (a) response outcome measures and (b) response process measures.

2. How does the type of information obtained by using fractionated reaction time differ from that obtained by using other types of reaction time measures?

3. Describe three task-related variables that influence how quickly a movement is initiated.

4. Identify the performance error measures that convey each of the following kinds of information about a performance.
   a. The total amount of error.
   b. Whether the performer undershot or overshot the target.
   c. The amount of variability observed in a task such as throwing.
   d. The accuracy with which a golfer putted a golf ball on five separate attempts.
   e. The accuracy with which a performer was able to track a moving object on a video screen.

5. Briefly explain what the term *speed–accuracy trade-off* means. In what type of movement situations is it likely to occur?

6. Briefly explain how the kinematic measures of limb displacement, velocity, and acceleration are derived from a high-speed film analysis of a performer's movements.

7. Compare the type of information obtained by using kinematic measures with that obtained by using kinetic measures.

8. Briefly describe how angle–angle diagrams and phase portraits contribute to our understanding of motor control. Provide examples of sports and/or clinical situations in which these two different types of measurement techniques have been used.

9. Identify neurological measures that are categorized as invasive techniques and those categorized as noninvasive.

10. What kind of information about brain function has been provided through the use of such brain mapping and scanning techniques as functional magnetic resonance imaging and transcranial magnetic stimulation?

## PRACTICAL ACTIVITIES

1. Calculate the mean absolute error (|AE|), mean constant error (CE) or mean absolute constant error (|CE|), mean variable error (VE), and total |Error| (E) for each individual shooter and the total group across the five shots recorded. Positive scores indicate that the shooter hit the target to the right of the bull's-eye, while negative scores indicate that the target was hit to the left of the bull's-eye.

   Shooter 1: −8, +6, −9, −9, −7
   Shooter 2: +6, +9, −5, +4, −8
   Shooter 3: −9, −7, −8, −10, +9
   Shooter 4: −4, −7, −4, −9, −7
   Shooter 5: −5, 0, +3, −4, +2

2. Calculate the radial error (RE) based on the scores of a golfer attempting to sink a putt from 15 feet away. The center of the hole is set at 0. Calculate the golfer's average radial error for the four putting attempts.

| Trial | $x$ Value | $y$ Value | Total RE = $(x^2 + y^2)$ |
|-------|-----------|-----------|--------------------------|
| 1 | 10 cm | 4 cm | |
| 2 | 8 cm | 2 cm | |
| 3 | 7 cm | 5 cm | |
| 4 | 4 cm | 2 cm | |
| | | | Average RE: |

# 3

# SOMATOSENSORY CONTRIBUTIONS TO ACTION

*Our sensory systems are the way in which we perceive the external world, remain alert,*
*form a body image, and regulate our movements.*

GARDNER & MARTIN (2000)

## CHAPTER OBJECTIVES

After studying this chapter, you should be able to:

- Understand and be able to identify the general properties of sensory receptors and afferent pathways and the processes by which they assist the various subsystems within the CNS to derive meaning from the many different types of sensations.

- Identify and describe the relative contributions of the various receptors that are associated with somesthesia—bodily sensations of touch, pain, temperature, and limb position.

- Describe how the various types of somatic sensations are relayed to the brain.

- Understand how knowledge about the processes underlying the reception, transmission, and interpretation of sensory information can be applied to practical settings.

- Identify the various afferent sources of kinesthetic sensations and explain how they can be exploited by the practitioner teaching different types of movement skills.

- Understand and be able to describe the multiple roles played by sensory feedback in both the planning and the moment-to-moment control of movement.

Our goal in this chapter and the one to follow is to describe how the various types of sensory inputs that are available to us from our surrounding environment are first received and then processed by the central nervous system. As you will learn, three sensory systems (somatosensation, vision, and vestibular) in particular provide us with a sophisticated ensemble of information about different aspects of the environment and our position in it. Once integrated and organized in specialized areas of the cortex, this information is used to guide the planning and execution of a variety of different movement responses. Although each of these three systems is unique in structure and function, certain principles related to the reception and transmission of sensory information are common to all sensory systems. In this chapter we will consider these general principles before proceeding with a more comprehensive discussion of the specific mechanisms that govern the processing of somatosensory information. Specifically, we will describe the processes occurring from the time receptors signaling the somatic sensations of touch, proprioception, temperature, and pain are activated to the first conscious perception that a significant environmental event has occurred. The visual and vestibular system will be discussed more fully in Chapter 4.

# General Properties of Sensory Receptors and Afferent Pathways

Sensory systems provide us with a sophisticated ensemble of information about the environment that can be used to guide the planning and execution of action.

Sensory receptors convert various forms of environmental energy into electrical impulses by a process called transduction.

Sensory receptors that monitor the external environment and continually apprise us of our position in space are located throughout the body. They are found in the retina of the eye, in various layers of the skin, and in other regions such as the joints and muscles. During the course of our discussion in these next two chapters, we will discover that different types of sensory receptors contribute specific information about the environment that is added to a larger ensemble of sensory information garnered from other sensory systems.

These sense organs, or sensory receptors, also serve as our windows to the external world through their ability to extract environmental information in its various forms (light, sound waves, and touch) and then convert it into a form that the CNS can understand. The process by which the various sensory receptors convert a particular form of energy into another form is referred to as **transduction.** In the case of the CNS, all environmental information is transduced into electrical impulses.

Three general properties of sensory receptors and their associated afferent pathways help the various subsystems within the CNS derive meaning from the various forms of energy available in the environment. These properties are adequate stimulation, intensity coding, and sensory adaptation. A discussion of each of these properties will be the focus of the next section.

## Adequate Stimulation

How do we know that a certain event has occurred in the environment? For example, how do we know that someone is tapping us on the shoulder or waving at us from across a room? A considerable number of sensory receptors that are designed to respond to particular kinds of sensory stimulation assist us in registering this information as it actually occurs. For example, sensory receptors located in the retina respond to changing patterns of light entering the eye, and sound waves that enter the ear stimulate specialized receptors for auditory sensations. In the case of the somatosensory system, cutaneous receptors respond to different levels of touch and pressure while the proprioceptors respond to other types of mechanical stimulation such as the stretching of a muscle or the increasing tension on a muscle as it contracts.

Although it is possible for other forms of energy to stimulate sensory receptors (for instance, high levels of pressure applied to the eyeball, perhaps as a result of being hit in the eye, result in a sensation of light), they are especially sensitive to particular kinds of sensory input. This latter property of sensory receptors is often called **adequate stimulation** and is exhibited when a particular sensory event or stimulus raises a receptor's resting level high enough to generate sensory impulses (Eyzaguirre & Fidone, 1975). In addition to informing the CNS that a particular sensory event has occurred, this characteristic of sensory receptors contributes to our ability to distinguish among the many types of environmental input available to us.

> Adequate stimulation is the process by which sensory receptors inform the CNS that a particular sensory event has occurred.

## Intensity Coding

Not only do the sensory receptors and the afferent pathways that carry the generated impulse into the CNS provide us with information about *where* and *when* an environmental event or stimulus occurred, but they also convey information about the *intensity* with which the event occurred. This second piece of information is carried in the form of an **intensity code** that begins at the level of the sensory receptors. This property of sensory receptors enables us to discriminate, for example, between sensations associated with a light tap and those resulting from a hard poke or a slap on the back.

The rate at which a particular sensory receptor or group of receptors is able to generate signals that are great enough to trigger an electrical impulse in the nearby sensory neuron largely determines how intensely we ultimately perceive a given stimulus to be. For example, a strong stimulus (such as a hard push) causes the stimulated receptors to fire at a much higher frequency than they would if a much less intense stimulus (such as a light tap) were applied to the skin's surface. This mechanism is referred to as **temporal summation.** Given that a stronger stimulus such as a hard slap also tends to affect a larger surface area, we can expect that a greater number of sensory receptors will also be stimulated. In fact, the number of sensory receptors that fire simultaneously provides another valuable clue to the nature and intensity of the stimulus. This second mechanism is called **spatial summation.** Sensations of high intensity generate larger **receptor potentials** (electrical signals produced by the stimulated receptors) that in turn generate a greater number and frequency of **action potentials** (electrical signals produced in the axons that lead away from the cell body, or soma, of the sensory neuron).

> The intensity code of a sensory event is conveyed to the CNS via temporal and spatial summation.

## Sensory Adaptation

Consider for a moment how you feel when you first dive into a mountain lake or outdoor pool. The first overwhelming sensation is probably one of being extremely cold as the water comes in contact with the thousands of cutaneous receptors lying close to the surface of the skin. Though it is often unpleasant initially, the sensation of coldness usually lasts for only a short time. Similarly, you can feel a pair of glasses pressing against your skin for a while after you put them on, but it is not long before the sensation subsides. In fact, some people become quite disturbed when they are unable to locate a pair of glasses they were wearing earlier, only to be told by a friend that

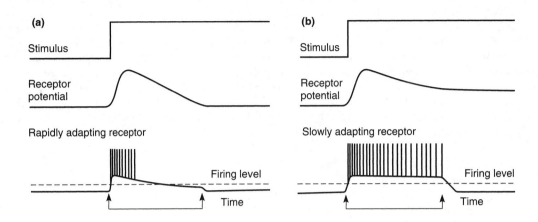

**Figure 3.1**   The sensory adaptation rates of these two sensory receptors are not the same, as indicated by the different firing patterns.

A sensory receptor adapts to a stimulus by reducing its level of firing soon after it is applied.

their glasses are perched on top of their heads. Why is it that we do not continue to be aware of these different cutaneous sensations until they are removed? A third property associated with sensory receptors, **adaptation,** provides us with the answer to this question.

As Figure 3.1 illustrates, shortly after a particular stimulus has been registered by a sensory receptor, the level of firing observed is greatly reduced. As you can also see by comparing the firing patterns of the two different types of sensory receptors shown, the rate of adaptation is not the same for all sensory receptors in the body. For example, receptors that transmit sensations of touch and pressure adapt rapidly, whereas pain receptors and certain proprioceptors adapt very slowly. Unlike rapidly adapting receptors that often cease firing immediately after a stimulus has been applied, slowly adapting receptors continue to respond throughout the duration of a sensory event.

Why is it advantageous for us to have these two types of sensory receptors with different adaptation rates? The existence of rapidly as well as slowly adapting receptors allows the sensory systems to detect differences in the pattern of sensory stimulation, with respect to both its temporal and spatial properties. For example, rapidly adapting receptors sense the temporal aspects of a given sensation (velocity and acceleration) because they fire rapidly when first activated but cease firing until the sensory stimulus either increases or decreases. These firing characteristics make them well suited for conveying information about changes occurring in the sensory environment to the brain (Gardner & Martin, 2000). In contrast, slowly adapting receptors, that are capable of signaling the magnitude of an applied stimulus for many minutes, are more likely to keep the brain apprised of the state of the environment at any given point in time.

# The Transmission and Integration of Sensory Input

Once the different types of sensory inputs have been converted to electrical impulses at the level of the sensory receptor, they travel via specialized pathways toward the cortex, where they are further analyzed and integrated with other sensory inputs. Before reaching the cortex, however, all sensory information except that provided by olfaction (smell) passes through an important group of nuclei located in an area of the brain called the **diencephalon.** It is here, within this group of approximately 50 nuclei, collectively called the **thalamus,** that a considerable amount of complex information processing takes place. While certain nuclei filter the incoming sensory information, gating out (blocking) irrelevant sensory inputs and directing those that are relevant to an impending or ongoing action toward specific areas within the primary sensory cortex, other nuclei participate in different types of motor functions, transmitting information received from the cerebellum and basal ganglia, for example, to motor regions within the frontal lobe. It is believed that as a result of these connections with the frontal lobe, the thalamus may play a role in cognitive functions such as memory (Amaral, 2000). Through its neural connections with the limbic system, a structure we will discuss in more detail in Chapter 5, the thalamus also influences our emotional responses to sensory experiences. Perhaps the best way to demonstrate how the thalamus influences our emotional responses to certain sensory events is to describe what happens when lesions form in the thalamus and disrupt its normal function.

*The thalamus acts as a sensory filter blocking out irrelevant sensory information and sending relevant information to the cortex.*

Patients with a disorder known as **thalamic syndrome,** that often results from an infarct in a small region of the thalamus known as the ventroposterolateral (VPL) area, experience sensations that are grossly exaggerated, distorted, and/or very unpleasant. Not only are sounds that were once pleasing to the ear perceived as extremely annoying, but even light touch induces painful burning sensations. In addition to the sensory problems experienced, patients with thalamic syndrome often suffer partial or complete paralysis of one side of the body. This is because certain nuclei within the thalamus connect with motor tracts leaving the cortex and the basal ganglia, which, as you will learn in Chapter 5, plays an important role in the planning of movements.

Once the sensory pathways carrying general sensory information about touch, temperature, pain, and proprioception finally terminate in specific areas within the primary sensory cortex, we become consciously aware of the many sensations that have impinged upon us. For example, once the various somatosensory inputs reach their primary sensory areas in the parietal lobe, we are able to recognize the source and intensity of sensations associated with pain and temperature, to discriminate between simple touch and light pressure applied to the skin, and to sense consciously the position of our limbs and their movement through space. Similarly, visual information reaching the primary visual area located in the occipital lobe enables us to detect brightness, light and shade, color, and the shapes of objects.

*Recognition of the source and intensity of sensations is possible once the sensory information reaches specific primary sensory areas.*

How is it that we are able to recognize the exact source of the sensation once the sensory information reaches the primary sensory areas of the cortex? The answer lies in the work of Penfield & Boldrey (1937), who discovered that the somatosensory cortex was **topographically** organized while performing brain surgery on conscious patients. What he found was that when he systematically stimulated different areas on the surface of the cortex, the patient

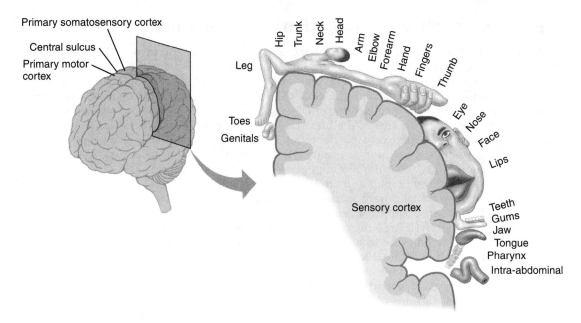

**Figure 3.2**   The amount of area on the sensory cortex devoted to sensory information coming from different regions of the body (e.g., lips, trunk, toes, legs) is not proportional to the size of the body parts relative to our total body mass.

experienced very distinct sensations occurring in different parts of the body. For example, if Penfield stimulated an area near the midline of the brain, the patient would experience sensations in the lower limbs, while if he stimulated areas in the lateral region of the somatosensory cortex, the patient experienced sensations in the upper body, hands, face, and lips.

The **sensory homunculus,** as it is called, provides a useful way of illustrating how the sensory inputs coming from different parts of the body are organized in the somatosensory cortex (see Figure 3.2). What Penfield and his colleague Jasper also found, as you can see in the figure, is that the degree of representation of each body part was disproportionate. Notice that the area devoted to the face and lips, in particular, occupy a much larger area on the cortex when compared to other body parts, such as the trunk and arm, even though these latter body parts constitute a greater proportion of our body mass. You will learn later in this chapter exactly why some regions of the body occupy more space in the somotasensory cortex than others—or have you already guessed why?

The meaningfulness of a sensory event is known once the sensory inputs reach their association areas.

Our final perception of what is occurring in the environment around us is achieved after all of these sensations are integrated and then interpreted by the **association areas** that lie adjacent to the various primary sensory areas associated with the different types of sensory input. Sensory information from a single sensory modality is first processed in **unimodal sensory association areas** that are immediately adjacent to the primary sensory cortex before being sent on to **multimodal sensory association areas** that are responsible for integrating sensory inputs from multiple sensory modalities (Saper, Iversen, & Frackowiak, 2000). Based largely on the clinical evidence provided by Hughlings Jackson (1932), these areas are collectively responsible for interpreting the meaning of the incoming sensory inputs and then associating them with prior experiences stored in memory to form a final perception of what has occurred.

In addition to their role in the sensory integration of sensory inputs, the association areas also perform cognitive activities for the purpose of associating the incoming sensory inputs with outgoing motor outputs. This second integrative function served by the association areas is made possible by the fact that these areas receive sensory information via pathways coming from higher-order sensory areas that are, in turn, sent to higher-order motor association areas responsible for transforming the sensory information into planned movements that are finally executed in the premotor and primary motor cortex. The specific roles played by the sensory and motor association areas, as well as the premotor and motor cortex, will be discussed in greater detail in Chapter 5.

> Association areas in the cortex are responsible for interpreting the meaning of incoming sensory inputs and associating them with prior experiences stored in memory to form a final perception of what has occurred.

Given the important interpretive role played by the association areas, one might expect that any damage to these areas is likely to severely impair our perceptual abilities. In fact, clinical observations have shown that damage to either the unimodal and/or multimodal sensory association areas makes it impossible to recognize familiar objects using one or more of the sensory modalities available to us. This disorder, which is called **agnosia,** may affect our ability to recognize familiar faces, to recognize the sound of a ringing telephone, and/or to identify known objects such as keys or utensils by handling them. Fortunately, an individual who suffers from agnosia caused by damage to the association area of one sensory system is able to compensate for the disorder by using other sensory modalities to derive meaning. For example, a person who has sustained damage to the association area that functions in the interpretation of auditory stimuli can learn to rely on other senses, such as vision. Visual devices can be installed that are activated when the doorbell rings or the oven timer sounds. In this way, an individual is able to function more effectively, at least, at home.

# Somatosensation

Now that we have identified some of the important characteristics of sensory receptors and some general principles associated with sensory transmission, we can begin to describe the three most important sensory systems that influence our perceptions and subsequent actions. The first of these three systems, the somatosensory system, is described in this chapter. In the chapter that follows, we will discuss the visual and vestibular systems and their role in the planning and execution of action.

> The term *somesthesia* means sensations of the body.

The receptors associated with **somesthesia**—bodily sensations of touch, pain, temperature, and limb position—are located in the skin, muscles, tendons, and joints. Collectively, they provide us with information we can use in a movement situation to distinguish between fine and gross tactile sensations, to keep track of the orientation of multiple body parts as they move in space, and to distinguish among different amounts of force applied to an object we are throwing at a target. These somatosensory receptors can be

> Somatosensory receptors can be divided into two categories: cutaneous receptors and proprioceptors.

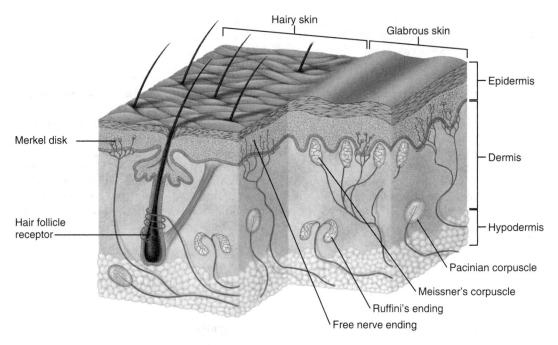

**Figure 3.3**   Cutaneous receptors located in different layers of the skin are responsible for providing specific types of sensory information based on their location and physical characteristics.

further subdivided into **cutaneous receptors** and **proprioceptors.** We will begin our discussion by identifying the various kinds of cutaneous receptors.

## Cutaneous Receptors

The distribution and density of cutaneous receptors determine the level of sensitivity in that area.

The skin contains a myriad of receptors that differ in structure, function, and distribution density. Specific tactile sensations occur when these different types of **mechanoreceptors,** located in different layers of the skin (see Figure 3.3), are physically deformed or the immediate area surrounding them is deformed. For example, Meissner's corpuscles and Merkel disk receptors located in the superficial layers of the skin respond to light touch and slow movement across the skin's surface, respectively, while Pacinian corpuscles located in deeper layers of the skin (dermis) are activated by deep pressure and vibration. The sensory adaptation properties of the different cutaneous receptors also vary. While the Meissner's and Pacinian corpuscles adapt rapidly following stimulation, the Merkel disks and Ruffini's endings, that sense stretch of the skin, are examples of slowly adapting receptors. Recall that earlier in this chapter we indicated that this important property of sensory receptors allows us to differentiate between different patterns of sensory stimulation. In the case of the somatosensory system, the different adaptation properties of the receptors allow us to differentiate between sensations that are quickly applied (such as a light tap) and those that are slow or sustained in nature (such as a stroking or stretching of the skin).

The distribution of cutaneous receptors throughout the body also varies, with the greatest number of receptors found in hairless skin regions such as the lips, fingers, palms of the hands, and soles of the feet. Of particular interest is the fact that Pacinian corpuscles, that respond to deep pressure and vibration, are found in their highest densities in the soles of the feet where they are believed to play an important role in different aspects of posture and locomotion (Quillian, 1975). The higher concentration of receptors results in greater tactile sensitivity in these regions of the body. In contrast, the number of cutaneous receptors in the arms, trunk, and legs is considerably lower. This disproportionate distribution of cutaneous receptors throughout the body explains why the representation of the various body parts within the primary somatic sensory cortex is also disproportionate in size. Recall from your review of the sensory homunculus in Figure 3.2 that the lips, fingers, and face occupied a much larger area than the arm, trunk, and leg. It is therefore the level of tactile sensitivity—not the size of the body part represented—that determines the degree of representation within the somatic cortex. As you have no doubt guessed by now, the different levels of tactile sensitivity associated with different body parts also influences the type of motor control possible. Those body parts with the highest level of tactile sensitivity are involved in the performance of movements requiring fine motor control, whereas other body parts are involved in more gross types of motor control. Just think how difficult the articulation of speech would be if the lips and tongue were not so well endowed with cutaneous receptors.

Although it was once believed that the somatosensory mapping of the body's surface was not amenable to being changed in any way, recent studies have shown that sensory cortical representations can be modified very quickly in some cases and over longer periods of time in other cases (Duchateau & Enoka, 2002). The availability of more sophisticated mapping and imaging techniques such as transcranial magnetic stimulation (TMS) and functional magnetic resonance imaging (fMRI) techniques, which were described in Chapter 2, have made it possible to observe these dynamic changes.

## Proprioceptors

Specialized mechanoreceptors located in the muscles, tendons, and joints provide us with uninterrupted knowledge about the position of body parts relative to each other and the general orientation of our body in space. Dancers and gymnasts use the sensory information provided by these receptors to sense, among other things, the changing and relative positions of their limbs in space throughout a routine. Similarly, a professional baseball pitcher can use this sensory information to determine how quickly his throwing limb is moving through the wind-up phase of the pitch. In the absence of vision, these proprioceptors become even more critical for even the most fundamental postures and movements. A good understanding of their respective functions is therefore warranted.

*Muscle Spindles.*   Muscle spindles, located within all somatic muscles, are considered the most important proprioceptive sense organs. Not only are they essential for the awareness of limb position and movement, but they are also key contributors to fine motor control. This dual sensory and motor function

Proprioceptors provide us with uninterrupted knowledge about the general position of the body in space prior to and during movements.

Muscle spindles signal the absolute length of muscles and the rate of change of muscle length during movement.

is made possible by the fact that the muscle spindle has both sensory and motor connections with the CNS. In this chapter we will discuss the sensory function of the muscle spindle; the motor function of the spindle will be addressed in Chapter 5. Specifically, it is the primary sensory role of the muscle spindle to detect and signal any changes in muscle length as well as the absolute length of a muscle so that we are constantly apprised of where the limbs are in space.

To better understand how muscle spindles can provide this type of sensory information to the CNS, it is important to consider the nature of their physical structure and how they are aligned with respect to the fibers of the extrafusal muscles in which they reside. As Figure 3.4 illustrates, the elongated structures of this proprioceptor, which actually resemble a spindle, lie in parallel with the **extrafusal muscle fibers,** the component of the muscle that produces force, and actually attach at both ends directly to the muscle sheath or the muscle tendon itself. This anatomical arrangement ensures that any change in muscle length is immediately sensed by the muscle spindles.

A closer look inside a single muscle spindle reveals the presence of two types of intrafusal muscle fibers: the **nuclear bag fibers** and **chain fibers.** The nuclear bag fibers are further subdivided into a static and dynamic fiber type. A typical muscle spindle contains two nuclear chain fibers for every four or five nuclear bag fibers. In addition to the two types of intrafusal muscle fibers, each muscle spindle also contains two different types of sensory endings: Ia and II afferents. It is by means of these sensory endings that the spindle is able to detect any changes that occur in the lengths of the extrafusal muscle fibers. As Figure 3.4 illustrates, the larger **Ia afferent,** also called the **primary afferent,** wraps its sensory endings around both the bag and chain fibers, whereas the **type II,** or **secondary afferents** attach to the nuclear chain fibers and static bag fibers but not the dynamic bag fiber subtype. As a result of this anatomical arrangement, the primary (Ia) sensory endings are sensitive to changes in muscle length and velocity, whereas the secondary (II) endings are sensitive only to muscle length.

Exactly how do these small muscle receptors first detect and then signal changes in muscle length to the CNS? During the actual stretching of a muscle, that might occur as a result of an external (such as an unexpected load added to a limb) or internal event (such as muscle fatigue during a movement), the intrafusal muscle fibers of the spindle are also stretched, causing the endings of both the primary (Ia) and secondary (II) afferents to be physically deformed. This deformation of both sensory endings gives rise to an afferent signal that is carried via the primary (Ia) and secondary (II) afferent neurons into the spinal cord and eventually to the higher levels of the CNS via one of the two ascending pathway systems we will discuss later in this chapter. It is interesting to note that the cell body of the afferent or sensory neuron that conveys the electrical impulses from the primary (Ia) and secondary (II) endings is located in the dorsal root ganglion just outside the spinal cord (see Figure 3.6 on page 73).

Although both sensory endings fire during the initial stretch of the muscle spindle, the primary (Ia) afferents fire more rapidly than the secondary (II) afferent endings. These different firing patterns demonstrated by the two types of afferents have been attributed to the different mechanical properties of the nuclear bag and chain intrafusal fibers. The central area (equatorial region) of

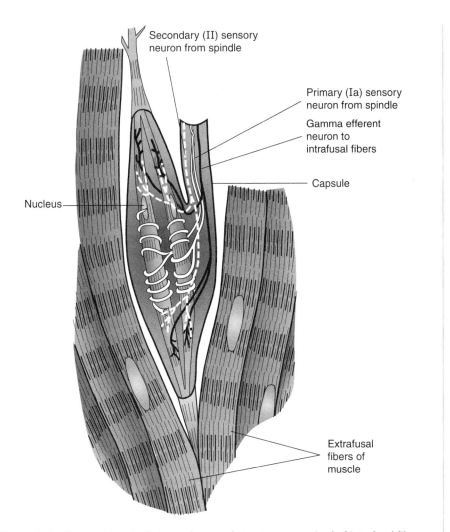

**Figure 3.4**   The muscle spindle is an elongated structure comprised of intrafusal fibers that lies in parallel with and directly attaches to the extrafusal muscles. The muscle spindle is served by two different types of sensory endings: a primary (Ia) and secondary (II) ending.

*Source: Human Anatomy and Physiology,* Second Edition, by Alexander Spence and Elliott Mason. Copyright © 1983 by The Benjamin Cummings Publishing Company. Reprinted by permission.

the nuclear bag fiber has a low threshold for stretch, whereas the chain fiber is stiffer and resists being stretched. Given that the sensory endings of the primary (Ia) afferents wrap around the more compliant bag fibers, it is not surprising that these endings are primarily responsible for informing the CNS about the speed with which the muscles are changing length in the limbs that are accelerating and/or moving through space as we execute a forehand stroke in tennis, swing a golf club, or begin to lift an object from the floor. In contrast, the secondary (II) afferents, whose sensory endings originate on the stiffer chain fibers, do not begin firing until some time after the muscle has begun changing in length. The slowly adapting properties of this second type of sensory receptor do, however, serve an important function by signaling the absolute length of the muscle. This is because they continue to send signals into the CNS long after the more rapidly adapting primary (Ia) afferents cease firing once the muscle stops lengthening.

The number or density of muscle spindles present in human muscles is very much dependent on the function of the muscle, that is, whether the muscle is involved in the performance of fine movements, such as following an object with the eyes or moving the fingers across piano keys, or more gross movements, such as those involved in throwing a ball or running to catch a football. The finer the movement that must be performed by muscles, the higher the densities of muscle spindles found within them. For example, it is estimated that at least 34 muscle spindles reside in the very small first dorsal interosseus, an intrinsic muscle of the hand, while as many as 320 reside in the larger biceps brachii, the muscle group responsible for flexing the elbow (Buchtal & Schmalbruch, 1980). Although the total number of receptors is higher in the biceps muscle, the actual density of receptors is greater in the small interosseus muscle because density is expressed in terms of the number of muscle spindles per gram of the muscle's mean weight (Jones, 1999).

What is interesting to note at this point is that, even though certain muscles in the body contain higher densities of muscle spindles than others, it does not mean that they have greater proprioceptive acuity. This was not the case for the cutaneous receptors just described; the higher the densities of cutaneous receptors, the greater the tactile sensitivity of that particular body region (including lips, tongue, sexual organs).

Golgi tendon organs signal rate of change and absolute amount of tension in a muscle.

*Golgi Tendon Organs.* A second important type of muscle receptor that also plays an important role in proprioception is the **Golgi tendon organ (GTO).** This specialized receptor type is situated at both the distal and proximal myotendinous insertions of skeletal muscle and is primarily responsible for signaling muscle tension and force produced by the contraction of extrafusal muscles. As Figure 3.5 illustrates, each GTO is innervated by a single axon referred to as a Ib axon. Once the myelinated axon enters the capsule surrounding the GTO, it branches into a number of very fine, unmyelinated endings that become intertwined among the collagen strands in the myotendinous junction. It is estimated that a tendon organ capsule has approximately 10 to 20 skeletal muscles housed within it (Bridgman, 1980).

Although it was once thought that GTOs only fired when the tension in a muscle reached a very high level, thus serving a protective role by preventing damage to a contracting muscle, it is now known that they are capable of signaling minute changes in muscle tension. This is no doubt because the axon endings of the GTO are so densely intertwined with the collagen fibers housing the receptor. As soon as the GTO is stretched, the collagen fibers straighten and exert pressure on the axon ending, causing it to fire (see the inset in Figure 3.5). In fact, it has been estimated that as little as one gram of force on the axons of a GTO is needed for them to fire. The fact that physical deformation of the GTO is required for it to fire also makes it a mechanoreceptor just like the cutaneous and muscle spindle receptors already described.

**Figure 3.5** The Golgi tendon organ is located at the junction of the tendon and muscle fibers. The axon endings are closely intertwined with the collagen strands which straighten as the muscle begins to contract, physically deforming the axon endings of the GTO and causing it to fire.

*Source:* Kandel, E. R., Schwartz, J. H., & Jessell, T. M., *Principles of Neural Science*, p. 723, 1985. McGraw Hill Companies. Reprinted by Permission.

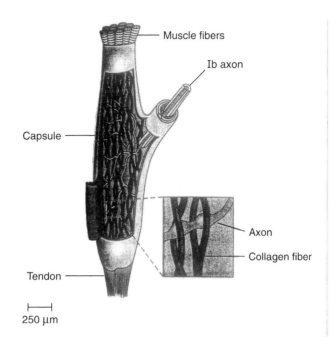

250 μm

From a motor control perspective, the sensory information provided to the CNS by this second important proprioceptor assists us, among other things, to monitor the moment-to-moment changes in muscle tension as we perform a variety of different movements. The sensory information signaled by the GTO also helps us estimate the weight of objects being held in the hands, such as a barbell or tray of food, or the force being applied to an object we are throwing or hitting during a game of baseball or softball.

***Joint Receptors.***   The joint capsules and ligaments of all synovial joints in the skeletal system are well supplied with proprioceptors. These receptors signal mechanical changes in the capsule and ligaments, including changes associated with painful stimuli. Four types of sensory endings, each with a different structure and physiological responsiveness, have been identified: these are Golgi-type endings, located in the ligaments of the joint; Ruffini endings, found in the joint capsule; paciniform endings, located in the periosteum near the articular attachments; and free nerve endings, also found in the joint capsule. These receptors are not uniformly distributed throughout the joint, which Gandevia (1996) suggests may reflect where stresses are applied to the joint during movement.

Given that the greatest percentage of joint receptors fire at the extremes of joint movement (at maximum extension and flexion) rather than during the midrange of joint movement, it is likely that joint receptors largely function as limit detectors, signaling the extremes of joint position and thereby protecting the joint from injury (Proske, Schaible, & Schmidt, 1988). In addition, free nerve endings respond to noxious stimuli that induce awareness of pain in the joint and surrounding area. Although they were once believed to be the primary source of *kinesthesis* (conscious awareness of limb movement), more recent research suggests a supportive rather than a leading role in the

Joint receptors protect the joint from injury by firing at the extremes of joint position.

conscious awareness of limb position and movement. The role joint receptors are believed to play in kinesthesis will be discussed in further detail later in this chapter (page 80).

Despite their reduced role in the conscious sensation of limb position and movement, the importance of joint receptors to normal function in the joint has been demonstrated experimentally and clinically. For example, when fluid is experimentally injected into the joint space of the knee joint to produce effusion of the joint, the maximum voluntary contractile capabilities of the quadriceps femoris are significantly reduced. In fact, depending on the volume of fluid added, maximum voluntary contraction of the quadriceps has been reduced by as much as 90% (Stokes & Young, 1984; Young, Stokes, & Iles, 1987). On the other hand, the removal of fluid from the knee joint during surgery (as in a meniscetomy) can lead to significant improvements in muscle function (Enoka, 2002).

## Transmission of Somatosensory Input

Somatic sensation is relayed to the cerebral cortex via one of two major ascending systems: the **dorsal column (DC) system** and the **anterolateral (AL) system.** Both systems relay afferent information to the brain for arousal, perception, and motor control. These systems are similar in anatomical organization: both involve three orders of neurons and three synapses in transmitting sensory input from the periphery to the cortex. The primary afferent, or first-order neuron, which is connected to the peripheral receptor, synapses with a second-order neuron in the spinal cord or lower brain, depending on the type of sensation. The second-order neuron then conveys information to the thalamus, where it synapses with the third-order neuron in an area of the thalamus called the ventroposterolateral (VPL) area.

From the thalamus, the third-order neuron then projects to the primary somatosensory areas in the cortex where perceptual processing begins. It is important to note that neurons within both ascending systems transmit somatosensory information that is modality and location specific.

### Dorsal Column System

The dorsal column (DC) system transmits sensory information that is important for the planning and execution of movements.

As Figure 3.6 illustrates, the DC system contains axons of primary sensory afferents from joint, skin, and muscle receptors. The primary afferents enter the spinal cord and immediately divide into long and short branches. The short branches terminate in the spinal cord, but the longer branches continue upward, without interruption, to synapse in one of two nuclei (the nucleus gracilis or the nucleus cuneatus) in the medulla at the level of the brainstem. The second-order neurons leave the medulla and immediately **decussate,** or cross, the midline to the **contralateral** (opposite) side before reaching the VPL area of the thalamus. The third-order neurons then convey the afferent information **ipsilaterally** (on the same side), terminating in the **primary sensory area** of the somatosensory cortex.

The nerve fibers of this system convey information about fine, discriminative sensations (such as light touch and vibrations), tactile pressure, and limb

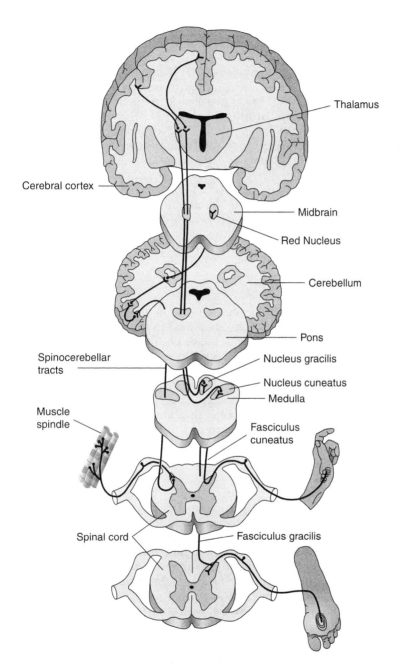

**Figure 3.6**   The dorsal column system pathways convey light touch, pressure, and proprioceptive information to the cerebral cortex.

*Source: Human Anatomy and Physiology*, Second Edition, by Alexander Spence and Elliott Mason. Copyright © 1983 by The Benjamin Cummings Publishing Company. Reprinted by permission.

proprioception. The DC system plays an important role in motor control because of its speed and fidelity of transmission. The heavily myelinated and wide-diameter axons within this system transmit at speeds of 80 to 100 meters per second (m/sec). This characteristic facilitates rapid sampling of the environment, which enhances the accuracy of motor actions about to be executed and of those already in progress. A second important characteristic of the DC system is that it is **somatotopically** organized. For example, sensory fibers entering the lowest levels of the spinal cord ascend in the most medial position of one of the two pathways comprising the system (fasciculus gracilis) while fibers entering at a thoracic level occupy a more lateral position in this pathway. Finally, fibers entering at the upper thoracic and cervical levels ascend in a lateral position in the second pathway (fasciculus cuneatus). This organization of fibers according to the part of the body from which they arise can help clinicians pinpoint exactly where damage has occurred within the system. This knowledge expedites the diagnosis and treatment of patients with different disorders affecting touch and/or proprioception.

## Spinocerebellar Tract

A large group of sensory fibers that comprise another important pathway called the **spinocerebellar (SC) tract** also ascend in the dorsal columns until they reach their final termination site in the cerebellum (see Figure 3.6). This pathway carries information about the position of muscles both directly and indirectly from the muscle spindles to the cerebellum. Unlike the DC system, these pathways do not synapse in either the thalamus or the cerebral cortex. As a result, the proprioceptive information conveyed by the spinocerebellar tract does not lead to the conscious perception of limb position or movement (kinesthesis). The afferent sources believed to contribute to kinesthesis will be discussed in more detail later on page 80.

## Anterolateral System

The anterolateral system transmits primarily sensory information related to pain and temperature.

The anterolateral (AL) system is comprised of three sensory pathways, two of which we will describe in this chapter. The pathways to be described here are the **spinothalamic (ST) tract** and the **spinoreticular (SR) tract.** In addition to carrying different types of sensory inputs, the two pathways terminate in different areas of the brain. The ST tract terminates in the primary somatosensory area of the cortex, while the SR tract terminates in the brainstem.

Primary sensory afferents from pain and temperature receptors located in the skin, muscles, joints, and viscera (heart, lungs, stomach, and so on) enter the spinal cord and immediately synapse with second-order sensory neurons located in the dorsal horn of the spinal cord (see Figure 3.7). Minute changes in temperature are signaled by unmyelinated free nerve endings called **thermoreceptors,** while **nociceptors** respond to noxious stimuli impinging on the body. These stimuli can be mechanical (puncturing of skin), thermal (extreme cold or heat), or chemical (resulting from tissue damage) in nature. In addition to pain and temperature, some secondary tactile input is also conveyed to the cortex via the spinothalamic tract. According to Jacobs and Lowe (1999), the transmission of touch information by this pathway, in addition to

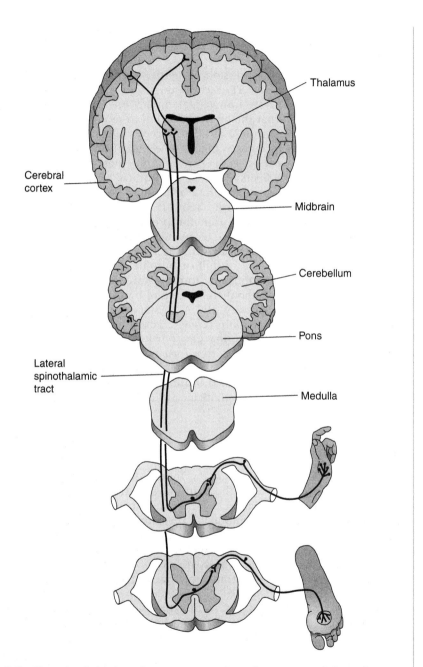

**Figure 3.7** The spinothalamic pathways convey pain and temperature information to the cerebral cortex.

*Source: Human Anatomy and Physiology*, Second Edition, by Alexander Spence and Elliott Mason. Copyright © 1983 by The Benjamin Cummings Publishing Company. Reprinted by permission.

that conveyed by the DC system, means that a person who experiences damage to the DC pathways will still be able to appreciate some level of tactile sensation from the skin.

In contrast to the transmission properties associated with the DC system, neurons that make up the ST tract conduct slowly (1 to 40 m/sec) and are small in diameter; some are unmyelinated. The anterolateral system therefore transmits information that the brain can afford to receive after delay. Once the information relayed from these different receptor types synapses with the second-order neuron, it ascends to higher levels via the ST or SR tract. Approximately 90% of the axons leading away from these second-order neurons decussate and form the fibers of the ST or SR tracts, whereas 10% of the fibers do not decussate but ascend ipsilaterally to the somatosensory cortex. ST neurons then synapse with third-order neurons in the VPL of the thalamus before terminating in specific areas within the primary somatosensory cortex (S-I). Unlike the ST tract, the SR tract terminates in a diffuse region of the brainstem called the **reticular formation.** The types of pain sensations conveyed by this sensory pathway are of dull or burning pain (Jacobs & Lowe, 1999). This pathway appears to contribute to our awareness of pain but cannot provide us with information about the source of the pain.

Similar to the DC pathway, the AL system is also somatotopically organized, although somewhat more crudely. Fibers in this sensory pathway are arranged such that fibers entering the spinal cord from the lower sacral and lumbar regions ascend to the cortex in a lateral and medial position, while fibers entering at the cervical level ascend in the most medial position of the pathway. The somatotopic organization of this pathway system also makes it possible for clinicians to both diagnose and treat different types of pain disorders.

## Somatosensory Cortex

Sensory information conveyed via the third-order neurons from the thalamus terminates in specific areas in the **primary somatosensory cortex (S-I)** that are modality specific (see Figure 3.8). Specific areas in S-I receive and process sensory information from cutaneous receptors, while other areas primarily receive inputs from proprioceptors in the muscles and joints. Higher-order sensory processing continues in the **secondary somatosensory cortex (S-II)** which, in turn, conveys the processed sensory information to certain regions within the temporal lobe that are important for tactile memory (Gardner & Kandel, 2000).

One additional area of the cortex that is involved in the processing of somatosensory inputs is located in Brodmann's areas 5 and 7 within the posterior parietal cortex. This area of the cortex also receives sensory inputs from the visual and auditory system that makes sensory integration between sensory modalities (visual, cutaneous, and proprioceptive inputs) possible. Any damage to this cortical area results in numerous sensorimotor problems, including poor eye–hand coordination during reaching and grasping movements. Lesions in this area also produce the perceptual problem called *agnosia,* which as you recall from an earlier discussion in this chapter, involves being unable to perceive objects even though the particular sensory pathway is functioning normally. Lesions in these association areas of the cortex can

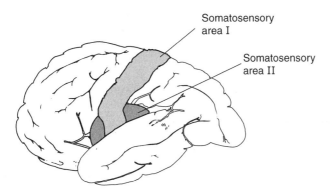

**Figure 3.8**   The processing of sensory information in the cerebral cortex begins in the primary somatosensory cortical area (S-I) and continues in the secondary somatosensory cortical area (S-II).

eventually result in different types of neglect syndromes ranging from the disownment of one side of the body (personal neglect) to the neglect of the immediate external space on one side of the body (spatial neglect).

## Disorders of the Somatosensory System

Any damage to the somatosensory system will result in sensory impairment. The type and extent of the impairment will not only be determined by the processing level at which the damage occurs, but by which of the two sensory pathways ascending to the cortex is affected. For example, any alterations to the somatosensory receptors that transmit information into the spinal cord via the first-order neuron will adversely affect the amount of sensory information received at higher levels in the processing chain. A reduction in the level of sensory reception is an inevitable consequence of the aging process as firing thresholds increase, particularly in the cutaneous receptors that signal vibration and fine discriminative touch (see highlight, Good Vibrations, on page 78). A variety of different sensory impairments also result from a number of different diseases, including diabetes, carpal tunnel syndrome, vitamin $B_{12}$ deficiency, spina bifida, and multiple sclerosis. The sensory loss experienced may be in the form of numbness, **paresthesia** (tingling, burning sensation), or elevated touch-pressure thresholds. When the sensory loss is profound (as in advanced diabetes), more serious tissue damage may result because the individual is unable to detect painful events (Cohen, 1999).

Some level of sensory impairment also accompanies disease or injury to the peripheral nerves or spinal cord, fractures, hemiplegia, multiple sclerosis, and cerebrovascular incidents. As one might expect, the nature of the sensory impairment depends on which of the two ascending *systems* is affected. For example, lesions of the ST tract (part of the AL system) generally result in the

The nature of the sensory impairment differs depending on which sensory pathway is affected.

# HIGHLIGHT

## Good Vibrations

Can increasing the amount of sensory information available from the feet positively influence postural stability? This research question was recently explored by Priplata, Niemi, Harry, Lipsitz, and Collins (2003) at Boston University in the Center for BioDynamics. Research had previously demonstrated that input noise could enhance sensory and motor function via a mechanism referred to as **stochastic resonance.**

One group of young adults and a second group of older adults were asked to stand quietly, with their eyes closed, on vibrating gel-based insoles as their postural sway was measured. The level of vibratory input was manipulated by the study participants until they could just feel the stimulation under each foot. The researchers then lowered the level of stimulation to a subsensory level—a level that the participants could no longer consciously detect. What the researchers found was that the random application of subsensory noise to the plantar surface of the feet resulted in a significant reduction in standing sway with the biggest changes evident in the older adult group.

Although Priplata and colleagues acknowledged that the results were preliminary in nature, they suggested that the use of vibrating insoles might also be effective in enhancing the perfor-

mance of more dynamic activities such as walking. As for the neurological mechanism thought to underlie the reductions in standing sway, the authors speculated that the additional noise input may have a priming effect on the sensory neurons innervating the Pacinian corpuscles, bringing them closer to the threshold for firing an action potential based on the weak signal. Bulsara and Gammaitoni (1996) define stochastic resonance as the maximum output signal strength that is achieved as a function of the noise generated.

Another research group (Maki, Perry, Norrie, & McIlroy, 1998) has also studied the issue of sensory loss and its possible impact on postural control and compensatory stepping, in particular, with some degree of success. Instead of vibrating insoles, this group has experimented with the use of mechanical devices (polyethylene tubing attached to the perimeter of the foot sole or tiny ball bearings imbedded in the supporting surface) to increase cutaneous sensitivity. Older adults using these devices were less likely to take multiple steps following a forward loss of balance. At a practical level, the collective results of these research findings may lead to the development of specialized footwear and/or insole devices designed to enhance the level of somatosensory feedback available to individuals with sensory loss.

loss of pain, temperature, and coarse tactile sensations, and the sensory deficits are usually felt on the side opposite that on which the lesion occurred. This is due to the early decussation of the nerve fibers composing this pathway in the spinal cord.

In contrast, lesions occurring anywhere along the dorsal column system result in partial or complete loss of discriminative tactile sensibilities in areas of the body served by the affected region. Discrimination between two points simultaneously applied to the skin is often severely affected, as is the ability to discriminate between different textures. Some kinesthetic sensations are also lost, such as the ability to recognize the direction of limb movement in space without visual or tactile cues. One particular sensory disorder that affects reception and transmission of sensory inputs in the DC system is called **large-fiber sensory neuropathy** and results in the loss of afferent input from muscles and cutaneous receptors. This disorder results in a human form of deafferentation, a phenomenon we discussed in Chapter 1. In the case of this disorder, sensory inputs from receptors in the muscles and skin are eliminated with complete loss of all kinesthetic sensibility occurring in the affected limbs. One frequently reported finding is an impaired ability to maintain the limb in a constant position in the absence of visual feedback (Rothwell et al., 1982). Individuals with this type of sensory disorder must rely heavily on vision to complete motor tasks in the absence of accurate proprioception.

Individuals with sensory neuropathy that is limited to the lower extremities are often encouraged to use an assistive device (such as a single point cane), particularly during locomotor activities. Important sensory information from the ground can be obtained through the unaffected hand holding the cane and used to enhance postural stability during gait. It is not uncommon for individuals with chronic diabetes to experience severe sensation loss in the toes and feet that also adversely affects their ability to use ground cues for maintaining balance. The use of an assistive device such as a cane is also regularly prescribed for this patient population for the same reason.

Finally, because this system also provides important sensory information for motor pathways involved in the performance of coordinated movements that are precise in nature, any interruption to the dorsal column pathways that reduces the amount of sensory information reaching the motor cortex will adversely affect the quality of the motor execution, particularly in the upper limbs. For many physical therapists, this is an important consideration in designing treatment programs for patients with motor problems that are sensory in origin.

## Application of Theory

Why is it important for practitioners to understand the seemingly intricate neuromotor processes underlying the reception, transmission, and processing of sensory information? Certainly, practitioners working in a clinical setting use their knowledge of how the human system receives, transmits, and finally gives meaning to sensory input as they devise and implement treatment programs. In view of the close relationship between sensory input and motor output, certain kinds of sensory disorders can be expected to influence motor performance negatively. For example, a patient who is experiencing decreased spatial awareness of a limb's position in space will surely find it difficult to perform a variety of movements that require accurate limb positioning. Any reduction in the level of sensory feedback available to us while we are planning motor actions can also be expected to compromise the quality of the movements produced. The more clinicians know about the healthy somatosensory system, the better equipped they are to make accurate diagnoses and implement effective treatment strategies.

Similarly, the physical educator or coach who understands how sensory information is processed and integrated within the CNS can learn to use cutaneous and proprioceptive cues to facilitate motor skill learning. For example, an instructor can apply this information to impart a better understanding of how a particular motor pattern should feel. In teaching aquatic skills, the instructor can encourage the learner to focus on the "feel" of the water against the forearm throughout the pull phase of a particular stroke or on the contrast in temperature as the arm and fingers leave the water at the start of the recovery phase. Similarly, a child's attention can be directed to the pressure of the ball contacting the fingers as it returns from the floor during dribbling. These somatosensory cues can be used to supplement visual demonstrations of a skill and to guide the learner's performance during practice.

Focusing the learner's attention on the somatosensory aspects of a movement contributes much to the learner's awareness of where the limbs are in space throughout the movement. It also provides the learner with a better understanding of the level of effort required. These sensory impressions of the movement can then be incorporated into the knowledge base the learner is developing about the movement being learned. The more knowledge a performer has about a particular movement pattern, the better he or she will recall the skill at a later time. The detection and correction of errors in performance will also be enhanced if the learner is aware of the somatosensory aspects of the movement.

## The Conscious Sensation of Movement

Knowing exactly where our limbs are moving in space is critical for successful performance in many sports and other activities that involve the intricate coordination of various body parts (gymnastics, diving, figure skating). Indeed, most activities that call for coordination of several body parts require that we understand this important piece of information. Fortunately, information about the movement of various body parts is available to us via peripheral receptors located within the skin, muscles, and joints throughout the body.

> Kinesthesis is a subcategory of proprioception that involves the conscious awareness of limb movement.

The subcategory of proprioception that includes *conscious* sensation of movement is often called **kinesthesis,** a term derived from the Greek words *kinein* ("to move") and *aisthesis* ("sensation"). We discussed the role of the proprioceptors in the subconscious control of action earlier in this chapter. Let us now consider whether these same proprioceptors provide information about movement control at a conscious perceptual level.

### Afferent Sources of Kinesthesis

Let us begin by briefly reviewing the literature identifying various afferent sources of kinesthetic sensations. Both the type and the number of afferent sources believed to be involved in kinesthesis have changed over the past 90 years as different research findings have emerged. Among the candidates still considered most likely to provide conscious sensation of limb position and other movement-related sensations are joint receptors, muscle spindles, Golgi tendon organs, and cutaneous receptors.

***Joint Receptors.*** Until recently, receptors in and around the joint were considered the primary afferent source of limb movement and position. The presence of slowly adapting receptors that continued to fire when a joint was maintained in a steady position, coupled with the finding that joint receptors sent signals to the higher cortical regions of the nervous system, seemed to establish a role for joint receptors in the conscious awareness of limb position. In addition, Adams (1977) proposed that these receptors performed two important feedback functions during movement. The first function was to regulate the dynamic aspects of limb movement; the second was to regulate static timing, or the sequence of action.

The conclusions of Adams and other theorists, however, were severely compromised by the results of neurophysiological experiments employing single unit recordings of joint receptors (Burgess & Clark, 1969; Clark & Burgess, 1975). Although joint receptors were shown to fire at the extreme range of joint rotation, they stopped firing when the limb was in midposition, a finding clearly incompatible with the idea that joint receptors continuously signal limb position. Because kinesthetic sensations continued throughout the range of motion, it was clear that other afferent sources were also being used to signal joint position.

*Muscle Spindles.*    From 1960 to 1970, muscle spindles were rejected as a possible afferent source of kinesthesis. They have since been shown to be the most important afferent source of kinesthesis available to us. A role for muscle spindle afferents in kinesthesis was finally confirmed by research conducted in three different areas: muscle vibration, tendon pulling, and elimination of joint and cutaneous signals.

> Muscle spindles have been shown to be the most important source of kinesthesis available to us.
>
> *Tonic vibration reflex:* A polysynaptic reflex elicited by vibrating muscle. Vibration activates muscle spindles, leading to activation of spinal motoneurons.

Perhaps the most conclusive evidence was provided in a series of experiments using percutaneous vibration techniques (Goodwin, McCloskey, & Matthews, 1972; McCloskey, 1973). When high-frequency vibration was applied through the skin over a muscle or its tendon, causing the level of spindle firing to increase (particularly the Ia afferents), the vibrated muscle contracted involuntarily. Surprisingly, the resulting **tonic vibration reflex (TVR)** was accompanied by an illusion of limb movement in the direction that would normally stretch the vibrated muscle. The blindfolded subjects in these studies were requested to keep the nonvibrated arm aligned with the vibrated limb, thus revealing their perception of the vibrated limb's position in space. Despite the fact that the vibrated arm was actually extending, the subject did not begin to move the tracking arm from its original position until the vibrated arm had already moved several degrees from its starting position. Once the vibration was stopped, however, the subjects were able to realign their arms quite accurately. When allowed to view the position of their arms at some point during the movement, subjects would appear surprised at the actual position of their limbs. It is clear from this observation that the subjects' perception of limb position was being severely distorted by the vibration.

Why would a subject experience a sensation of movement in a limb that was not moving? Brooks (1986) suggests that the brain is unable to distinguish between artificially induced sensory input and that which arises from actual changes in muscle length. In the absence of information suggesting otherwise, the brain simply adds the two types of input in estimating limb position. Depending on the original position of the limb and on the level of vibration, subjects report sensations ranging from mild hyperextension to broken limbs!

Further support for muscle spindle involvement in signaling joint position was provided by experiments in which surgically isolated tendons were stretched (McCloskey, Cross, Honner, & Potter, 1983; Moberg, 1983). As a

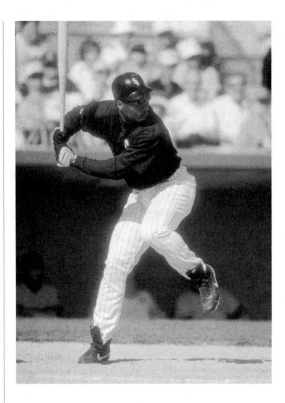

Despite hip replacement surgery, Bo Jackson maintained a high level of kinesthetic awareness in his artificial hip joint.

consequence of having their tendons pulled, subjects experienced direct sensations of joint rotation rather than specific muscular sensations, which indicated that sensory stimulation of the muscle spindle was being directly referred to the joint and translated into position sense.

Advancements in prosthetic medicine during the 1960s, which enabled surgeons to replace diseased joints with artificial ones, also provided clinical evidence that further discredited the involvement of joint receptors while providing further support for muscle spindle involvement in kinesthesia. Patients who receive total hip replacements do not suffer kinesthetic anesthesia and are able to detect small movements (5 degrees per second) of the artificial hip with little difficulty. Consider the difficulties Chicago White Sox player Bo Jackson would experience if he were unable to sense the position of his limbs during movements such as batting, a skill that requires heightened kinesthetic awareness. Jackson made history by returning to professional baseball, however briefly, after successful hip replacement surgery.

*Golgi Tendon Organ.*   The Golgi tendon organ (GTO) has also been identified as a possible source of kinesthesis, particularly because it is also located within skeletomotor muscle. As you will recall from our earlier discussion of this proprioceptor, the GTO conveys information about muscle tension, whereas the muscle spindle signals changes in muscle length. Despite the fact that tendon organs are excited when a muscle is vibrated or actively contracted, a kinesthetic role for the tendon organ has not been clearly established. The consensus among researchers, as summarized by Matthews (1981) in a comprehensive review of the issue, is that tendon organs may work cooperatively with other proprioceptors in the muscles and joints to signal other movement-related sensations, such as the forces acting on the body during movement.

***Cutaneous Receptors.***   Although cutaneous receptors are inevitably excited as a result of movement in a nearby joint, the possibility that cutaneous afferents provide an important afferent source of kinesthesia has received little support on the basis of studies in which the skin was anesthetized (Clark, Matthews, & Muir, 1979). Kinesthetic sensation of joint movement was not significantly affected by eliminating cutaneous signals. The conclusion that cutaneous afferents do not contribute significantly to kinesthesis must be tempered, however, in light of other research involving anesthesia (Goodwin, McCloskey, & Matthews, 1972). In contrast to the limited effects on kinesthesis observed at the hip joint, kinesthetic judgment of limb position was significantly impaired after the elimination of cutaneous signals from the hand and fingers. These contradictory findings suggest that the kinesthetic contribution of cutaneous afferents varies across joints in the body, becoming increasingly more important in distal joints involved in the performance of more finely graded movements.

# The Conscious Sensation of Muscular Effort

Having now described the afferent sources that contribute to the conscious sensation of limb movement, let us now turn to a discussion of the mechanisms that contribute to the conscious sensation of effort of muscular force. Not only is it important to know where the limbs are in space during the performance of a movement, we must also know how much effort or muscular force must be applied to achieve a successful outcome.

Jones (1999) has identified two primary sources that contribute to the conscious sensation of muscular effort. Not surprisingly, the primary afferent source of this perception is the Golgi tendon organs (GTOs). You will recall from our earlier discussion of the proprioceptors that the GTO signals the amount and magnitude of tension on a contracting muscle. This sensory information is then relayed to the primary somatosensory cortex via the dorsal column system. The second source that gives rise to the conscious perception of muscular effort is actually central in origin. Specifically, the **sense of effort,** as Jones refers to it, is believed to result from a copy of the descending motor commands being sent to higher-order sensory centers (such as the somatosensory cortex). This **corollary discharge,** as it is called, is believed to provide the sensory centers with information about the magnitude of the descending motor commands sent to the spinal cord (McCloskey, 1981). As the magnitude of the motor signal increases, so too does the magnitude of the corollary discharge sent to the sensory cortex.

Under normal conditions, the level of GTO firing also increases with increased muscular tension and is proportional to the magnitude of the corollary discharge produced by the descending motor commands. It is therefore difficult to determine the relative contribution of the central and peripheral sources of the sensation unless the matching relationship that exists between the level of GTO firing and the magnitude of the corollary discharge changes. When the muscle is fatigued, however, it becomes possible to better understand the relative contributions of these two different sources of information. In order to fatigue the muscle, researchers require study participants to sustain a constant force against a load applied to a test limb until the point of maximal endurance is reached (Cafarelli, 1988; Jones, 1995; Jones & Hunter, 1983; McCloskey, Ebeling, & Goodwin, 1974). Periodically during this time, participants are asked to estimate how much effort they are exerting against the load by contracting the muscles of the contralateral limb until they think they have matched the level of contraction in the loaded limb.

What the researchers observe as the experiment progresses is that study participants increase the level of contraction in the contralateral limb to a level that no longer matches that of the loaded test limb. The participants consciously perceive that the level of muscular force has increased in the fatiguing limb even though the actual level of muscle contraction has not changed in the test limb. The general conclusion emerging from these experiments is that the conscious perception of muscular force or effort is predominantly signaled by the corollary discharge, while the feedback from the GTO contributes more to sensations of heaviness or muscle tension (Enoka, 2002). Jones (1999) suggests that the preference for centrally generated perceptions of effort or muscular force may serve a protective function. By monitoring the magnitude of the descending motor signals, the CNS can detect an imminent failure in the muscle's capacity to generate force and take corrective action before injury to the muscle occurs. Similar changes in the perception of force and heaviness have also been observed when muscle weakness is artificially induced (Gandevia & McCloskey, 1977) and among patients with certain CNS disorders (cerebellar disease and upper motoneuron paresis, for example).

## Practical Applications

Movements that require us to maintain a given posture or consciously direct our limbs to a particular point in space in a controlled fashion depend on our ability to utilize kinesthetic information efficiently, particularly in the absence of vision. The application and ongoing adjustment of just the right amount of muscular force and effort are also critical for successful completion of a movement.

A teacher or therapist who encourages an individual to focus on the feelings associated with a particular movement is acknowledging the importance of proprioceptive and cutaneous information in the control and learning of movement. The knowledge that certain proprioceptors provide information that can be used to sense the movement and position of joints in space can be exploited by the instructor, particularly in the teaching of skills that demand an acute sense of spatial positioning and rapid error correction while they are being executed. For example, skills such as ballet dancing and gymnastics are well suited to the use of kinesthetic cues to guide learning.

In movement situations where visual input is absent or distorted, as it is in swimming and discus throwing, the performer is highly dependent on the kinesthetic cues provided by the cutaneous and intramuscular receptors. Just as the swimmer derives sensations of muscular force as the arm moves against

Skills such as ballet dancing and gymnastics are well suited to the use of kinesthetic cues to guide learning.

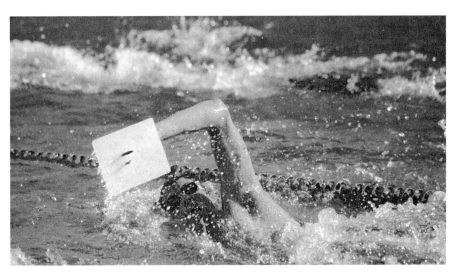

The kinesthetic "feel" of certain swimming movements can be heightened with the use of devices such as hand paddles or webbed gloves.

the resistance created by the water, the discus thrower uses the kinesthetic sensations associated with the movements of the body and outstretched arm as he or she is rotating rapidly to optimize the release angle of the discus. Directing such performers' attention to the kinesthetic aspects of the performance should significantly enhance their immediate perception and ultimate memory of the skill.

It is interesting to note that coaches often employ devices that are designed to accentuate the kinesthetic feel associated with certain movements. Hand paddles or webbed gloves may be provided to swimmers. Weighted rings may be added to a baseball bat to give the batter a heightened feel of the bat's movements throughout the swing.

Can our ability to use kinesthetic information during movement be improved? This question was the focus of a series of studies conducted by Laszlo and Bairstow (1983). It was well known that kinesthetic perception improved with age, but little attention had been directed to investigating whether kinesthetic perception and memory could be improved with training. In addition to finding that children ranging in age from 6 to 8 years could be trained to improve their level of kinesthetic sensitivity, the authors also demonstrated that once kinesthetic awareness had been established, the ability to use the kinesthetic information was retained.

The knowledge derived from early muscle vibration studies has also been successfully applied in clinical settings to facilitate accurate diagnoses and improved rehabilitation. The *tonic vibration reflex (TVR)*, elicited by muscle vibration, has been used to evaluate muscle tone, the integrity of certain stretch reflexes, and higher cortical function. As Brooks (1986) reports, the TVR has also been used in the clinical setting to assist in the rehabilitation of hemiplegic patients who would otherwise ignore their affected limbs, to inhibit undesirable motor patterns resulting from spasticity, and to provide a valuable source of biofeedback for patients with reduced skin sensations.

# The Role of Feedback in Controlling Actions

It is important that the CNS receive an uninterrupted flow of sensory information if movements are to be performed effectively.

The important role played by sensory (afferent) information in both the planning and the moment-to-moment control of movement should now be evident. In fact, if we are to perform movements effectively, it is essential that the nervous system receive an uninterrupted flow of sensory information. The performer uses this sensory information in a variety of ways; we will consider three important uses here. Sensory information (a) provides us with information about the body's spatial position before, during, and after the action, (b) guides the planning and modification of action plans, and (c) helps us learn or relearn movement patterns.

## Knowledge of Body Position

The first important function sensory feedback serves is to provide us with information about the position of our many body parts in relation to each other (proprioception) and about the orientation of the whole body to the surrounding environment (exproprioception). This information is useful to a batter trying to adopt the appropriate stance before the pitch and to the gymnast performing a difficult maneuver on a balance beam. In this latter movement situation, sensory information provided by the visual and proprioceptive senses enables the gymnast to monitor the changing positions of her limbs and body frequently throughout the routine. In this way, she can check the correctness of her movements and make minor adjustments in limb and body position to optimize her performance. Movement-related sensory feedback that is available after a movement has been completed can also serve an important error-correcting function. Knowing the final position of the limbs and/or body following a movement can often give us valuable information about the performance and provide clues to why the intended outcome was not achieved.

## Planning and Modification of Action Plans

A related function of sensory feedback is to guide us in the action-planning process by helping us construct the plan of action that best suits the demands of the environment. The rich network of interconnecting pathways between the various neural task systems ensures that feedback from a variety of internal and external sources can be used to elaborate and/or modify an action plan throughout the planning process. Given sufficient time to execute the action plan, we can also use sensory feedback to make numerous minor adjustments to the movements to ensure their success.

To illustrate this point, consider a tennis player who is preparing to follow up an attempted deep forehand return to his opponent with a short, angled volley stroke. In this movement situation, the player uses the available visual and proprioceptive feedback to determine whether a volley stroke is, indeed, the most suitable action. If the player fails to strike the ball with sufficient force or observes the opponent speeding into the net immediately after his own stroke, it is likely that the player would consider altering that proposed course of action. This would not be possible, however, if the player were

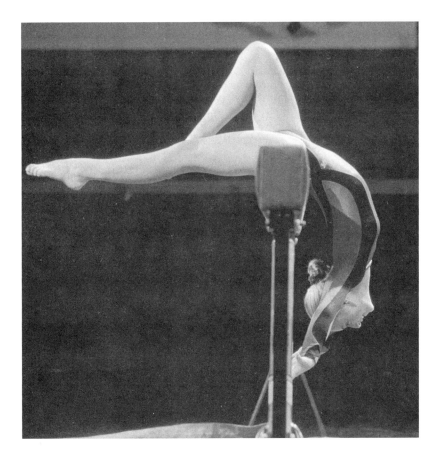

Sensory feedback provides information about the relative positions of the various parts of the body and about the body's orientation relative to other objects in space.

unable either to observe the movements of his opponent or to feel the impact associated with striking the ball.

## Learning or Relearning of Movements

The third, and perhaps most important, function of sensory feedback is to facilitate the learning of new movement skills and the relearning of existing movement patterns that have become dysfunctional through trauma and/or disease. The novice performer attempting to learn how to hit a baseball uses the feedback derived from physically practicing the skill to make adjustments in subsequent attempts. This trial-and-error approach continues until the goal of hitting the ball is consistently achieved. Similarly, patients attempting to relearn how to walk after a stroke must depend on visual feedback to guide their legs through the action.

# Errors in Performance

Despite the cooperative efforts of the various neural subsystems and despite the availability of sensory feedback, various types of performance errors are inevitable. These errors may arise as a consequence of incorrectly evaluating the environmental display and thus developing an inappropriate plan of action; developing an appropriate plan of action but applying the wrong movement dynamics (such as force, velocity, timing); sensory conflict that results in a misperception; or many other unexpected factors that lead to inappropriate motor behavior.

The degree to which errors affect a performance depends on the time required to complete the movement and on the quality of the feedback.

Although these errors are sometimes unavoidable, the degree to which they affect performance is largely determined by how much time it takes to complete the movement and by the quality of the feedback mechanisms available to the performer. Movements that must be performed ballistically, such as firing a pistol, give the performer little opportunity to use the available sensory feedback to change the plan of action or modify the movement in progress. In contrast, movements that last for several seconds can be continuously modified on the basis of the feedback arising from the action itself and on the basis of changes observed to occur in the environment.

The level to which the various feedback mechanisms are developed within the performer clearly determines the degree to which errors influence performance outcomes. Given that the quality of these mechanisms is strongly influenced by experience, it is to be expected that the performance of less-skilled performers will be most affected by the types of errors we have described.

# Summary

Sensory receptors help the various subsystems in the CNS derive meaning from the external world. They not only tell us when a sensory event has occurred (adequate stimulation), but also code the intensity of that event by means of their temporal and/or spatial firing patterns. These same receptors are also able to block out redundant or irrelevant sensory information by reducing their firing levels shortly after an event occurs. This property of sensory receptors is called sensory adaptation.

Sensory information is conveyed by specialized afferent pathways to primary sensory areas distributed throughout the cortex. It is then further processed and integrated with sensory information from other senses. Before reaching the cortex, however, all sensory information (except that derived from smell) passes through the thalamus, which serves as a "sensory filter." Our final perception of what is occurring in the environment is achieved once the integrated sensory information reaches the association areas of the cortex. This final perception forms the basis of future voluntary actions.

The cutaneous receptors and proprioceptors that make up the somatosensory system give rise to sensations of touch, pain, temperature, and limb position and movement. These sensations are conveyed to the cortex by one of two primary sensory pathways: the dorsal column (DC) system and the anterolateral (AL) system.

Disorders of the somatosensory system can be expected to compromise our ability to perform many activities of daily living because of the close relationship between sensory input and motor output. The treatment programs prescribed for patients are influenced by this relationship.

Somatosensory cues can be used in motor skill settings to enhance a learner's understanding of a skill's spatial requirements and of the amount of effort needed to accomplish the goal of the movement.

Muscle afferents, primarily muscle spindles, are the most important peripheral source of kinesthetic sensations related to joint movement and position in space. The primary (Ia) afferents signal the dynamic and static aspects of limb position and perhaps velocity of limb movement, whereas the secondary (II) afferents contribute to awareness of static limb position. Conscious sensation of effort or muscular force come from two primary sources: the Golgi tendon organ receptors that signal changes in muscle tension and from corollary discharges that inform sensory centers in the brain about the magnitude of the descending motor signals. Corollary discharges serve as the preferential source of conscious sensations of muscular effort of force, while GTO discharge levels are more likely to give rise to conscious sensations of heaviness or tension.

Cutaneous receptors contribute to kinesthesis primarily by supporting and enhancing signals generated by muscle receptors, and their contributions are more important in distal joints involved in fine movement control. Joint receptors, once considered the only afferent source of kinesthesis, probably play no major role in the conscious sensation of movement.

Sensory feedback has many functions in the control of action. We discussed three: knowledge of body position, the planning and modification of action, and the learning and relearning of movements. The degree to which the individual is able to utilize her or his internal sensory feedback mechanisms determines the magnitude of the errors made in the performance of any movement.

## IMPORTANT TERMINOLOGY

After completing this chapter, readers should be familiar with the following terms and concepts.

| | |
|---|---|
| action potentials | Ia afferent |
| adaptation | intensity code |
| adequate stimulation | ipsilateral |
| agnosia | kinesthesis |
| anterolateral (AL) system | mechanoreceptors |
| association areas | moreceptors |
| chain fibers | multimodal sensory association areas |
| contralateral | nociceptors |
| corollary discharge | nuclear bag fibers |
| cutaneous receptors | paraesthesia |
| decussate | primary afferent |
| diencephalon | primary sensory area |
| dorsal column (DC) system | primary somatosensory cortex (S-I) |
| extrafusal muscle fibers | proprioceptors |
| fiber sensory neuropathy | receptor potentials |
| Golgi tendon organ (GTO) | reticular formation |

*continued*

secondary somatosensory cortex (S-II)
sense of effort
sensory homunculus
somatotopically
somesthesia
spatial summation
spinocerebellar (SC) tract
spinoreticular (SR) tract

spinothalamic (ST) tract
temporal summation
thalamic syndrome
thalamus
tonic vibration reflex (TVR)
transduction
type II or secondary afferents
typographically
unimodal sensory association

## SUGGESTED FURTHER READING

Cohen, H. (Ed.), (1999). *Neuroscience for rehabilitation.* Philadelphia, PA: Lippincott Williams & Wilkins.

Kandel, E. R., Schwartz, J. H., & Jessell, T. M. (Eds.) (2000). *Principles of neural science* (4th ed.). New York: McGraw-Hill.

## TEST YOUR UNDERSTANDING

1. Identify the specific characteristic(s) of a sensory receptor that do each of the following:
   (a) Help(s) us know when a particular sensory event occurred.
   (b) Assist(s) us in distinguishing between sensations of light touch and heavy pressure applied to the skin.
   (c) Prevent(s) us from becoming irritated by clothing against our skin.

2. Briefly describe the specific routes that electrical impulses follow from receptor to cortex for each of these somatosensory sensations:
   (a) Fine, discriminative touch.
   (b) Pain.
   (c) Proprioception.

3. Describe the disorder known as agnosia that is caused by damage to the association area in the cortex.

4. Identify the two categories into which somatosensory receptors have been divided. Briefly explain the sensory contribution that each category makes to perception and action.

5. Briefly describe the different types of sensory information provided to the CNS by the primary (Ia) afferent and the secondary (II) afferent in the muscle spindle.

6. What type of information is provided to the CNS by the various types of joint receptors located throughout the body?

7. Explain how the nature of the sensory impairment differs depending on which of the two major ascending pathways is affected.

8. Briefly describe ways in which knowledge about the somatosensory system can be utilized in a practical setting. Provide examples to illustrate your answer.

9. Briefly explain what the term *kinesthesis* means.

10. Identify the afferent sources that contribute to the conscious perception of limb position and movement.

11. Describe the two primary sources of conscious perception of muscular force or effort. Which of the two sources appears to be preferred by the CNS and why?

12. Discuss the various clinical and practical implications of the fact that certain proprioceptors can be used to sense the position of limbs in space.

13. Identify the various functions served by sensory feedback in the planning and execution of movements.

14. Identify the various factors that may lead to errors in performance.

## PRACTICAL ACTIVITIES

1. Clinicians use a variety of different methods to test somatosensation. Examples of these different methods are described below. Review the descriptions of each test (with a partner) and discuss which sensory receptors are being stimulated and the processes occurring in the CNS that lead to conscious awareness of the different sensations.

| Test | Tools | Procedures |
| --- | --- | --- |
| **Discriminative Touch** | | |
| Touch awareness | Cotton ball, feather, blindfold | Person being tested indicates *when* stimulus is felt against skin. |
| Touch localization | Same as above | Person points to *where* skin was touched. |
| Two-point discrimination | Paper clips (×2) | Two points of paper clips are applied to the skin starting 5 mm apart. Points are gradually moved closer together. Person being tested indicates whether "one" or "two" points are touching skin. |
| **Proprioception** | | |
| Vibration | Tuning fork | Tuning fork is applied to bony points of big toe or ankle. Respondent indicates when vibration is first felt. Speed of response monitored. |
| Joint position | Blindfold | Limb is passively moved to a position in space. Respondent must match position with opposite limb. |
| Joint motion | Blindfold | Limb is passively flexed or extended. Person being tested must indicate nature of limb's movement (e.g., bending, extending). |

*continued*

| | Temperature | |
|---|---|---|
| Temperature awareness | Cold stimulus (40°) | Hot or cold stimulus is applied to skin. |
| | Hot stimulus (115°) | Person being tested must indicate whether "hot" or "cold." |
| | Blindfold | |
| | **Pain** | |
| Pain sensation | Safety pin, blindfold | Sharp or dull end of pin is applied to skin. Person being tested indicates whether stimulus is "sharp" or "dull." |

2. Discuss how a person's performance on selected tests might be affected if the following sensory disorders were present: (a) large-fiber sensory neuropathy affecting both legs below the level of the knee; (b) a lesion affecting the dorsal column system at the midbrain level; (c) a lesion affecting the spinothalamic tract in the cervical area of the spinal cord.

# 4

# VISUAL AND VESTIBULAR SYSTEM CONTRIBUTIONS TO ACTION

*The interconnectedness of the visual and vestibular systems is demonstrated by the vestibular ocular reflex, which functions to stabilize the eyes when the head moves.*

## CHAPTER OBJECTIVES

After studying this chapter, you should be able to:

- Understand and be able to describe the different types of sensory information provided by the visual system in the control of movement.

- Understand and be able to explain how the visual system is functionally organized to receive and interpret incoming visual information.

- Identify the functional differences between the two visual systems and their respective contributions to various aspects of motor control.

- Become familiar with the two contrasting theories of visual perception and the different underlying assumptions associated with each theory.

- Understand and be able to describe how vision is used as a feedforward mechanism in certain movement situations and as a feedback mechanism in others.

- Understand and be able to describe how vision can be used to predict time-to-contact with another object and/or person.

- Describe the relationship between basic visual function and sport performance and how visual training is used to improve sport vision.

- Understand and be able to describe how the vestibular system is anatomically and functionally organized to receive incoming sensory information relative to head movements.

- Describe the respective roles of the ascending and descending vestibular pathways in motor control.

- Describe how the various diseases and/or disorders of the vestibular system affect motor control.

- Understand and describe how the vestibular and visual systems work together to signal the movement of self or the surrounding environment.

Though an important source of information for controlling and coordinating movement, **proprioception** is not the only means by which we successfully interact with our environment. As you will learn in this chapter, the visual and vestibular systems also provide two additional sources of sensory information for the control and learning of many motor skills. We begin our discussion here with the visual system.

Many consider the visual system to be the richest source of information about the world in which we live. Not only do we use our eyes to monitor the position of objects of interest in the visual field, but we also rely on vision to maintain an upright position in space and to navigate safely. In the context of sport, vision is also critical for the successful interception or avoidance of objects and the advanced planning of subsequent actions. As you will also come to learn later in this chapter, it is the primary means by which we evaluate the quality of our performance.

According to Lee (1978), vision provides three very important types of sensory information in the control of movement. These are exteroception, proprioception, and exproprioception. First, vision provides **exteroceptive** information by informing us about the layout of surfaces and the relative positions of objects in the environment. The monitoring of events occurring in a given movement situation is also made possible by vision. This information can be used to assist us to plan new actions or adapt an ongoing movement in response to changes occurring in the environment. Vision is therefore integral to **perception** (adding meaning to an event that has occurred). Although we tend to think that information about the relative position and/or movement of body parts is derived solely from the somatosensory receptors in the skin, muscles, and joints, vision has also been shown to serve a **proprioceptive** function.

As we will see when we discuss posture and balance, vision is an integral component of the control system used to maintain an upright stance because of its ability to extract important sensory information from the changing optic array. This third type of sensory information provided by vision is called **exproprioception.** Unlike proprioception, this type of information provides us with knowledge about the position of the body and its various parts relative to the surrounding environment. It therefore helps us to intercept moving objects, avoid obstacles in our path, and perform other activities associated with daily life.

In this section of the chapter we will once again adopt a multilevel discussion of vision and the many important contributions it makes to the planning and execution of movement. Our discussion will begin at the neuromotor processing level of analysis, where we will focus on describing how the visual system is functionally organized to receive and process incoming visual information. Then we will move to a psychological level of analysis and describe two theories of visual perception that view perception and action quite differently. Finally, we will consider the role of vision in the control of action.

> Vision provides three types of sensory information: exteroceptive, proprioceptive, and exproprioceptive.

## Neuromotor Processing of Vision

### Reception of Visual Input

Light enters the eye through the cornea and proceeds through the **pupil** and **lens** before reaching the **retina** (see Figure 4.1). In contrast to the somatosensory receptors (such as cutaneous receptors and proprioceptors) described in

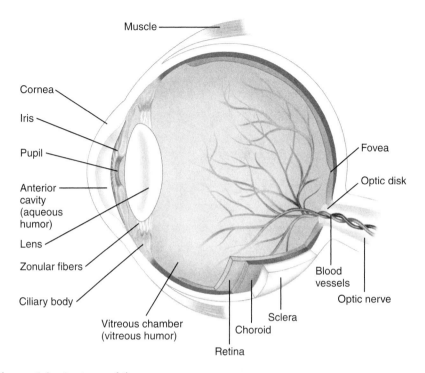

Muscle

Cornea

Iris

Pupil

Anterior
cavity
(aqueous
humor)

Lens

Zonular fibers

Ciliary body

Vitreous chamber
(vitreous humor)

Retina

Choroid

Sclera

Blood
vessels

Optic nerve

Fovea

Optic disk

**Figure 4.1**   Anatomy of the eye.

the previous chapter, the retina, which serves as the primary sensory organ of the visual system, is not considered a peripheral receptor. Instead, it forms part of the CNS (Tessier-Lavigne, 2000). Light-sensitive receptors then convert the light waves to electrical impulses. This process of *transduction,* which we first discussed in Chapter 3 as it operates in the somatosensory system, prepares visual input for further processing in various subsystems within the CNS. Two types of photoreceptors, located in different parts of the retina and serving different functions, are responsible for this first stage of visual processing.

The photoreceptors called **rod** cells tend to be heavily concentrated in the peripheral retina, nearest the lens. They are absent from the center of the retina (fovea centralis). These rod cells, by virtue of their sensitivity to very low levels of illumination, act as our primary photoreceptors in conditions of poor lighting and for night vision. In contrast, the **cone** receptor cells are stimulated only at very high levels of illumination. They are therefore more suited for day vision. Cone receptors not only contain photopigments that enable us to see objects in fine detail (such as the seam of a baseball in flight and the variations of texture in an oil painting), but also allow us to detect colors. Unfortunately, colorblind individuals lack the types of cone cells that contain the photopigments necessary to detect red and green light and are therefore "blind" to these colors.

Rod and cone cells transduce light waves into electrical impulses, preparing them for further processing in other subsystems.

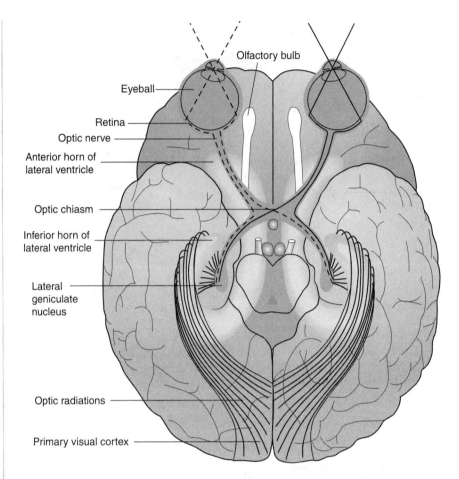

Olfactory bulb

Eyeball

Retina

Optic nerve

Anterior horn of
lateral ventricle

Optic chiasm

Inferior horn of
lateral ventricle

Lateral
geniculate
nucleus

Optic radiations

Primary visual cortex

**Figure 4.2**  Anatomy of the visual system.

## Transmission to the Brain

After further processing in progressively deeper layers of the retina, electrical impulses leave the eye via the **optic nerve,** which transmits impulses directly to the brain. Just as somatosensory input received by receptors on one side of the body is transmitted via nerve pathways that eventually terminate in the opposite cortical hemisphere, impulses arising from the portions of the retina that serve the left visual field are sent to the right hemisphere of the brain, and impulses derived from viewing objects in the right visual field terminate in the left hemisphere. The point at which this crossing of nerve fibers takes place is called the **optic chiasm.** The partial crossing of optic nerve fibers at the optic chiasm is also a requirement for the binocular vision that enables us to see the world in three dimensions.

As Figure 4.2 illustrates, the greatest percentage of optic nerve fibers synapse in a specialized area of the thalamus known as the **lateral genicu-late nucleus (LGN).** From here, visual impulses are relayed via optic radiations to the *primary visual cortex, or striate cortex.* This area is located in the most posterior portion of the occipital lobe. It is not until this stage in the transmission process that the spatial organization of a visual scene is detected. This ability is made possible through the functioning of specialized cells located in the primary visual cortex that enable us to identify such characteristics of objects as shading, brightness, and form. Once the visual information sent to the primary visual cortex is processed, it is then conveyed to the association area of the visual cortex (Brodmann's areas 18 and 19). Although most of the visual processing occurs within the visual cortex, there are additional areas outside the visual cortex that are involved in some form of visual processing. These additional areas are located in the frontal lobe and are referred to as the frontal eye fields. These areas are integrally involved in oculomotor control.

A smaller percentage of impulses also travel via other nerve pathways and terminate in the *superior colliculus* located in the midbrain. In the superior colliculus, vision is integrated with other incoming sensory inputs from the somatosensory and auditory systems. This integration of the senses enables other sensory responses to be coordinated with movements of the head and eyes toward events occurring in the environment. Although the superior colliculus is primarily involved in the reflex control and regulation of many eye and head movements, it also plays an important role in attention and visual perception.

> Two anatomically distinct pathways convey visual input to two separate areas in the brain.

## Topographic Organization in the Visual System

The topographic organization of subcortical and cortical areas that was evident in the somatosensory system is once again observed in the visual system. Neurons in the visual system are arranged such that specific regions of the retina project to clearly defined areas within the thalamus and the visual cortex. The degree of representation is once again determined by the level of receptive sensitivity in the area of the body being represented. The foveal region of the retina permits the highest level of visual acuity, and almost 50% of the representational area in the thalamus and visual cortex is devoted to the fovea and the immediate area surrounding it. The much larger and less sensitive peripheral areas of the retina are significantly less well represented. Such a topographic arrangement of neurons provides us with a map of the retina that can be recreated in the visual cortex. The final interpretation of what has been seen occurs in the visual association areas of the visual cortex, giving rise to a perception of the external world.

> The final interpretation of what has been seen occurs in the association areas of the visual cortex.

## The Control of Eye Movements

Six extraocular eye muscles attached to different parts of the eye are responsible for producing coordinated eye movements once stimulated. These muscles have very few muscle fibers and a single nerve fiber innervating each muscle fiber. This one-to-one innervation ratio ensures that the eye movements generated will be very accurate. Each extraocular muscle is also richly endowed with muscle spindles that provide information relative to the position and velocity of eye movements.

Five types of eye movements are possible, two of which are reflexive in nature and three that are voluntarily controlled. The goal of the two reflexive eye movements is to keep a visual image or images fixed on the foveal

The vestibular ocular reflex (VOR) and optokinetic reflex (OKR) both function to keep a visual image fixed on the fovea of the retina.

area of the retina. The first is called the *vestibular-occular reflex (VOR)* and is primarily driven by the vestibular system. We will discuss the physiology of this reflexive eye movement in more detail on page 119. The second type of reflexive eye movement is called the **optokinetic reflex (OKR).** This reflex utilizes visual information in a manner that is complimentary to the VOR. Its primary goal is also to maintain a stable visual image on the fovea when the entire visual field moves. In contrast to the VOR, this reflex has a longer latency and is most responsive at lower frequencies of head movement (below 0.1 Hz). The OKR works in combination with the VOR in lighted conditions, making it possible for us to respond more accurately to movement of the visual environment or ourselves when the head is moving at different speeds.

Smooth pursuit eye movements are used to track slow moving objects through space.

Three types of voluntary eye movements can also be generated for the purpose of (a) tracking objects that are moving slowly through space, (b) shifting our gaze quickly from one point of interest in space to another, and (c) fixing our gaze on objects at different depths within the visual field. The first of these voluntary eye movements is called **smooth pursuit,** and, as just mentioned, is called upon to assist us to keep a moving object fixed on the fovea. The velocity of smooth pursuit eye movements can be changed to track objects moving at different speeds in the environment up to a maximal velocity of 100 deg/sec. As the lead changes in a 200-meter race, for example, the observer can speed up his/her smooth pursuit eye movements to move from watching the first place runner who is about to be overtaken by a faster moving runner in the adjacent lane.

Saccadic eye movements help us shift our gaze quickly between points of interest in space.

Vergence makes it possible to bring objects at different depths relative to the eyes into focus using binocular vision.

In contrast, the velocity of **saccades,** the second type of voluntary eye movement, cannot be controlled. We use saccades, for example, when watching an overhead volleyball or tennis serve so we can quickly see if the receiving player successfully intercepts the ball. In the case of this type of eye movement, the angular distance between the two objects of interest determines the speed of the eye movement. The further apart the objects of interest, the faster the eye movement that is generated. Saccadic eye movements are both quick and accurate, reaching a maximum velocity of approximately 900 deg/sec (Goldberg, 2000). The last of the three types of voluntary eye movements is **vergence.** In order to achieve vergence, the eyes must now move in opposition to each other rather than together, as was the case for each of the four other eye movements described. That is to say, each eye rotates in the opposite direction so that objects at different depths relative to the eyes can be bought into focus using binocular vision (both eyes). When the eyes converge on an approaching visual target, the eyes rotate toward the nose whereas the eyes rotate away from the nose and back toward their normal parallel position when the eyes diverge on a target that is receding into the background.

Although the exact mechanisms involved in the neural control of eye movements are not well understood in some cases, several regions within the midbrain (including the pons and medulla), frontal eye fields, and the parietal lobe are associated with the neural control of some eye movements. The vestibular nuclei also play an important role by sending the processed signals to cranial nerves III, IV, V, and VI that innervate the different extraocular eye muscles. The superior colliculus also participates in the generation of saccadic eye movements.

# Two Visual Systems?

The existence of two structurally distinct visual pathways that terminate in different areas of the brain has prompted several researchers to advance the idea of two separate visual systems that are functionally different from each other. The terms *focal* and *ambient* are generally used to describe these two systems. The **focal system,** which is served by the fovea of the eye and where visual acuity is high, is thought to be responsible for identifying objects primarily in the center of the visual field. The fact that identifying objects requires conscious thought also suggests that the visual pathway that terminates in the primary visual cortex is responsible for this type of visual processing. Unlike the focal system, the **ambient system** is used for detecting space around the body while providing information about where objects are located in space. The major advantage of ambient vision is that it is served by the whole retina and so is not degraded in conditions of poor lighting. It is this second system that helps us navigate through space at night.

Empirical evidence supporting the existence of two visual systems has been provided in controlled animal studies (Trevarthen, 1968) and case study reports of patients with damage to the visual cortex. In one such case study, Weiskrantz and colleagues (Weiskrantz, Warrington, Sanders, & Marshall, 1974) observed patients in whom partial destruction of the visual cortex caused blindness in certain areas of the visual field. Their report indicated that even though patients were unable to identify an object presented in the affected part of their visual field, they were able to point to it accurately. Patients were also able to orient their eyes toward the object when asked to guess where it was presented in space. It appears that patients were able to use their functioning ambient system to *locate* the object even though damage to the area of the brain responsible for focal vision prevented them from being able to *identify* it.

## Two Visual Systems and Motor Control

How do these two systems contribute to the various aspects of motor control? Although the two visual systems serve different functions, it is likely that both systems operate in parallel in most movement situations. The focal system helps us identify objects in space, and the ambient system is used to locate objects in space at a subconscious level. This parallel operation of the two visual systems is particularly useful in situations such as downhill skiing and even just walking along a busy street. In both of these situations, it is important to orient the body with respect to objects in the peripheral field of vision in order to avoid potential collisions, but there is no need to identify the particular object.

The focal system operates concurrently to identify important changes in terrain or objects in the center of the visual field that may pose a more immediate problem. In this way, one system can be used to attend to one type of visual input while the other system guides the orientation of our body as we move through the complex environment. Indeed, the parallel organization evident in the visual system is often cited by theorists as evidence for the distributed model of motor control described in the first chapter of this section.

The focal visual system identifies objects; the ambient system locates objects in space.

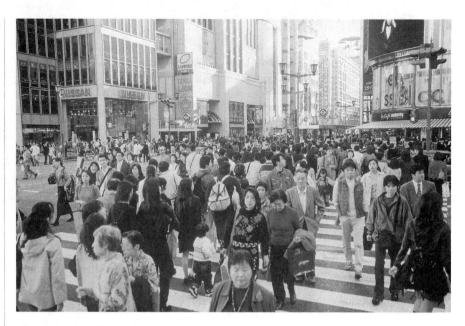

Whereas the focal system assists us in identifying objects in space, the ambient system is used to locate objects in space at a subconscious level. The second system is particularly useful in helping us avoid collisions with others when walking on a busy street.

# Psychological Studies of Perception and Action

## Contrasting Theories of Visual Perception

Now that we have outlined the neuromotor processes of vision, let us turn to the psychological level of analysis and begin to explore how our perceptions of the external world can be used to plan and guide our actions in a variety of movement contexts. Unfortunately, considerable disagreement exists among researchers striving to understand the relationship between perception and action. The primary issue dividing researchers is related to whether or not inferential, or cognitive, processes are necessary for perception. This section is devoted to a discussion of this controversial issue and how it has influenced the way the perception–action relationship has been investigated by the different groups of researchers.

Central to tradi-
tional theories of
visual perception is
the idea that infor-
mation received
from the environ-
ment is not imme-
diately meaningful.

At present, two seemingly different theories of visual perception are being put forward to explain how perception is coupled to action. These may be described as the **cognitive,** or **indirect** (Shallice, 1964; Sharp & Whiting, 1974; Smyth & Marriott, 1982), and the **ecological,** or **direct** (Gibson, 1979; Michaels & Carello, 1981), theories of visual perception. Central to cognitive theories of perception is the assumption that information received from the environment is not perceived as meaningful by the performer until a series of inferential processes has been completed internally. These cognitive processes are considered necessary to elaborate the flat, two-dimensional visual image falling on the retina and to determine its potential relevance by making a comparison with existing mental representations. The assumption of cognitive theories that perception is indirect would certainly appear reasonable in light of our discussion of the neuromotor processing aspects of vision. Recall that identification of a visual scene did not occur until the incoming visual information reached the level of the occipital cortex.

In contrast to this cognitive or indirect view, proponents of the ecological, or direct, theory of perception argue that visual information can be directly extracted from the environment without the need for any intervening cognitive processes to render it meaningful. Cognitive mediation is considered unnecessary because of the direct relationship between perception and action. The assumptions governing this theory were founded on the early work of J. J. Gibson (1966, 1979), who argued that the optic array alone provides the observer with all the visual information necessary to guide action. Moreover, this visual information can be directly extracted from the environment with no need for any mediating processes.

> Ecological theorists argue that visual information can be directly extracted from the environment.

The cognitive and ecological theories of perception differ both in their theoretical assumptions and in the types of investigative procedures and experimental settings that have been used to test them. The proponents of the cognitive or indirect view have chosen to conduct experiments in carefully controlled laboratory settings, whereas advocates of the ecological or direct perception theory have attempted to study the relationship between perception and action in more natural movement settings.

As appealing as the ecological perception theory of visual perception appears because of its inherent parsimony, it is not devoid of shortcomings. These were addressed in an excellent review article (Williams, Davids, Burwitz, & Williams, 1992). One of the more important shortcomings is the use of realistic skills, which actually makes it more difficult to determine exactly what type of perceptual mechanisms are being used to guide action. In fact, Williams and colleagues suggest that in natural conditions, subjects have the opportunity to estimate "time-to-contact information by both direct and computational methods" (p. 176).

Whether our perception of sensory events is direct or indirect also appears to be strongly influenced by the movement context itself. For example, van Wieringen (1988) has suggested that direct perception strategies may be best suited to situations wherein a direct fit between perception and action exists. Examples of such movement situations include those in which we are maintaining an upright posture, locomoting through space, or attempting to intercept a moving object in a stable, nonchanging environment. In contrast, actions performed in more variable movement environments that are governed by a set of abstract rules appear to demand additional cognitive processing. These additional cognitive processes are thought necessary in order to compare what is seen with what is known about the rules of the game. Williams argues that during the course of a game of soccer, for example, simply seeing a ball approaching at head height does not provide enough information on which to base subsequent action. In this situation, the player must refer to the rules of the game before knowing what action is appropriate. As those familiar with the rules of soccer know, it is not legal for a player, other than the goalkeeper standing in the penalty area, to intercept the ball with his or her hands. Given that these rules governing action cannot be discerned simply by watching the approaching ball, the player must use additional cognitive processing to guide action.

> The movement context appears to influence strongly whether our perception of sensory events is direct or indirect.

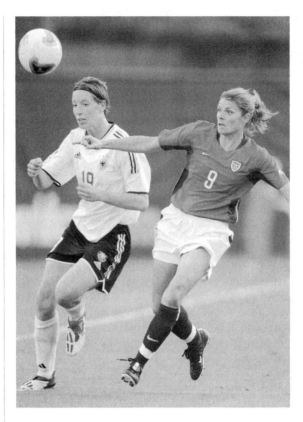

Direct perception theories cannot explain actions performed in sports environments that are governed by abstract rules (such as when a ball may not be touched by a player's hands). In these situations, there is no longer a direct fit between the perception and action.

Direct perception explanations also appear to be inadequate to explain actions that occur in time-constrained movement contexts. In these contexts, a performer attempts to extract advance cues by watching an opponent's movements just before or shortly after movement begins. Cognitive or indirect perception theorists argue that performers first derive meaning from these advance cues by referring to an existing knowledge base stored in memory and then act accordingly. The very speed with which the visual scene is unfolding would seem to limit the use of the optic array alone to guide action.

Even though the ecological perception theory of visual perception cannot adequately describe how perception and action are coupled in certain movement situations, this alternative approach has challenged researchers to study perception and action in more natural movement settings where the perceptual processes are directly coupled to action. Ecological theorists have also helped us to understand other forms of human action (such as jumping, locomotion, and stairclimbing) that have been largely ignored in cognitive theories of perception and action.

Perhaps the best compromise between the two theories is offered by Williams and colleagues (1992) in the concluding section of their review article. They suggest that an ecological theory of visual perception may be best suited to describing how vision is used during the visual control of gait and

Direct perception theories may be best suited to describing how vision is used in movement contexts where there is a direct fit between perception and action.

the performance of interceptive actions such as catching and striking objects. Conversely, in movement situations where meaning is not readily apparent from the visual scene, or where decisions to act must be made on the basis of advance visual cues, it may be necessary to refer to a computational, or indirect, view of perception. Examples of movement contexts in which indirect theories of perception seem better able to account for the relationship between perception and action include rule-bound sporting environments, time-constrained movement contexts, and the appreciation and/or expression of movement aesthetics typical of many dance and mime performances.

# Visual Guidance of Action

## Reaching and Grasping

Research in motor control has provided strong support for the role of vision in the performance of aiming, reaching, and grasping skills. Goal-directed voluntary movements that require endpoint accuracy are particularly affected when the availability of visual feedback is either removed or degraded (Jeannerod, 1984; Prablanc, Echallier, Komilis, & Jeannerod, 1979; Woodworth, 1899). The availability of vision prior to the performance of such movements also appears to be important because of the fact that proprioception is limited to personal space and is therefore unable to tell us where the limb is relative to the target. To demonstrate the important premovement role played by vision, Prablanc et al. (1979) compared the accuracy of hand-pointing movements when vision of the hand was available prior to the movement only and when it was not available at any point prior to or during the trial. What the researchers found was that the performance of their study participants was significantly better when the position of the hand could be seen prior to the pointing movement when compared to the no vision condition. These findings suggest that vision is serving an exproprioceptive function prior to limb movement by signaling limb position relative to the body and the target. In this way vision is used to calibrate position sense and provide the CNS with information relative to the location, distance, size, and orientation of the target relative to the body that can be used to plan the movement phase of the action.

As far back as the late 1800s, considerable importance has also been placed on the role of visual feedback during the performance of aiming movements (Woodworth, 1899). It has been argued that vision is particularly important during the final phase of an aiming movement when minute corrections to the limb's trajectory are needed to ensure that the target is successfully reached. When these final visual adjustments cannot be made, the movements are not only less accurate, but there is also a tendency to undershoot the target position (Prablanc et al., 1979).

More recent studies have further demonstrated that a tight coupling exists between vision and the movements of the hand that is both temporal and spatial in nature. Using three-dimensional motion analysis synchronized with eye tracking equipment, Helsen and colleagues (1998, 2000) have not only confirmed the critical role played by vision prior to the initiation of an aiming movement, but also during the final phase of the movement when the

Goal-directed reaching movements requiring accuracy are adversely affected when visual feedback is removed or degraded.

performer is attempting to correct both the spatial trajectory and speed of the limb movement in order to accurately reach the endpoint target.

How much time do we need to use visual feedback to successfully reach an endpoint target in space? To address this question, Keele and Posner (1968) trained their study participants to move a stylus from a starting position to a target in different amounts of time—150, 250, 350, or 450 milliseconds (ms). On a random number of the movement trials, the lights in the room were turned off as soon as the movement began, making it impossible for the participants to use vision to control their movements. What the results indicated was that only those movements that required 200 ms or longer to complete were adversely affected by the removal of vision. Keele and Posner concluded that at least 200 ms is required to make visually based movement corrections to ensure endpoint accuracy. Although the results of later studies suggest that the time required to make visually based corrections is much lower, it has been estimated that at least 100 ms is needed for visually based corrections in movement (Carlton, 1981; Zelaznik, Schmidt, Gielen, & Milich, 1983).

Jeannerod (1984) has divided movements that require reaching to grasp an object into two phases. The first phase is called the **transportation phase,** during which the hand moves quickly to the vicinity of a target, and the second phase is called the **manipulation phase.** During this second phase, the final adjustments are being made to the aperture of the grasp just prior to contact with the object. Picking up a pencil, for example, would require a much smaller grasp aperture than lifting a glass from a table. The results of a number of research studies have also shown that our ability to grasp objects is also compromised when vision is not available during the movement. In these types of movements, vision is needed to prepare the distal muscles in the hand and fingers for generating the grip aperture needed to grasp the object, in advance of the object being contacted. Greater performance errors in grasping have also been observed when grasping movements must be performed quickly (Wallace & Weeks, 1988). Again, it would appear that a minimum amount of time is needed to use vision to ensure the precision of the grip aperture during the manipulation phase.

## Standing Balance

A balanced and upright posture can be achieved using a variety of sensory inputs. These include cutaneous and proprioceptive inputs from the feet and ankle joints, vestibular input, and, of course, vision. Among adults, vision is generally used to supplement the information provided by proprioceptors to maintain an upright posture. Not so for children, however, who tend to rely more on visual inputs when first learning to stand. This preference for visual input at an early age is believed to be due to the infant's inability to integrate the various proprioceptive inputs necessary for successful balance control. Infants' visual system tends to be more advanced developmentally, and therefore more reliable, than their proprioception function. Continued experience with tasks requiring postural control, however, eventually enables the growing child to take full advantage of the multiple sensory inputs available and rely less on visual cues.

---

At least 200 ms is needed to make visually based movement corrections to ensure endpoint accuracy.

In children, vision plays a greater role in standing balance than it does in adults.

An important proprioceptive role for vision in the control of balance has been demonstrated by Lee and colleagues (1974, 1975) in their innovative series of "moving wall" experiments. The researchers were able to manipulate visually the environment in which they placed their study participants by constructing a three-sided room that was suspended slightly above a stable floor surface. Movement of the wall in a forward or backward direction produced an optic flow field and provided visual information that convinced the participant that he or she was swaying in the opposite direction. Despite the fact that the information coming from the mechanical proprioceptors was in conflict with the visual information, participants attempted to correct their perceived postural sway with varying levels of gusto. The loss of upright posture was most visible among infants, who had not yet acquired the adult degree of fine tuning in the mechanical proprioceptors. The findings of these studies suggest that vision plays a major role in maintaining upright posture because it provides us with a higher level of proprioceptive sensitivity than do the mechanical proprioceptors.

## Locomotion

The role played by vision in controlling locomotion clearly varies as a function of the movement situation. When the surface is smooth, the locomotor pattern appears to be largely controlled by the spinal system (see Chapter 5). Similarly, running in daylight conditions poses little problem, given our ability to use the visual system to monitor and anticipate changes in the environment. We are also able to use vision in these lighted conditions to tell us what direction we are traveling in, to avoid colliding with objects in our path, and to identify the type of terrain ahead. In addition to providing us with important exproprioceptive information in these movement situations, vision also serves an important feedforward function by preparing the motor system in advance of the actual movement.

> Vision serves an important feedforward function by preparing the motor system in advance of the actual movement.

Our ability to use vision in this way is particularly important when we are moving over irregular terrain. In this movement situation, proper footing is achieved by visually regulating step length, primarily by varying the vertical impulse applied to the ground during the stance phase of the step cycle. This temporal regulation of the step cycle occurs before the foot strikes the ground, ensuring a secure footing once it does so (Warren, Young, & Lee, 1986). A feedforward role for vision has also been demonstrated in situations in which we are required either to change directions on the basis of visual cues while walking or to step over obstacles placed in our path (Patla, Prentice, Robinson, & Neufeld, 1991).

Visual feedforward is also evident in locomotor activities that require a change in the dynamics of posture at a certain point in space. The performer must not only judge the distance involved but also predict, on the basis of the speed at which she or he is moving, when to begin altering body position. Thus these activities comprise both a spatial and a temporal component. In long jumping, for example, the athlete must strike a take-off board at a predetermined point in space while running at maximum speed. As soon as the board is contacted, the performer must forcefully project his or her body upward, adopting a position that will maximize distance through the air.

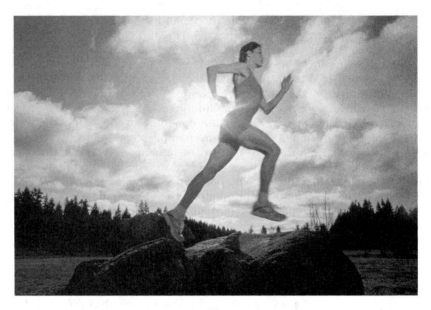

The feedforward role played by vision enables this runner to prepare the movement system in advance of her performance, ensuring a secure footing when her foot strikes the ground.

Contrary to the opinion of many coaches, however, who argue that successful striking of the board is achieved by developing a standardized approach run, the filming of highly skilled athletes suggests the use of a different strategy—one that employs vision to estimate time-to-contact, particularly during the final strides before the board. Lee, Lishman, and Thomson (1982) filmed the approach runs of three highly skilled female athletes. The temporal regulation of stride length via vision was particularly evident when the early phase of the approach run was compared to the last few strides before contacting the take-off board. Stride length began to vary quite dramatically during the final three strides as the performer attempted to compensate for the inconsistencies in stride length that occurred during the early phase of the approach run. These results provided support for the idea that the athletes were using vision to adjust the flight time of the final few strides in order to zero in on the take-off board. The findings of Lee et al. have also been supported by Hay (1988), who studied a larger number of highly skilled male and female long-jumpers, and by Meeuwsen and Magill (1987), who observed similar variability in foot placement among female collegiate gymnasts approaching the vault.

Berg, Wade, and Greer (1994) have since replicated and extended the findings of Lee et al. (1982) to a group of novice long-jumpers. Similar to the earlier findings with elite performers, the authors found that vision was again being used to regulate step length in the final approach steps to the board. They concluded that the visual control of gait during the long jump was not the result of specific skill training but rather the preferred means of controlling gait during this type of activity.

## Jumping from Different Heights

Vision also enables us to prepare the appropriate muscle synergies in advance of a landing to absorb the shock of impact and prevent injury to our joints and muscles. This feedforward role for vision is particularly important for gymnasts attempting to perform difficult dismounts from various apparatus and for parachute jumpers, who are traveling at very high speeds just before contacting the ground.

Sidaway, McNitt-Gray, and Davis (1989) demonstrated how vision can be used to prepare the motor system in advance of a landing during a jumping activity. The authors recorded the level of EMG activity in the rectus femoris muscle of a group of young adults required to jump from a platform set at three different heights (0.72 m, 1.04 m, and 1.59 m) above a force plate. The research question was whether the study participants used a computation process based on such parameters as distance to the floor, velocity, and acceleration, or simply used the readily available visual information to predict time-to-contact. A comparison of the EMG data with the force plate trace indicating foot contact provided support for the idea that participants were using vision to determine exactly when the muscles should be activated in preparation for landing from the different heights.

## Catching Objects

Many motor activities require that we not only regulate the movements of our body as we locomote through space but also make our movements coincide with those of an object or another person. Consider, for example, the timing sequence involved in an outfielder's attempt to catch a fly ball in a game of baseball or softball. As soon as the ball leaves the bat, the outfielder visually locates the ball and begins to move the whole body to the position in space where the ball is predicted to be at a given time. As the fielder continues to move, the catching hand is oriented to coincide with the path of the ball, and the fingers begin to close in anticipation of the ball's contact with the glove.

In order for the catch to be successful, the outfielder must complete this sequence of movements *before* the ball reaches the catching hand. In fact, a cinematographical study of one-handed catching conducted by Alderson, Sully, and Sully (1974) has shown that orientation of the catching hand must begin between 150 and 200 ms before the ball contacts the palm, and that closure of the fingers around the ball must begin as early as 50 ms before ball contact, if the catch is to be successful. This study also demonstrated a smaller margin for error with respect to the timing of these movements when the velocity of the ball was greater.

The precision with which the outfielder executes this sequence of movements also demands a precise visual assessment of the ball's flight characteristics. Once the player's eyes locate the ball in space, its flight must be monitored long enough to predict where the ball will be at any given time. Continuous monitoring of the ball's entire flight is not necessary for successful timing of the catch, but good vision of the ball becomes critical in the final 200 to 300 ms. In fact, a number of catching studies (Fischman & Schneider, 1985; Smyth & Marriott, 1982; Whiting, Gill, & Stephenson, 1970) have demonstrated the importance of seeing the ball and/or the catching hand

In anticipation timing skills such as catching, vision is used to make the movements of the body and/or its parts coincide with those of an object or other person.

during the final moments of the ball's flight. According to indirect theories of visual perception, the predictive information provided by the visual system early in the ball's flight ensures that the outfielder's movements to intercept the ball begin well before its arrival.

## Hitting Objects

A second coincident timing skill in which vision plays an important role is that of hitting. Although studies have shown that even professional baseball players are unable to keep their eyes on the ball until it hits their bat, sight of the ball early in its trajectory enables the batter to predict the ball's location as it crosses the plate (Bahill & LaRitz, 1984). Hubbard and Seng (1954) have also shown that batters use vision to synchronize the timing of their forward step with the release of the ball from the pitcher's hand and that they regulate the duration of their step as a function of the ball's speed. This use of vision enables skilled batters to keep the duration of their batting swing relatively constant from pitch to pitch.

A group of researchers at the Free University in Amsterdam (Bootsma & van Wieringen, 1990) have also investigated the role of vision in timing a forehand stroke in table tennis. Although they too found that highly skilled players demonstrated a high degree of temporal consistency and accuracy at the moment of ball-paddle contact, it was not due to the players' adopting a standardized movement pattern. Instead, their ability to compensate for variability occurring in one movement parameter (time at which the stroke was initiated) by adjusting a second movement parameter (speed with which the paddle was swung) as the ball approached the paddle differentiated their performance from that of their novice counterparts. The authors concluded that the players were continuously using the visual information present in the visual display to guide their actions prior to ball-paddle contact.

## Time-to-Contact Information

Just how are we able to use vision to regulate our actions temporally in each of the movement situations discussed? According to cognitive, or indirect, theories of visual perception, our ability to alter the position of our body at a given point in space and to intercept a moving object depends on our ability to process a number of movement variables (including distance, velocity, and acceleration) during the early stages of execution. This early processing of visual information involves taking discrete retinal "snapshots" of the visual array that then form the basis for predicting when the body or an object will arrive at a certain location. How accurately the performer is able to predict where an object or the body will be at a given time is largely determined by his or her existing knowledge of the movement situation and by the speed with which an appropriate action plan can be retrieved from memory and then executed.

The advocates of ecological or direct perception theories offer an alternative interpretation. They argue that time-to-contact information can be gleaned directly from the changing optic array, eliminating the need for the performer to compute other flight-related variables that would appear to make the predictive process much more complex. For example, Lee and Young (1985, p. 7) believe that computing time-to-contact from such variables as distance and velocity introduces multiple sources of error that would not exist if contact point were directly perceived. According to these and other authors, a single optical variable provides us with an estimate of time-to-contact.

This optical variable, referred to as **tau,** has been mathematically defined by Lee (1976, 1980) as the inverse of the rate of dilation of an image on the retina. Simply put, the faster an approaching object fills the visual field, the faster the object will contact a particular point in space (such as a ball contacting a bat or a vehicle contacting another vehicle). Performers can therefore use tau to time their actions simply by determining how quickly the size of an approaching object fills the visual field. This explanation has been invoked to interpret the experimental findings of many of the studies discussed in the previous section. Unfortunately, as easily as many experimental findings can be used to support this alternative explanation, many of the results can be explained just as well in terms of the performers' using a computational process to predict time-to-contact. Future research will need to focus on devising experimental situations and methods of testing that clearly demonstrate the use of one strategy rather than the other.

> Tau is an optical variable used to predict time-to-contact.

Moreover, we do not know at this point whether tau can also be effectively used to predict time-to-contact when the object to be intercepted is coming from different trajectory angles other than directly in front of the performer. In more complex catching situations such as we encounter when playing sport, the effective interception of an object is also likely to require that we also predict where the limb must move in space prior to contact. This would require a spatial as well as temporal prediction on the part of the performer.

To address this issue, Todd (1981) conducted a series of experiments that investigated whether a person could accurately predict where an approaching object would land relative to him/herself. Using two time-to-contact components (time-to-contact with a vertical plane through the point of observation and time-to-contact with the horizontal plane through the point of observation), he developed a ratio that could be used to predict whether an object would land in front of or behind the observer. For example, if $T_c$ vertical (time-to-contact in the vertical direction) and $T_c$ horizontal equal 1, then the object could be expected to land at the point of observation. Conversely, when the ratio of the $T_c$ vertical component relative to the $T_c$ horizontal component is greater than 1, the ball will land behind the point of observation, and if it is less than 1, the ball will land in front of the point of observation. Lee (1980) has further speculated that the direction of an object's flight can be specified quantitatively by studying the displacement of the center of expansion relative to the point of observation. Fitch and Turvey (1977) have also studied how the changing texture of the background might also provide additional information relative to the path of the ball's flight. They argue that if the texture of background surrounding the approaching object is lost equally in all directions relative to the object expanding on the visual field then the object is approaching from directly in front of the observer. If, however, the background texture is being asymmetrically lost relative to the expanding object, then it is likely that the object is approaching the observer from a different angle of trajectory. They argue that catching objects against a richly textured background enhances the amount of information provided in the optic array.

> It is hypothesized that the direction of an object's flight can be quantified by studying the displacement of the center of expansion relative to the point of observation.

# HIGHLIGHT

## Grasping Tau

Perhaps the strongest empirical evidence supporting the use of the optical variable tau to predict time-to-contact information has been provided by a group of creative researchers at the Free University in The Netherlands (Savelsbergh, Whiting, & Bootsma, 1991). During the course of two experiments, subjects were required to catch different-sized balls suspended from an aluminum pendulum (see the figure) that was released from an electromagnet. The unique feature of these experiments was that the size of the approaching ball could be altered during its flight. How was this possible? A luminous balloon was used to form a "skin" around the enclosed ball that could be inflated prior to its release and then progressively deflated, by as much as 2 cm in diameter, during flight. In fact, the deflation of the ball was so subtle that it was not perceptually noticeable to the subjects.

The authors hypothesized that if performers rely on time-to-contact information to time their actions, they would be able to adjust their hand movements to accommodate the changing ball size. The variables measured included the time at which the grasping movement was initiated after release of the ball pendulum and the time elapsed between the initiation of the grasp and the moment of ball–hand contact.

As the results show (see the figure below), subjects were clearly adjusting the timing of their grasping movements right up to the moment that the deflating ball contacted the hand. On the basis of this finding, in particular, the authors concluded that the subjects were using the optical expansion rate of the oncoming ball to time their grasping movements, particularly in the final 200 ms before ball contact.

This study was published in the *Journal of Experimental Psychology: Human Perception and Performance, 17* (2), 315–322.

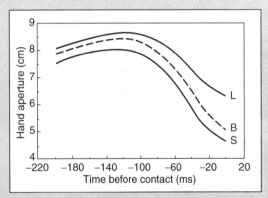

The hand aperture was affected by the nonveridical, or illusory, visual information, particularly during the final moments before the ball contacted the hand.

(L = large; B = deflating; S = small)

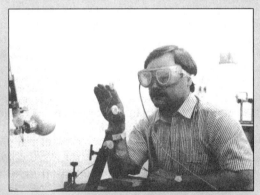

The experimental set-up.

## Visual Dominance

Although the foregoing discussion might lead us to conclude that vision always contributes significantly and positively in a wide variety of movement situations, there are times when our reliance on vision leads to errors in performance. In situations of **sensory conflict,** for example, our preference for visual information can often result in slowed or even incorrect responses. Even when contradictory sensory input is available from receptors in the skin, muscles, joints, and inner ear, we still tend to rely on vision to guide the action. For example, have you ever found yourself quickly reaching for the brake in the car while you waited at a traffic light only to realize it was the neighboring car, not yours, that was moving? In this situation, seeing movement in the periphery has convinced you that you are the one moving, even though other sensory inputs suggest otherwise. The moving wall experiments discussed on page 105 also demonstrate how easily postural stability can be influenced by manipulating vision alone.

The predominance of vision over other sensory systems has also been demonstrated to affect performance negatively in movement situations that require rapid responses. For example, Jordan (1972) trained a group of novice fencers to respond as quickly and efficiently as possible to the deflection of a mechanical blade. He manipulated the availability of visual and proprioceptive information in the following ways: group I (vision only) could see the mechanical blade prior to its deflection but not make contact with it prior to the start of the trial; group II (vision + proprioception) were able to see the mechanical blade and also place their own blades against it prior to the start of each trial; group III (proprioception only) positioned their blades so they were in contact with the mechanical blade prior to each trial, but participants were blindfolded.

What Jordan found over the course of the first 10 training sessions was that the fencers who were only able to feel the mechanical blade in contact with their own prior to each trial responded significantly faster to the movement of the mechanical blade when compared to either group permitted to see and/or touch the mechanical blade prior to it being deflected. In the absence of vision, the fencers were utilizing the faster somatosensory cues provided by the cutaneous receptors in order to quickly respond to the deflected blade. When vision was available, however, responses were significantly slower by comparison.

## Role of Vision in Performance of Sport Skills

It is clear from the previous sections in this chapter that vision not only plays an important role in all aspects of motor control (including movement planning, execution, and evaluation), but is the preferred modality for sensory information, even though other sensory systems are capable of providing sensory information more quickly and, in some situations, more accurately. What has also been a topic of considerable research interest over the years is the contribution of vision to the performance of sport skills. Two research questions that have been investigated in a number of published studies are whether basic visual functions are related to sporting performances and whether training the visual system will result in enhanced sporting performances.

In situations of sensory conflict, our preference for vision can result in slowed or incorrect responses.

Moderate relation-
ships do exist be-
tween certain basic
visual functions and
sport performance.

Basic visual functions studied have included those of static and dynamic visual acuity, peripheral vision, depth perception, and divergence/convergence (see Blundell, 1985 for a review). In general, the results have demonstrated moderate relationships between athletic ability and dynamic acuity (Beals et al., 1971), peripheral vision (Stroup, 1957; Tergerson, 1964), and depth perception (Blundell, 1984; Tatem, 1973) but a number of concerns have been raised concerning the methodology and/or instruments used to measure the different visual parameters and/or how the different skill levels were defined across studies.

A second question that has been studied by a number of researchers is whether sporting performance can be significantly improved by training the visual system. On the strength of the moderate amount of evidence that certain visual parameters are related to sporting performance, a number of general vision training programs have become commercially available. The developers of these self-help training programs claim that substantial improvements in the performance of sport skills can be realized following relatively short periods of training (Revien & Gabor, 1981). Once again, a small number of studies have provided support for the beneficial effects of these training programs on sport performance. For example, Vedelli (1986) reported a significant improvement in the training group's ability to hit a tennis ball for accuracy, while West and Bresson (1996) found that the cricket batsmen they studied were better able to judge the flight of the ball following a general vision training program. One major criticism of these studies has been the failure to include a placebo group, in addition to a standard control group, as a means of determining whether factors other than improved vision (improved confidence, modifications in technique, greater knowledge of the sport, and so on) could account for the significant differences observed between groups. A second criticism raised has been that the eye exercises performed are very similar to the eye tests used to measure visual function, and therefore improvements could also be attributed to test familiarity (Abernethy & Wood, 2001).

Limited evidence
exists that general
vision training pro-
grams enhance
sporting perfor-
mances.

The results of two studies conducted by Abernethy and colleagues (Abernethy & Wood, 2001; Wood & Abernethy, 1997) in which a placebo group was included did not demonstrate significant improvements in sporting performance following four weeks of general vision training. The results from these more carefully controlled experiments suggest that general vision training programs may not yield the significant improvements in sporting performance found in previous research studies nor provide support for the use of commercially available sport vision training programs by coaches. In a review article, Abernethy and Wood (2001) further conclude that general visual training programs should be applied cautiously because basic visual function may not be the limiting factor in the performance of sport skills. Rather, it may be more related to how the specific visual information provided in a particular sporting context is interpreted and used to guide action. Simply put, the differences between expert and novice performers may be better elucidated by studying the central processes related to visual perception rather than the capabilities of the visual system alone.

# Disorders of the Visual System

Because we rely so heavily on vision to interact with the world, any damage to the visual system will compromise our ability to function efficiently. In fact, a reduction in vision ranks third, behind heart disease and arthritis, as the most often cited reason that people give for limiting their activities of daily living (Fox, 1999). This comes as no surprise given that 90% of all spatial information we receive is derived from vision. Compromised vision can occur as a result of age-related eye diseases such as cataracts (impairs clarity of vision), glaucoma (leads to visual field loss), or macular degeneration (involves loss of central vision) or as a secondary consequence of diseases such as arteriosclerosis, diabetes, or multiple sclerosis. Any damage to the visual pathways projecting into the midbrain or cortex will also cause partial blindness in the visual field. If damage occurs to the retina or optic nerve leading away from the eye, the visual deficit will be unilateral, whereas the visual loss will usually be bilateral if damage occurs at the chiasm or in the visual pathways beyond the chiasm. Many individuals with higher cortical damage (particularly damage to the parietal lobe of the brain) may also experience a lack of awareness of the body's structure and of the relationship among body parts. This body scheme impairment can make it impossible for such patients to distinguish among body parts or imitate movements. In order to offset these problems, physical therapists often adopt a **sensorimotor approach.** This type of treatment may involve asking the patient to stimulate the ignored body part, perhaps by rubbing it with a rough cloth as the therapist either names or points to it.

> A sensorimotor approach is often used to offset a patient's inability to distinguish among body parts or imitate movements.

Visual deficits are also a common form of sensory loss among hemiplegic (stroke) patients. These deficits may result in poor visual acuity, partial blindness, or eye movement disorders. Visual-perceptual dysfunction may also be evident when damage occurs to the higher cortical areas responsible for recognizing and attaching meaning to visual input. Total failure to appreciate incoming visual information caused by damage to the cortex ultimately results in cortical blindness. Even though the retina and lower visual pathways are receiving and transmitting the visual information, the person with cortical blindness cannot interpret it at a cortical level and is therefore considered to be functionally blind. A person with cortical blindness, for example, can reach for a cup located to his/her left when given an instruction to do so but cannot visually identify it. For those hemiparetic patients who do not suffer from any visual impairment, vision can be used to assist them in the temporal sequencing of muscular activity. How is this possible? Lee, Lough, and Lough (1984) hypothesized that vision provides extrinsic timing information that can serve as a substitute for the information derived from such intrinsic sources as joints and muscle receptors.

In order to test their hypothesis, Lee et al. studied the ability of four left-hemisphere stroke patients to reach for a stationary soccer ball and intercept a soccer ball moving down an inclined track toward them with one or two hands. When they compared the quality of movement in the affected arm when the ball was stationary with the quality of arm movement when the ball was moving, the authors found significant differences in performance. Not only did the patients reach for the moving ball more smoothly, but they were also able to reach for it more quickly. These results would appear to

> Vision can be used to drive the motor system when intrinsic sources of sensory input are disrupted.

provide support for the authors' original idea that vision can be used to drive the motor system when intrinsic sources of sensory information are disrupted. Findings such as these have important implications for the physical therapist's work with hemiparetic patients during the recovery phase.

# Vestibular System

The second special sense that we will describe in this chapter is the vestibular system. This system also contributes to the ensemble of sensory information we need to plan and execute actions successfully. Specifically, this gravitoreceptor signals the orientation and movement of the head in space and tells us which way is up as a function of its sensitivity to the effects of gravity. In conjunction with other somatosensory inputs, the vestibular system also plays an important role in multiple facets of posture and gait. We will discuss this topic in greater detail later in this section of the chapter.

## Anatomy of the Vestibular System

Five sensory organs within the vestibular system signal where and how the head is moving.

The vestibular apparatus, as it is often called, resides in the innermost compartment of each ear in an area referred to as the vestibule that is located behind the medial wall of the middle ear and deep within the temporal bone (see Figure 4.3). Five sensory organs located within each vestibular system are designed to convert movements of the head into electrical signals that the brain can interpret. The three **semicircular canals** are responsible for measuring angular accelerations of the head or body while two **otolith organs** called the *utricle* and *saccule* measure linear accelerations that are produced by gravity and/or the movement of the body. The otolith organs also help us sense how the head is oriented with respect to gravity due to the fact that gravity exerts a constant linear acceleration on the head. How is it that these different sensory organs can accomplish these different functions?

The three semicircular canals signal the angular acceleration of the head in different planes.

The ability of the three semicircular canals to measure angular acceleration of the head in different planes is made possible by the fact that they sit at right angles to each other in each vestibular labyrinth (see Figure 4.3). The three canals are also named according to their orientation relative to the head. For example, when the head is anatomically positioned, the lateral, or horizontal, canal is tilted approximately 25 degrees above a horizontal axis, the posterior, or inferior, canal points toward the nose, and the anterior, or superior, canal points away from the nose (Cohen, 1999). What is important to note here is that the semicircular canals on the right and left sides of the head do not work independently during head movements but actually work in combination with each other. For example, turning the head to the right or the left stimulates one pair of canals, while pitching (neck flexion or extension) or rolling (right or left side bending of the head) the head in a certain direction activates another pair of semicircular canals. Because the two sets of semicircular canals work in combination, a certain amount of sensory redundancy results, so that if one vestibular system is damaged, the intact semicircular canals on the other side can still provide the CNS with information about head motion (Allison & Fuller, 2001). We will discuss a number of different disor-

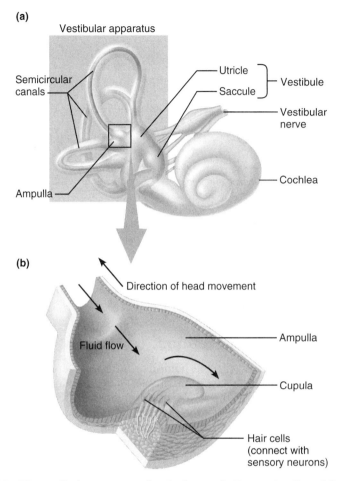

**(a)**

Vestibular apparatus

Semicircular canals

Utricle

Saccule

Vestibule

Vestibular nerve

Cochlea

Ampulla

**(b)**

Direction of head movement

Ampulla

Fluid flow

Cupula

Hair cells (connect with sensory neurons)

**Figure 4.3**   The vestibular apparatus signals changes in the acceleration of the head via three semicircular canals (anterior, posterior, and lateral) and the utricle and saccule.

ders that affect one or both vestibular systems and how the brain learns to adapt to the altered or lost information in the vestibular disorders section (pages 121–123).

Similar to the semicircular canals, the utricle and saccule are aligned at almost right angles to each other and also work in a complementary way with the contralateral utricle and saccule. The sensory surface of the utricle lies in a near horizontal position, and the saccule is positioned in a more vertical orientation. By virtue of their different anatomical positions, the utricles are sensitive to the magnitude and direction of head movements that occur in a horizontal plane while the saccules are more responsive to vertical accelerations of the head, particularly those that are gravity induced. Activities such as riding in a car that is accelerating away from the curb stimulates firing of the sensory receptors housed in the utricles, whereas the saccules are more

The saccule is sensitive to acceleration of the head in a horizontal plane while the utricle is more sensitive to vertical head accelerations.

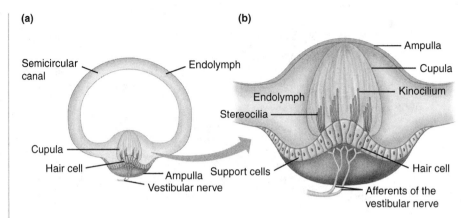

**Figure 4.4**   Clusters of hair cells reside in an area called the ampulla which is located at the widest region of each semicircular canal. These hair cells are deformed when the head accelerates.

likely to be stimulated when we ride in elevators or go up or down a flight of stairs (Herdman, 2000).

## Peripheral Sensory Reception

The process of transducing the mechanical stimuli (acceleration of the head) into receptor potentials begins with the physical deformation of clusters of **hair cells** that reside in each of the five sensory organs of the vestibular system. In the case of the semicircular canals, the clusters of hair cells reside in an area called the **ampulla** located at the widest region of each semicircular canal (see Figure 4.4). The hair cells then project into a gelatinous area called the **cupula.** When the head accelerates in an angular direction, endolymphatic fluid in this region of the canal moves against the cupula housing the hair cells, causing it to bow and the hair cells within to depolarize.

In the otolith organs (utricle and saccule), similar clusters of hair cells are located in an area called the macula and project into a gelatinous otolithic membrane (see Figure 4.5). Embedded within and on top of that membrane are calcium carbonate crystals called **otoconia** that are free to move across the membrane surface. The presence of otoconia on the otolithic membrane also adds mass so the **vestibular hair cells** within can respond to the effects of gravity as well as head movements (Allison & Fuller, 2001). Unfortunately, during space travel, the otolith organs become unloaded due to the lack of gravity. Spatial orientation is adversely affected by this unloading with astronauts losing the ability to detect where "up" is in space (see highlight, Mixed Up in Space, on page 118 for a more in-depth discussion of the effect of space travel on the vestibular system).

When the head accelerates in a linear direction, the otoconia move across the membrane, which in turn shifts the otolithic membrane, causing deformation and firing of the hair cells within.

It is estimated that the cupula of each semicircular canal is penetrated by almost 7,000 hair cells, while the utricle and saccule contain approximately

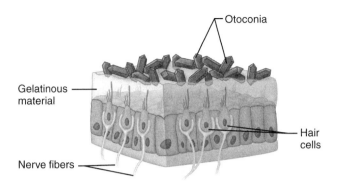

**Figure 4.5**   The otolith organs contain clusters of hair cells that are located in the macula and project into a gelatinous otolithic membrane.

30,000 and 16,000 hair cells, respectively (Goldberg & Hudspeth, 2000). The hair cells in each of the vestibular organs are extremely sensitive to head movement and are capable of detecting movements as small as 0.1 deg/sec. Even the smallest head movements that occur during standing sway are sufficient to trigger the hair cells in this sensitive set of sensory organs.

## Ascending Pathways

The signals leaving the peripheral component (labyrinths) of the vestibular system travel via as many as 20,000 myelinated axons that comprise the vestibular portion of cranial nerve VIII (Goldberg & Hudspeth, 2000). This nerve can be further divided into two parts: a superior and inferior nerve. The superior vestibular nerve innervates the utricle and the anterior and lateral semicircular canals while the inferior vestibular nerve innervates the saccule and posterior semicircular canal. The cell bodies associated with each part of the vestibular nerve are located in an area called **Scarpa's** (or **vestibular**) **ganglion** (see Figure 4.3). The vestibular nerve transmits signals to vestibular nuclei in the brainstem (medulla and pons). The vestibular nuclei are then responsible for integrating the signals coming from the vestibular organs with other signals arriving from the visual system, cerebellum, and even the spinal cord.

The vestibular nuclei in the brainstem are responsible for integrating signals coming from the vestibular organs with other signals arriving from the eyes.

Once the incoming signals are integrated within the vestibular nuclei, these signals are then sent on to several different areas within the CNS, including the vestibular regions of the thalamus, somatosensory cortex, cerebellum, spinal cord, and the oculomotor nuclei (Goldberg & Hudspeth, 2000). This sophisticated network of vestibular connections helps us spatially orient our bodies relative to gravity and know where we are in space as the head and body rotate. Just imagine how difficult it would be for figure skaters or springboard divers to detect where their body was in space during the many difficult spinning, jumping, and somersaulting maneuvers they perform in their respective sports if the vestibular system were not operating effectively. In fact, in the highlight on page 122 you can read about the story of Mary Ellen Clark, an Olympic medalist in platform diving who developed a serious vestibular problem while training for the Olympic games in Barcelona, Spain, in 1992.

## HIGHLIGHT

### Mixed Up in Space

A common problem, particularly for astronauts undertaking their first space mission, is adapting to being in a world that is now devoid of gravity. They become quite "mixed up"' in this situation, no longer able to distinguish which way is now up or sense where their arms and legs are in space. In fact, many astronauts experience a form of space sickness very much like many people experience when they try to read while traveling in a moving vehicle. Because the vestibular system, and the otolith organs in particular, rely on the pull of gravity for determining our spatial orientation, once it is no longer available, this part of the system becomes befuddled because inputs from the inner ear no longer match those generated by the visual system. To counter the sensory conflict problem that astronauts experience in space, the space modules are designed to create a consistent "up" orientation. Even the writing on the module walls points in the same direction. Virtual reality training tools are also being used to help astronauts learn preflight strategies they can apply in space.

Fortunately, the vestibular system is also capable of rapidly adapting to new weightless surroundings, and the brain learns to reinterpret the conflicting information coming from the vestibular and visual systems. Unfortunately, once the astronauts return to earth, the confusion returns as the astronaut becomes disoriented again. Now they have to readjust to the return of gravity. According to NASA (National Aeronautics and Space Administration) scientists, recovery of spatial orientation

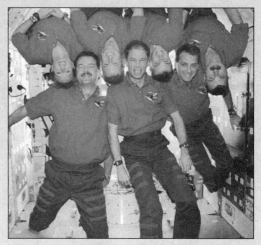

In the absence of gravity, the vestibular system no longer provides the brain with information about the body's position relative to "up" or "down."

following a return to earth can take anywhere from hours to days, depending on the length of the space mission. Balance is also severely compromised in returning astronauts and can take up to two weeks to return to normal. NASA scientists are currently working on developing in-flight treadmill training systems to help astronauts readapt to gravity environments more quickly.

For more information about research being conducted to improve vestibular system function in space, the reader is encouraged to log onto Science@NASA at http://science.nasa.gov.

## Descending Pathways

In addition to the ascending pathways that carry vestibular signals to higher order centers within the brain, two pathways leaving the vestibular nuclei within the brainstem descend to the spinal cord. These pathways are important for postural control, particularly in reactive situations when balance is unexpectedly lost and must be restored. The lateral and medial **vestibulospinal tracts (VST)** synapse directly and/or indirectly (via interneurons) with motoneurons at various levels of the spinal cord that innervate extensor muscle groups. These antigravity muscles, as they are aptly named, are responsible for counteracting the effects of gravity so we can maintain an upright posture in space.

The vestibular system, through these pathways, plays an important role in both mediating and facilitating the development of automatic righting and equilibrium reactions in young children (Shumway-Cook, Horak, & Black, 1987). These reactions occur when the utricles and semicircular canals are stimulated in response to changes in the center of gravity. To counteract these changes, the antigravity extensor muscle groups are activated to oppose the altered head, trunk, and limb positions that are perturbed, thus restoring the body to its upright position.

## Vestibular-Visual Interactions

Although the vestibular system provides an array of unique sensory information to the CNS, its accuracy and capabilities are enhanced through its interactions with other sensory systems, and the visual system in particular. One vestibular reflex that nicely demonstrates the interconnectedness between the vestibular and visual system is the **vestibular ocular reflex (VOR).** The primary function of this reflex is to stabilize the eyes when the head moves. For example, it assists us to see clearly when we are moving our entire bodies or during rapid head movements. It becomes particularly important to us when we walk or ride a mountain bike over uneven terrain or turn quickly to see who has called our name.

The vestibular system signals the speed of the head's rotation and the oculomotor system then uses the information to stabilize the eyes. When the vestibular system is operating normally, the eyes move at the same velocity as the head (a ratio equal to one), albeit in the opposite direction. Simply put, when the head turns to the left, the eyes actually move to the right in an effort to stabilize the image on the retina. This creates what is called the **gain** of the VOR. The gain can be altered with any disturbance to the visual or vestibular systems. The gain of the VOR has also been demonstrated to decline with aging, making it more difficult for older adults to maintain a stable image on the retina when the head is moving in space (Wolfson, 1997).

In other situations, such as when we wish to slowly track an object through space, the activation of the VOR must now be canceled so the head and eyes now move in the same direction rather than in opposite directions. Individuals who are unable to effectively cancel the VOR in these situations will not be able to smoothly track objects with the eyes. In fact, the eyes may periodically jump in order to catch up with the moving target and bring it back into focus.

## Adaptability of the Vestibular Ocular Reflex

The vestibular ocular reflex is a highly adaptable mechanism and has been used to study the neural mechanism of motor learning extensively over the years. Through the use of magnifying glasses, researchers are able to observe the gain of the VOR change very quickly. Although initially disrupted because the size of the retinal image is now larger, within a week of beginning to wear

*Through its descending pathways, the vestibular system plays an important role in restoring the body to its upright position following a perturbation.*

*The VOR is a highly adaptable reflex and has been used to study the neural mechanisms of motor learning.*

the magnifying glasses, the gain of the VOR has been similarly increased to compensate for the larger visual image. Similarly, researchers have been able to study the plasticity of the VOR by studying the behavior of people asked to wear inverting prisms that turn the world upside down. After a short adaptation period involving active movement exploration designed to recalibrate the visual and vestibular systems, the person was not only able to accurately pour water from a glass into a jug, both of which look inverted, but could even successfully ride a bicycle in what appeared to be an upside-down world.

One hypothesis that has been proposed by Ito (1984) to explain the adaptive capabilities of the VOR involves the excitatory and inhibitory pathways that connect the vestibular labyrinth with the cerebellum and the cerebellum with the vestibular nuclei. According to Ito, the observed adaptation occurs as a result of the relative strength of the excitatory and inhibitory pathways being altered during the adaptation period. Although Ito's hypothesis has been challenged by other researchers (Lisberger, 1988), who propose a different mechanism for the adaptability, the involvement of the cerebellum is common to both theories.

## Vestibular Contributions to Equilibrium

The vestibular
system collaborates
with the visual
system to stabilize
vision when the
head is moving.

The vestibular apparatus, in collaboration with the visual system discussed earlier in this chapter and the somatosensory system described in the previous chapter, plays an important role in multiple dimensions of balance and gait. Not only does it provide the brain with the information needed to orient the body in space, but through its descending pathways it exerts both direct and indirect influences on the extensor muscle groups for the maintenance of upright stance and the reflexive control of balance when it is unexpectedly perturbed. The vestibular system then collaborates with the visual system to help us stabilize vision when the head is moving through the VOR mechanism. This becomes an important mechanism for maintaining normal gait postures. Finally, in situations of sensory conflict, the vestibular system acts as a "referee" when information provided by the visual and somatosensory system is not congruent (in agreement) (Allison & Fuller, 2001). Recall the example provided earlier of reaching for the brake in your car at a stop light because a vehicle next to you has begun to move. Despite the fact that your somatosensory inputs are telling you that you and the car are perfectly stationary, the visual system has tricked you into thinking that you are moving. This feeling of disorientation can also occur when standing on a moving or compliant surface with your eyes closed or engaged in the performance of a second task (such as reading, reaching for an object); in this situation we must rely totally on the information provided by the vestibular system, because the somatosensory information provided at the ankles is no longer accurate, and vision is no longer available for gaze fixation and spatial orientation.

Individuals who are unable to utilize vestibular inputs to reconcile this conflict, whether it arose as a result of disease or underutilization that is often associated with aging, will avoid situations or activities likely to introduce sensory conflict. They will avoid negotiating stairs, escalators, or crowded malls and will never arrive late to a movie or leave before the last credit has left the screen for fear of losing balance and falling. Certain central sensory processing deficits that often result from cerebrovascular trauma can also make it difficult for individuals to successfully integrate visual, vestibular, and somatosensory inputs to maintain an upright position in space.

In summary, the vestibular system provides the CNS with information that is critical for the performance of the following perceptual–motor tasks:

1.  Perception of spatial orientation as a function of the vestibular organs monitoring the absolute position of the head and the direction of gravity (otoliths) and also signaling changes in head position (semicircular canals).
2.  Gaze stabilization during movement made possible through the operation of the vestibular ocular reflex.
3.  Maintenance or restoration of upright balance. This task is achieved through the generation of vestibulospinal reflexes that compensate for changes in the center of gravity and restore the head to an erect position.

## Disorders of the Vestibular System

In addition to a number of different metabolic and immune disorders that can affect the normal function of the vestibular system, physical trauma such as a blow to the head can also seriously impact the functioning of one or both vestibular systems. In some cases, the problem is confined to the vestibular labyrinths or peripheral component of the vestibular system, while for certain other disorders it will involve the central pathways of the vestibular system. Depending on the type and location of the disorder, the effects can be quite small or completely disabling. Let's consider in a little more detail some of the more common vestibular disorders and how they are likely to affect motor control.

Unlike the disorders that affect only one of the two vestibular systems, individuals with bilateral disorders rarely experience symptoms of **vertigo** (an illusory sensation of motion) although their ability to maintain balance, particularly when the eyes are closed, is severely compromised. One general complaint of individuals with bilateral disorders is **oscillopsia** (apparent movement of objects in the visual field), particularly when the head is moving at a high frequency (Cohen, 1999). Due to the absence of the VOR, people with this disorder cannot maintain gaze stabilization when they are moving. Severely compromised vestibular function can also result from ototoxic medications (such as gentamicin, streptomycin) taken in large doses. These medications selectively destroy the hair cells within the vestibular system, causing severe balance and visual problems. People with this type of vestibular problem find it extremely difficult to gaze-stabilize while moving and must stop to read signs. They also make very few spontaneous head movements, even while carrying on a conversation, to avoid their vision becoming blurred.

Perhaps the most common peripheral vestibular disorder that affects one of the two vestibular systems is *benign positional vertigo (BPV)*. In this condition, otoconia, the tiny calcium carbonate crystals that sit on top of the otolithic membrane, become dislodged and fall, in the majority of cases, into the posterior semicircular canal (Baloh & Hornrubia, 1990). When a person with BPV turns the head quickly or pitches the head up or down as normally happens many

Depending on the type and location of the vestibular disorder, the effects on motor control can be quite small or completely disabling.

Vertigo is the illusory sensation of motion.

# HIGHLIGHT

## "Vexed by Vertigo"

The title of the *Sports Illustrated* article was "Vexed by Vertigo." Mary Ellen Clark, one of the nation's best 10-meter platform divers, was the subject of the story. She was struggling with severe bouts of dizziness that were severely affecting her ability to perform what were usually routine backward 2½ revolution somersaults from the 3-meter springboard. In fact, as she tells it in the story, she would become so disoriented that "sometimes she would swim to the bottom of the pool rather than the top after a dive." She had to make sure that her friends were watching her after each entry in case she swam the wrong way and needed their physical help to get out of the pool.

In her determination to keep diving at an international level and qualify for the Olympic games that were to be held in Barcelona in 1992, she underwent all kinds of testing ranging from EKG to caloric and rotary chair testing to find the cause of her dizziness. She also explored every possible treatment option in the years leading up to the games. She tried antidizziness medication, craniosacral therapy, acupuncture, and alternative herbal remedies in her efforts to resolve the problem. Following further testing at the Dizziness and Balance Center at the University of Miami she was diagnosed with benign positional vertigo (BPV), a peripheral vestibular condition that results from otoconia becoming dislodged from the otolithic membrane and falling into the posterior semicircular canal, in the majority of cases.

To address the problem she underwent a mechanical procedure called canalith repositioning in which a physical therapist, with specialized training in vestibular disorders, rotated her body and head that were hanging off the end of the treatment table on which she was lying, through a series of positions designed to return the otoconia to their original position. The treatment worked, at least for a period of time, but given the regular physical head trauma a platform diver experiences on every dive, it was not likely to be a permanent solution to her problems. She underwent the procedure many times over the next few years.

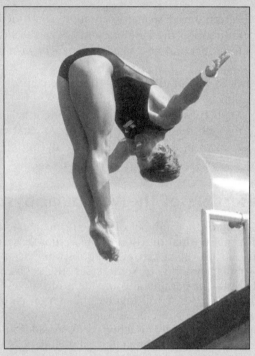

Mary Ellen Clark, U.S. Olympic diver, triumphed over her dizziness to win a bronze medal in the 10-meter platform event at the 1992 Olympic games.

Despite her continued bouts of dizziness, which really only bothered her when she dove, Mary Ellen qualified for the Barcelona Olympic games and went on to win a bronze medal for the United States in the 10-meter platform event. She, unlike other elite athletes who have suffered from similar problems with dizziness and vertigo and have never been able to return to competing at high levels in their sport, had triumphed in spite of her disabling condition.

"Vexed by Vertigo" was written by Leigh Montville and appeared in an issue of *Sports Illustrated* on August 7, 1995, pp 25–51.

times during the performance of daily activities (as in tilting the head back to wash the hair in the shower, bending down to pick up an object from the floor), they become severely dizzy and lose balance easily. The most prominent cause of the disorder is head trauma (see highlight, "Vexed by Vertigo"), but other conditions can trigger the problem. Many older adults also suffer from this disorder and often sustain falls as a result of the condition.

Another vestibular disorder that generally affects only one of the two vestibular systems is called *Ménière's disease*. This poorly understood vestibular disorder is characterized by intermittent attacks of vertigo that can range from mild to debilitating in their severity. It also causes distorted hearing during the attacks. In its most severe form, it is necessary to surgically destroy the affected vestibular system so that the erratic vestibular signals can be eliminated, making it easier for the brain to accurately interpret the vestibular signals coming from the intact vestibular system (Goldberg & Hudspeth, 2000).

## Summary

The contributions of the visual and vestibular systems to different aspects of motor control were described in this chapter. Both systems provide us with answers to important questions on which to base our movement responses. Answers to questions such as "Where is it?" and "What is it?" are provided by the visual system while the vestibular system tells us which way is up and where we are going in space. The two systems also work together to facilitate the control of head and eye movements. Because we rely on vision to not only orient ourselves to objects in space, but also identify them, vision also plays an important role in the guidance of human actions. It not only provides important feedback information for evaluating and modifying actions but it can also be used to anticipate, and therefore accommodate to, changes occurring in the environment. This feedforward function of vision guides us in a variety of postural and locomotor activities as well as in those that involve interaction with objects or other persons.

One particular optical variable that appears to guide our performance in situations that require high levels of spatial and temporal accuracy is called tau. Based on how quickly an approaching object fills the visual field, we are able to determine when time-to-contact with an object (ball, car, take-off board, and so on) will occur. Research findings reveal that it is used to regulate stride length temporally, prepare muscle response synergies in advance of a landing, and to intercept objects moving at constant or accelerating velocities.

Two different theories of visual perception have been advanced to account for the relationship between visual perception and action. Cognitive, or indirect, theories assume that a number of inferential processes are necessary to render incoming visual information meaningful to the performer, whereas direct, or ecological, theories maintain that seeing is knowing. That is, visual information can be directly extracted from the optic array without the need for any mediating processes. Neither theory has been shown to account for the relationship between perception and action in all movement situations.

Although the quality of the sensory information provided by vision far exceeds that of the other sensory systems, our overreliance on vision to guide actions can often lead to slowed responses and/or errors in performance.

Despite the availability of often contradictory sensory input from the various somatosensory receptors, the performer continues to rely on visual inputs to guide movement. Our susceptibility to making errors is greatest in situations of sensory conflict.

Five sensory organs located within each vestibular apparatus of the ears comprise the peripheral component of the vestibular system and are particularly responsive to head accelerations in multiple planes of motion. These receptors signal both the magnitude and direction of head movements in space. Vestibular information that projects to the cerebral cortex via its ascending pathways provides information about our vertical orientation in space, while the vestibular pathways that descend to the spinal cord contribute to our ability to restore upright balance following a perturbation. The vestibular system also works collaboratively with the visual system to maintain gaze stabilization when the head is moving. This is accomplished via the vestibular ocular reflex (VOR). Because of the plasticity of this reflexive mechanism, it has also been used to study the neural mechanisms of motor learning.

## IMPORTANT TERMINOLOGY

After completing this chapter, readers should be familiar with the following terms and concepts.

| | |
|---|---|
| ambient system | proprioceptive |
| ampulla | pupil |
| cognitive theory of perception | otoconia |
| cone | otolith organs |
| cupula | retina |
| direct theory of perception | rod |
| ecological theory of perception | saccades |
| exproprioception | Scarpa's ganglion or vestibular |
| exteroception | semicircular canals |
| feedforward | sensorimotor approach |
| focal system | sensory conflict |
| gain | smooth pursuit |
| hair cells | superior colliculus |
| indirect theory of perception | tau |
| lateral geniculate nucleus (LGN) | thalamus |
| lens | topographic organization |
| manipulation phase | transduction |
| optic chiasm | transportation phase |
| optic nerve | vergence |
| optokinetic reflex (OKR) | vertigo |
| oscillopsia | vestibular hair cells |
| perception | vestibular ocular reflex (VOR) |
| proprioception | vestibulospinal tracts (VST) |

## Suggested Further Reading

Elliot, D., & Lyons, J. (1998). Optimizing the use of vision during motor skill acquisition. In J. P. Piek (Ed.), *Motor behavior and human skill,* pp. 57–72. Champaign, IL: Human Kinetics.

Horak, F., & Shupert, C. (2000). Role of the vestibular system in postural control. In S. Herdman (Ed.), *Vestibular rehabilitation* (2nd ed.), pp. 25–51. Philadelphia, PA: F. A. Davis.

## Test Your Understanding

1. Briefly describe the three types of sensory information provided by the visual system in the control of movement. Provide an example to demonstrate your understanding of each type.

2. Briefly explain why researchers believe there are two separate visual systems that serve different functions. Identify the two systems, and describe their respective roles in motor control.

3. In what way(s) does the ecological theory of visual perception differ from cognitive theories?

4. In what type of movement situations is vision most likely to serve a feedforward function? Explain your answer.

5. Briefly describe how balance is affected in situations of sensory conflict. Why is balance affected in this way?

6. Define the term *tau.* What role does tau appear to serve in the visual control of movement?

7. Briefly describe the type of research evidence that suggests that vision can provide time-to-contact information.

8. Why does our reliance on vision to guide action often lead to unsatisfactory motor performance?

9. Explain why physical therapists use a sensorimotor approach to treating patients with damage to the visual areas in the cortex.

10. Identify the five sensory organs located within the vestibular system, and briefly describe the sensory function of each organ.

11. Briefly describe how the vestibular system contributes to equilibrium.

12. Briefly describe how the vestibular ocular reflex (VOR) works, and provide three examples of movement situations in which it is used.

13. Describe the phenomenon of sensory conflict.

14. Identify three important perceptual–motor tasks that require the availability of sensory information from the vestibular system.

15. Describe one disorder of the vestibular system that is particularly problematic for athletes who participate in sports requiring complex somersaulting or spinning maneuvers.

## PRACTICAL ACTIVITIES

1. Become familiar with the different types of eye movements by engaging in the two activities described below.
   a. Two different types of eye movements are used to track moving objects. The first of these two eye movements is called slow pursuit tracking eye movements, which are used to maintain eye fixation on objects moving slowly through space (as with a fly ball in baseball). Practice moving a visual target (such as a pen or pencil) slowly through your field of view while keeping the head still. Move the target in a vertical, horizontal, and diagonal direction. Now repeat the activity but move the head and eyes as you move the target in different directions. What mechanism are you using to successfully track the visual target (a) when your head is stationary, and (b) when your head and eyes are moving?
   b. The second type of eye movements are used to quickly move and then focus the eyes on a new target of interest (for example, a player moving into your peripheral field of view as you dribble the ball toward the goal). Practice these eye movements by extending your arms at shoulder height with thumbs in a vertical position and no more than 4–6 inches apart. Practice quickly moving the eyes only between your two thumbs. Notice that you are able to rapidly move the eyes from one thumb to the next and bring it into focus. Use your knowledge of the visual system to explain how these eye movements are possible.
2. To better understand how the vestibular and visual systems work together to stabilize your gaze, try the following activity: Read a paragraph in this textbook while shaking your head. Did you encounter any problems reading the text? Explain the mechanism that you use to accomplish this task.

# 5

# DEVELOPING AND EXECUTING A PLAN OF ACTION

*It has become increasingly clear that motor control is not localized within the brain but is distributed throughout the central nervous system.*

## CHAPTER OBJECTIVES

After studying this chapter, you should be able to:

- Understand and be able to describe the cognitive and neuromotor processes involved in the planning and execution of goal-directed actions.

- Understand and be able to describe the various mechanisms available in the spinal system for the ongoing control and modification of movement.

- Understand and be able to describe the primary mechanisms by which the appropriate amount of force for a given motor action can be generated.

- Understand how the musculoskeletal system influences the production of force.

- Understand and be able to describe how movements can be controlled and/or modified at a subconscious level.

- Identify the three variables that constrain action and how they influence motor control.

Interaction with our environment is achieved through a variety of goal-directed postures and movements. Consider an infant attempting to take those first uncertain steps or a prima ballerina performing a virtuoso sequence of dance steps. The observable motor behavior of both requires the cooperation of the nervous and musculoskeletal systems. Whereas the nervous system is largely responsible for orchestrating the plan of action, the musculoskeletal system is ultimately responsible for its execution.

Despite the fact that we still do not know exactly *how* information flows between the two systems or *what* movement variables are controlled by the CNS, it has become increasingly clear that motor control is not localized within the brain, but rather is distributed throughout the CNS. Various cortical, subcortical, and spinal centers work together to produce coordinated movement, and cooperation among the neural centers is made possible by a rich network of feedback loops. These reciprocal connections facilitate communication, comparison, and correction at all levels of the CNS.

This chapter is intended to provide the reader with a general understanding of how we plan and execute goal-directed actions. We will conduct our discussion at both the cognitive and the neuromotor level of analysis in order to achieve a more comprehensive understanding of the action-planning process. We will begin with a brief description of the types of cognitive processes involved in the planning and execution of action plans. Then we will consider the areas of the nervous system that appear to be involved in carrying out these cognitive processes. Although our discussion of the processes involved in the planning and execution of action will be sequential, always remember that many cognitive processes are occurring simultaneously and that other areas within the CNS are also active at various times during the planning and execution of action. Much is known about the operations of the CNS, but much more remains to be discovered.

## Planning the Action

### Making the Decision to Act

The action planning process begins with a decision or intention to act.

At a cognitive level, the action-planning process begins with a decision or intention to act. This decision may be the result of an internally generated goal or may occur in response to changes in the surrounding environment. During this aspect of the action-planning process, illustrated in Figure 5.1, the performer receives and analyzes a myriad of inputs from the various senses within the body but also acknowledges a large amount of information from the external environment. These inputs may then be matched with an existing goal for action or used to develop the goal the performer thinks will best fit the constraints imposed by the surrounding environment. For example, during the course of a game, a tennis player may decide to return the ball as close to the baseline as possible so that she or he can run in close to the net and prepare to follow up with a short, angled volley return to win the point (the goal).

Before acting on the goal, however, it is important for the player to monitor carefully all the associated sensory input, such as the opponent's position on the court, the movement of the ball off the opponent's racket, and the player's own responding movements and court location. In this way, the player can best determine, on the basis of the incoming sensory input, whether the intended goal is realistic. It is quite likely that the player who does not attend to certain relevant cues in the environment will develop a less-than-optimal plan of action. This would certainly be the case if the opponent's return forced the player to run deep into the corner of the court and make a weak return stroke that barely passed over the net. Given this change in the environmental conditions, it would be necessary to rethink the goal of the action.

THE ENVIRONMENT

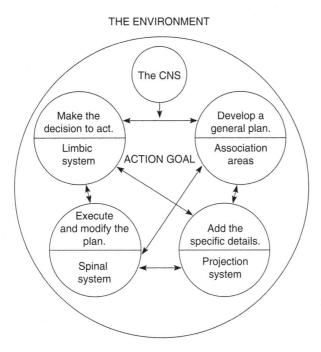

**Figure 5.1**  A multilevel view of the cognitive operations and multiple subsystems involved in the planning and execution of goal-directed actions.

## Developing a General Plan

Once the decision to act has been made, the planning process continues with the development of a very general plan of action. The appropriateness of the plan of action that is subsequently developed will be determined by a variety of factors. Important among these are the performer's previous experience with the movements to be executed and how well the movement situation was initially evaluated. If the performer has experienced the same or a similar movement situation before, then it is likely that his or her evaluation of the environment and choice of action will be more accurate. Experienced players of golf, for example, are more likely to choose the most appropriate approach shot to the green because they have experienced a similar situation on many previous occasions. In contrast, the novice player has little idea what stroke or golf club is most appropriate for the situation.

The quality of the action is influenced by the performer's previous experience and by how well the movement situation was initially evaluated.

## Adding Details to the Plan

Once the general plan of action has been developed, the individual begins to add the specific details of the action. These details involve selecting the various movement parameters (e.g., force, velocity, displacement) necessary to accomplish the original goal of the movement. The decision to propel a ball at a particular target, for example, is not sufficient to prompt or ensure a successful outcome. Before this is possible, the performer must also decide which

Specific details must be added to the general plan in order to accomplish the movement goal.

body part will be used to propel the ball, what level of force is needed, and the direction and amount of limb displacement.

In addition to considering the goal of the movement itself, the performer must also consider the existing environmental constraints. These might include the distance from the target, its overall size, and whether it is fixed or moving in space. Unless all these variables are accounted for during the planning process, it is unlikely that the emerging action will adequately reflect the intended goal. Having said this, however, we must also recognize that many actions fail to achieve the intended goal because of factors outside the control of the individual. For example, the environment may be changing too quickly as the action is being planned to allow sufficient time for the performer to make the necessary modifications.

## Executing the Plan of Action

The specific plan of action is finally performed by various parts of the musculoskeletal system, and a movement outcome is produced. The process does not stop here, however, because it is important to know whether the movement outcome adequately reflected the original goal. This all-important evaluation is made possible by feedback derived from sources that are either internal or external to the performer. Examples of internal sources include the various subsystems involved in the planning and execution of the action and the various muscles and joints performing the action. The surrounding movement environment also provides an extremely important source of feedback to the performer and, very often, determines the shape of the movement outcome. The ability to recognize the available sensory feedback and prioritize its use often distinguishes the skilled from the novice performer because it is on the basis of this movement-based feedback that the performer is able to elaborate and/or modify aspects of the action plan at all stages of its development and implementation. As we will also see in the section of this textbook on motor learning, movement-based feedback is essential for helping us develop knowledge about our movement-based experiences that is then used to make the learning of new motor skills or the refinement of existing skills easier.

## The Neuromotor Level of Analysis

The skilled performer develops the action plan that produces the best match between the goals of the task to be performed and the environmental constraints.

As informative as it is to describe the cognitive processes involved in the formulation and implementation of action plans, descriptions based only at a cognitive level do not tell the whole story. Not only do they fail to identify the actual mechanisms responsible for transforming our many thoughts into action, but they also leave us with the impression that information follows a specific and unidirectional route through the four cognitive processes shown in Figure 5.1. One has only to observe skilled actions to realize that there are many ways in which a movement goal can be achieved. Instead of producing a specific movement pattern on each attempt, the skilled performer chooses the action plan that produces the best match between his or her own performance goals and the constraints of the environment in which the movement is to be performed. Moreover, it is rare that only one action plan is being developed at any given moment. In reality, the performer is often planning

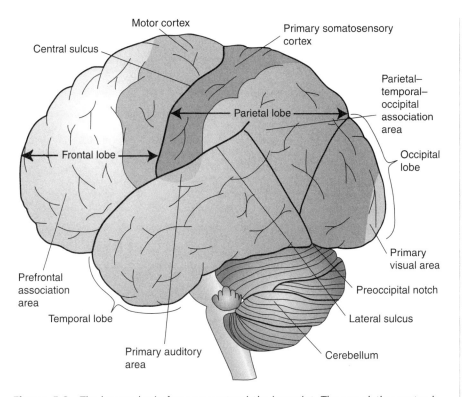

**Figure 5.2**   The human brain from an anatomist's viewpoint. The association cortex is comprised of a number of specialized areas in each lobe of the brain.

*Source: Principles of Neural Science,* 4th ed., by Eric Kandel and James Schwartz. Copyright 2000 by McGraw Hill Companies. Reprinted by Permission.

future actions while still implementing earlier ones. Any or all of the systems illustrated in Figure 5.1 could be active at any moment in time.

In order to better understand how goal-directed behavior is accomplished, it is necessary to describe the action-planning process at the neuromotor processes level. Describing action at this level helps us begin to identify the actual neurological mechanisms that are involved in the planning and execution of any particular action. As is evident in Figure 5.2, the human brain can be divided into several anatomical regions that serve different but complementary functions. Some regions are primarily responsible for vision, hearing, speech, and higher intellectual thought, whereas others are intricately involved in the orchestration of movements. It is to these movement-related areas of the brain that we now direct our attention.

Let us begin by identifying the various neural centers that have been shown to be involved in some aspect of the planning and/or execution of action. To guide us in this discussion, a review of Figure 5.1 is in order. Four areas within the CNS appear to be actively involved in the cognitive processes underlying the planning and execution of action. These include the limbic system, the association cortex (composed of the various association areas shown in Figure 5.2), the projection system, and the spinal system. These areas are identified not in

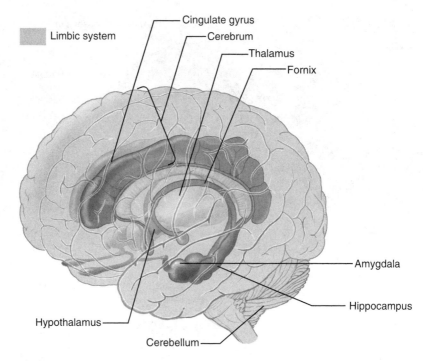

**Figure 5.3**   The limbic system is comprised of a number of cortical and subcortical structures that surround the hypothalamus.

terms of their anatomical location within the CNS but, rather, according to the way they function during the planning of actions. Brooks (1986) has collectively described these areas as functional neural "task systems" (p. 19).

## The Limbic System

The motivation or desire to act is generated in the limbic system.

The intention to act is associated with a set of interconnected neural structures that surround the upper brainstem area within the cerebrum. The **limbic system** helps us fulfill our desire to act in response to the demands of the environmental context. The motivation or desire to act that is generated within the limbic system is then analyzed and transformed into an idea or general plan for action in the association cortex (that is, frontal, temporal, parietal, and occipital lobes) (Iyer, Mitz, & Winstein, 1999). The limbic system is comprised of a number of cortical and subcortical structures that surround the hypothalamus. Important structures included in this system include the fornix, amygdaloid complex, hippocampus, and the cingulate gyrus of the cerebral cortex (see Figure 5.3).

In addition to its important role in providing the motivation or desire to act, specific neural circuits within the limbic system are integrally involved in declarative learning and memory (the acquisition and storage of factual knowledge). The role of the hippocampus, in particular, will be discussed in Chapter 10 with the discussion of how motor skills are remembered.

# The Association Cortex

Because the association areas distributed throughout the cortex receive partially processed sensory inputs from other areas within the CNS, it is likely that these areas play an important role in the planning of actions. A second look at Figure 5.2 confirms the distributed nature of the **association cortex;** association areas are located in the frontal, temporal, and parietal lobes of the brain. Among the primary functions attributed to these areas are the recognition, selection, and integration of relevant sensory inputs reaching the higher levels of the cortex. A sophisticated network of nerve pathways that connects the limbic system with the association cortex also provides the means by which the decision to act or not act can be communicated to the entire association cortex. It is within this widely distributed area of the cortex that a general plan for action is thought to be first formulated. Of course, the development of this plan is also influenced by the incoming sensory inputs that receive their final processing in the association cortex. In this way, the association cortex has information relevant to the needs of the performer and to the state of the environment in which the action will be executed.

> The general plan of action is developed within the widely distributed association areas of the cortex.

# The Projection System

Yet another set of cognitive processes related to the planning and execution of action resides in a set of midbrain and cortical structures that make up the **projection system.** A large body of neurological research has indicated that one of the primary functions of this system is to determine how the action is to be carried out. The projection system is responsible for adding the movement dynamics necessary to shape the general action plan into one that best fits the performer's goal and the environmental constraints of the moment. The projection system consists of both the sensory and motor areas of the cortex in addition to various other subcortical nuclei. Two subcortical structures and one cortical structure—the basal ganglia, the cerebellum, and the motor cortex, respectively—are integral to the successful functioning of this task system. In light of the fact that these three components are thought to be instrumental in the development of more specific action plans, a discussion of their respective roles in the formulation of action plans is warranted.

> Structures within the projection system determine how the action is to be executed by adding the details needed to make the general plan more specific.

***Basal Ganglia.***   The basal ganglia (BG), a subcortical structure involved in the projection system, are comprised of four major nuclei that send their efferent signals to the cerebral cortex, thalamus, and certain other nuclei within the brainstem. The four important nuclei include the striatum (caudate nucleus, putamen, and ventral striatum), globus pallidus, substantia nigra, and subthalamic nucleus (DeLong, 2000) (see Figure 5.4). Through a set of parallel pathways that directly or indirectly connect the basal ganglia with the motor and sensory areas of the cortex, in particular, the basal ganglia are thought to play an important role in the planning and initiation of internally generated movements and the application of complex movement strategies to the executed movement (Flowers, 1976).

> The basal ganglia are thought to play an important role in the planning and initiation of internally generated movements and the application of complex strategies to the executed movement.

The specific roles played by the BG in motor control have been examined using a variety of research methods. These have included intracellular recordings of selected BG nuclei in awake animals trained to produce certain

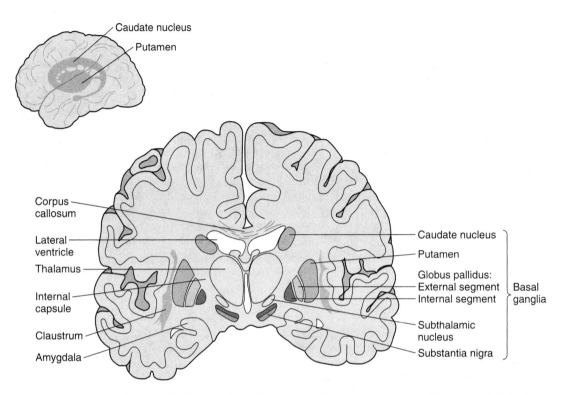

**Figure 5.4**   The basal ganglia are comprised of four major nuclei that send their efferent signals to the cerebral cortex, thalamus, and certain nuclei within the brainstem.

voluntary movements (DeLong, 1972; Neafsey, Hull, & Buchwald, 1978), lesion studies (Stern, 1966; Denny-Brown, 1962), and clinical studies that track the progression of diseases specific to the basal ganglia (Hallett, 1993; Hoehn & Yahr, 1967; Sotrel et al., 1993). Collectively, the research findings emerging from these studies suggest that the BG are not only involved in the preparation and control of movement but also contribute in a meaningful way to a number of different cognitive and perceptual tasks.

*Motor set:* Involves preparing the CNS in advance of initiating a goal-directed movement.

Their role in motor control is made possible through complex neural circuitry that connects the motor and sensory cortex with the BG which, in turn, send processed information back to the motor cortex via the thalamus and then onto the muscles involved in the movement. The "gain" (ratio of signal input to signal output) of the system is thought to be adjusted within the processing units of the BG for the purpose of appropriately scaling the size of the intended movement and the level of postural stability needed (Melnick, 2001). The results of single-cell recording studies also suggest a role for the BG in establishing an appropriate motor set (DeLong, 2000). A **motor set** involves altering the firing patterns of motor neurons within the CNS in advance of initiating a goal-directed movement. This may result in the activation of the muscles in the trunk and legs in preparation for pulling open a door or the adoption of a particular posture as you brace yourself for a wave that is about to hit you as you stand at the water's edge.

In addition to motor functions, the BG are also believed to play a role in a variety of different cognitive activities. In addition to the neural circuitry that connects the BG with the motor and sensory cortex, additional neural pathways that connect the BG with the prefrontal and limbic regions of the cortex suggest a role for select areas of the BG in the performance of "executive processing functions." According to DeLong (2000), these executive functions "include cognitive tasks such as organizing behavioral responses and using verbal skills in problem-solving" (p. 866). Buchwald et al. (1975) further hypothesize that the BG are involved in establishing a **cognitive set** which they define as the "ability to discriminate a situational context and make an appropriate response to a given signal" (p. 175). Graybiel (1998) has also hypothesized that the BG provide behavioral flexibility and variety in the preplanned action so that it is as appropriate as possible for the environment in which it must be performed. Each of the functions attributed to the BG, whether they are of a motor or cognitive nature, suggest that this complex set of nuclei is integral to the successful functioning of the projection system.

*Cognitive set:* Ability to discriminate a situational context and make an appropriate motor response to a given signal.

***Basal Ganglia Disorders.***   Diseases of the basal ganglia are generally of two types: **hypokinetic** (abnormal decrease in motor activity) disorders or **hyperkinetic** (abnormal increase in motor activity) disorders. The most well-known hypokinetic disorder that affects the BG is Parkinson's disease (PD). This disease is progressive in nature and characterized by impaired initiation of movement, a reduction in the velocity and amplitude of movements referred to as **bradykinesia,** muscular rigidity (resistance to passive displacement), and a resting tremor. Individuals with this disorder experience progressively more serious disturbances in their posture and gait and fall frequently as the disease progresses. Ineffective sensory processing has been advanced as an explanation for the postural instability observed in individuals with PD (Jobst, Melnick, Byl, Dowling, & Aminoff, 1997).

Basal ganglia disorders are of two types: hypokinetic or hyperkinetic.

Individuals with PD also develop what is referred to as a **festinating gait** pattern (short, hurried steps) that is thought to be associated with a decline in equilibrium reactions or abnormal motor unit firing patterns (Melnick, 2001). A number of different therapeutic strategies are used to assist patients with PD in maintaining as close to normal function as possible (Formisano, Pratesi, Modarelli, Bonefati, & Meco, 1992; Miyai et al., 2002). Specific emphasis is placed on having patients with PD repeatedly practice a variety of different functional movements in varied environments (Palmer, Mortimer, Webster, Bistevins, & Dickinson, 1986). The use of rhythmic exercise, visual instruction, and mental rehearsal prior to performing movements has also been shown to be beneficial in the treatment of patients with PD. We will discuss the application of motor learning principles in much greater depth in Chapters 6 through 11; these are believed to be of critical importance when designing treatment programs for this population (Melnick, 2001).

In contrast to the signs and symptoms associated with hypokinetic disorders of the BG, hyperkinetic disorders of the BG such as Huntington's disease and hemiballismus are characterized by excessive motor activity. Involuntary movements, or **dyskinesia,** are evident in the trunk, face, and extremities and a decrease in muscle tone is also observed in patients with hyperkinetic disorders. Gait velocity is severely compromised in this patient population, with a wider base of support being adopted. The performance of fine movements also becomes slow and clumsy. In addition to motor dysfunction, this disease is

*Dyskinesia:* Production of involuntary movements.

also associated with signs of dementia and emotional disorders which become significantly more debilitating as the disease progresses. Group exercise programs that include resistance, aerobic, and balance activities as well as some treatment techniques used for the treatment of PD (such as rhythmical auditory cueing) have been shown to be reasonably effective in the early stages of the disease (Peacock, 1987; Thaut et al., 1996).

***Cerebellum.*** The cerebellum (or "little brain," as it is often called because it, like the larger cerebrum, is composed of two hemispheres) has also been shown to play a vital role in the control of action. What is perhaps most interesting about the cerebellum is that it contains over half the total number of neurons in the brain and receives 40 times the number of inputs as outputs.

The specific roles played by three functionally distinct regions in the cerebellum are of particular importance to our discussion here. These regions include the cerebrocerebellum, spinocerebellum, and vestibulocerebellum. The cerebrocerebellum receives its input exclusively from the cortex and sends its output back to the motor, premotor, and prefrontal cortices via the dentate nucleus. The results of imaging studies (e.g., Ryding et al., 1993) suggest a role for the cerebrocerebellum in the planning and mental rehearsal of complex motor actions as well as the conscious evaluation of movement errors (Ghez & Thach, 2000).

Conversely, a direct role for the spinocerebellum in the regulation of limb and body movements is made possible by virtue of it receiving afferent inputs, both directly and indirectly, from proprioceptors in the muscles and joints of the lower body. The direct pathway to the cerebellum via the spinocerebellar tract was previously described in Chapter 3. These incoming sensory signals can be compared with outgoing signals associated with the intended movement to determine whether they match. Because the output signals from this region project to descending motor pathways (e.g., rubrospinal and corticospinal tracts), it is possible to alter movements, thus correcting any mismatch that exists between the intended and actual movement.

The third region, or vestibulocerebellum, receives inputs from the semicircular canals and otoliths of the vestibular apparatus, which (as you learned in Chapter 4) provide us with information about the position and movements of the head relative to gravity. The same region also receives inputs from the superior colliculus, which you have also learned is involved in the reflexive control of head and eye movements. This region of the cerebellum is believed to be involved in the regulation of balance and eye movements. Specifically, output signals from this region influence the vestibulospinal tracts responsible for the control of important postural muscles (e.g., axial and extensor muscles) involved in the maintenance of upright stance and stability during gait and also influence the control of head and eye movements via the medial vestibular nucleus located in the brainstem. Its vital role in postural control is further evidenced by the increase in postural sway and the delayed equilibrium reactions that are observed following damage to the vestibulocerebellum (Melnick & Oremland, 2001).

Researchers have also proposed a role for the cerebellum in the learning of motor skills because of its strong reciprocal connections with the cerebral cortex (Marr, 1969; Albus, 1971; Ito, 1970). The Marr-Albus-Ito model, as it has been termed, describes a central role for the climbing fibers (afferent fibers

The cerebrocerebellum is believed to play a role in the planning and mental rehearsal of complex motor actions and conscious evaluation of movement errors.

A role for the cerebellum in the learning of motor skills has also been proposed.

that convey somatosensory, visual, and cerebrocortical information to the cerebellar cortex via Purkinje neurons) that they believe are able to detect errors in a movement and change the ensuing movement plan. Through trial-and-error practice, the cerebellum is able to gradually reduce the amount of error produced. Considerable support for the cerebellum's role in learning has been provided by studies in which prism glasses were used to distort the individual's view of the world (Thach, 1996, 1998). Although behavior was initially maladaptive, with repeated practice the individual was able to adapt very well to the altered input–output relationship. Further support for the cerebellum's role in learning has been provided by the results of clinical studies and observations of patients with cerebellar disease who demonstrate an impaired ability to make adaptive motor changes despite repeated practice (Lang & Bastian, 1999; Martin, Keating, Goodkin, Bastian, & Thach, 1996).

***Disorders of the Cerebellum.***   Three distinct categories of signs and symptoms have been identified that significantly influence the quality of motor control possible following lesions or diseases affecting the different functional regions identified earlier (Holmes, 1939). These signs and symptoms include **hypotonia** (reduced resistance to passive displacement of the limb), **ataxia** (lack of coordination or impaired ability to execute voluntary movements), and **tremor** (oscillations of the limb that may occur during movement [kinetic tremor], during the performance of a postural task [postural tremor], or as the limb approaches a desired endpoint [intentional tremor]).

Hypotonia, ataxia, and tremor are three categories of signs and symptoms associated with cerebellar disorders.

Hypotonicity is believed to result from decreased excitation of deep nuclei in the cerebellum that project to brain regions responsible for controlling alpha and gamma motoneurons. Individuals with this symptom will find it very difficult to hold the limb out against gravity without directing a significant amount of attention to the task; and, if the limb is suddenly dropped, it will fall rapidly without correction (Melnick & Oremland, 2001). For individuals with ataxia, one can expect to observe increased reaction times when the affected limb must initiate movements. Moreover, they will be unable to accurately define the extent, force, and relative timing required when performing complex multijoint movements. These errors will manifest themselves in a tendency to overshoot targets and an inability to perform movements that require quick bursts of speed or to sustain the rhythm of rapid, alternating movements. Postural stability during gait will also be adversely affected in patients with ataxia that is caused by cerebellar disease. Finally, symptoms of tremor, depending on its severity, will make it difficult to terminate movements due to the oscillating limb and require a series of corrective movements. Performing tasks that require precision of limb placement and steadiness, such as reaching for and drinking from a cup filled with liquid, putting on makeup, or putting a key in a lock, will be very difficult.

***Motor Cortex.***   As early as 1870, Fritsch and Hitzig discovered that the direct application of electrical current to a particular area of the cortex resulted in movement. Unfortunately, this discovery led a number of researchers to conclude erroneously that the area known as the motor cortex controlled the execution of all voluntary movements. Current research suggests that the motor areas of the cortex play an integral part in the planning and execution of movements, but their role is considerably more specialized than was previously thought. In this chapter, we will discuss the functions of three relatively distinct areas within the motor cortex: the primary motor area (M1), premotor area (PMA), and supplementary motor area (SMA). Not only does each of these areas receive inputs from different cortical and subcortical areas, but they also serve different functions related to the preparation and execution of action. We will discuss each area in a little more detail here.

*Primary Motor Area (M1).*   The primary sensory inputs to M1 come from the primary somatosensory cortex (Brodmann's areas 1, 2, and 3a) and the posterior parietal cortex (area 5) first discussed in Chapter 3. The inputs received from area 3a of the somatosensory cortex provide the M1 with information about the position of the body in space and the amplitude, velocity, and direction of movements in progress, while the inputs from areas 1 and 2 carry information about events signaled by the cutaneous receptors (e.g., texture, shape, and edges of objects) (Porter, 1999). This information is then supplemented by inputs from area 5 in the postparietal cortex, which, you may remember, is responsible for integrating visual, auditory, and proprioceptive inputs. This sensory information is critical for the accurate planning of reaching and grasping movements that require hand–eye coordination. In addition to these cortical inputs, M1 also receives input from the basal ganglia and cerebellum via the thalamus. Just as the somatosensory cortex was somatotopically organized, so too is the motor cortex. Once again, the various parts of the body are disproportionately represented in this area with the body parts responsible for more precise movements occupying a larger area on the surface of the motor cortex.

Intracellular recordings and brain-mapping techniques (such as transcranial magnetic stimulation) have been used to elucidate the role of M1 in the planning and execution of action. Collectively, the findings of a number of different studies have revealed that M1 is involved in the actual execution of movements because the neurons in this area fire just before movement begins (Porter, 1999). Neurons in this area also appear to be involved in controlling the speed and force of muscle contraction. This is an important feature of slow movements that demand precision and of those that entail controlled acceleration and/or deceleration, such as lifting and lowering a free weight.

The evidence further suggests that selected neurons in M1 are involved in coding the direction of a movement (Georgopoulos, Kalaska, Caminiti, & Massey, 1982). Finally, M1 neurons appear to be selectively involved in the execution of skilled movements of the distal musculature (e.g., hand). This ability can be observed in a skilled seamstress threading a needle or in a musician performing a musical piece on a classical guitar.

Lesions of M1 usually result in weakness, or **paresis,** in the limb on the opposite side to the lesion. Over time, gradual improvement in movements requiring the proximal muscles is observed, but more precise movements, particularly of the fingers, are never regained. It is believed that the recovery of proximal movements is made possible by the ability of undamaged premotor areas to assume at least some of the lost functions of the M1 (Porter, 1999).

*Premotor Areas (PMA).*   The premotor areas of the motor cortex not only receive sensory inputs from the posterior parietal cortex (Brodmann's areas 5 and 7), but also from association areas in the prefrontal cortex. This second source of sensory input is linked to working memory, making it possible for

---

*Sidenotes:*

The motor cortex area is somatotopically organized.

The primary motor area (M1) is involved in the actual execution of movements as well as the control of speed and force in the contracting muscles.

The premotor areas (PMA) appear to play a role in the advance planning and coordination of complex bilateral movement sequences.

the premotor areas (which are also well connected) to influence certain aspects of motor planning that involve memory (specifically, the temporary location of objects in space to guide reaching movements (Krakauer & Ghez, 2000). The PMA also appears to play an important role in the advance planning and coordination of complex bilateral movement sequences. This hypothesis is based on the fact that neurons in this area are activated during the planning phase of a movement but less so during the movement itself (Porter, 1999). Of particular interest is the fact that the mental rehearsal of a movement gives rise to the same pattern of activity of neural activity in the PMA and posterior parietal cortex as occurs when the movement is actually being performed. As Krakauer and Ghez (2000) point out, this finding shows how important it is for skilled performers to engage in mental imagery as well as physical practice.

***Supplementary Motor Area (SMA).***   As part of the motor cortex, the SMA is also involved in the preparation for movement. Neural activity is particularly high when the movements to be performed are internally generated as opposed to being triggered by sensory events. PET (positron emission tomography) scanning studies have also demonstrated increased activity in this area when participants are asked to imagine that they were performing a movement instead of actually performing it (Roland, Larsen, Lassen, & Skinhöf, 1980).

> The supplementary motor area (SMA) appears to be involved in the preparation of internally generated movements.

Lesions in the premotor areas have greater consequences for movement execution. Movements are slow and clumsy, some weakness is evident in the proximal joints, and the ensuing movements appear uncoordinated. **Apraxia** (difficulty performing purposeful movements) is a motor disorder that results from damage to both the PMA and posterior parietal lobe (Carr & Shepherd, 2003). In addition to the deterioration of already learned movement sequences, patients with lesions of the PMA also find it much more difficult to learn to execute new and complex movement sequences (Porter, 1999). SMA lesions also result in serious disturbances to complex motor functions. A lack of motion, or **akinesia,** on the side opposite the lesion is observed as well as increased difficulty performing bilateral tasks that require coordinated hand movements. Unlike patients with PMA lesions who can no longer learn to initiate movements in response to sensory cues, patients with lesions in the SMA experience more difficulty performing internally generated movement plans.

Although the specific functions of the basal ganglia, cerebellum, and motor cortex have been highlighted in this section, it is important to remember that the motor behavior we observe cannot be attributed solely to any one of these three components—or even to the larger projection system to which they belong. As already discussed in Chapters 3 and 4, the unimodal and multimodal association areas of the somatosensory, visual, and vestibular systems analyze and integrate the incoming sensory information that underlies our perception of the world around us. In some cases, the flow of sensory events will be sufficient to trigger action, while in other situations action will follow an internal desire to act—which is provided by the limbic system. As we said earlier, the emerging motor behavior is the result of an interaction among the many subsystems within the nervous system, and no single subsystem is able to produce the movement or even to dictate how it is to be performed. The nature of the emerging motor behavior will be further influenced by the goals of the task to be performed (e.g., quickly throw a fielded softball to the first base fielder before the runner arrives at the base) and the constraints imposed

> The emerging motor behavior is the result of an interaction among the many subsystems within the CNS that is further shaped by the goals of the task and the environmental constraints.

by the environment in which the task is to be performed (e.g., a strong wind is blowing in the direction of the fielder attempting to throw the ball). The knowledge that multiple systems interact to produce movement and that both the goals of a task and the environment will further shape the emerging motor behavior has important implications for the physical therapist who helps patients relearn functional movement patterns that can no longer be accessed or organized in the ways they were before.

## Motor Pathways

The motor areas of the cerebral cortex (M1, PMA, and SMA) discussed in the previous section of this chapter can influence the spinal system either directly or indirectly via descending motor pathways that originate in the cerebral cortex or from three motor centers located within the brainstem. Once the information is conveyed to this system, it becomes the responsibility of specialized neurons (alpha, or skeletomotor, neurons) to carry the information out to the various muscle response synergies (a group of muscles constrained to act together) that will ultimately perform the action. The alpha motoneuron therefore serves as the final pathway linking the CNS with the musculoskeletal system.

The descending pathway that exerts a direct influence on the spinal system is called the **corticospinal** (ventral and lateral), or **pyramidal, tract,** while two main systems of pathways in the brainstem exert a more indirect influence on the emerging motor control. The first of these two indirect systems is called the **medial brainstem system** and is comprised of three major tracts: the **vestibulospinal tract,** the **reticulospinal tract,** and the **tectospinal tract.** The second indirect system of pathways is referred to as the **lateral brainstem system** and includes one major descending pathway called the **rubrospinal tract** (Ghez & Krakauer, 2000). Let's begin our discussion here by describing the corticospinal tract and its role in the control of voluntary movements.

*Corticospinal Tract (CST).*   As Figure 5.5a illustrates, this large descending pathway, comprised of more than one million fibers, features some of the longest axons in the human CNS. Most of the neurons associated with the CST originate in M1, with some cells also originating in the SMA, PMA, and the somatosensory cortex. The axons that comprise this tract descend uninterrupted to the spinal cord where they synapse indirectly, and sometimes directly, with motoneurons distributed across several segments of the spinal cord. The fact that the CST has large-diameter axons, the majority of which are myelinated, and no synaptic connections between its origin and termination sites ensures that movement-related information reaches its final destination in the spinal system with considerable speed.

What is also noticeable in Figure 5.5a is that a large majority (approximately 75%) of this pathway's axons cross midline, or **decussate,** at the level of the medulla in the brainstem and descend to the spinal cord (SC) via the lateral CST. These axons finally terminate on interneurons and motoneurons within the spinal cord that control the distal musculature on the **contralateral** (opposite) side of the body. The remaining axon fibers descend on the **ipsilateral** (same) side of the body via the ventral CST. These axons terminate mostly on interneurons in segments of the spinal cord that control the axial muscles on both sides of the body (Enoka, 2002).

The corticospinal tract exerts a direct influence on spinal system function.

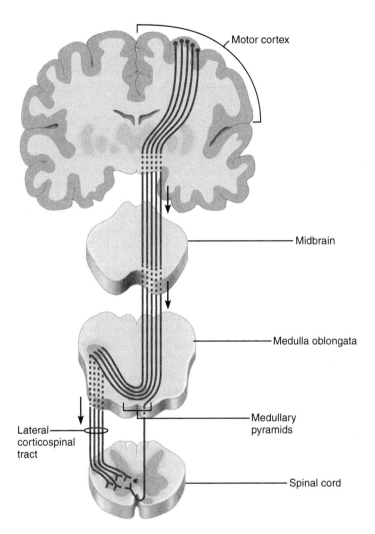

Motor cortex

Midbrain

Medulla oblongata

Medullary pyramids

Lateral corticospinal tract

Spinal cord

**Figure 5.5a** The corticospinal (ventral and lateral) tract carries motor impulses to the spinal cord where they synapse indirectly, and sometimes directly, with motoneurons distributed across several segments of the spinal cord.

CST neurons that project to the upper cervical levels of the spinal cord innervate motoneurons that are involved in the control of distal arm movements, while those terminating in lower cervical segments are involved in the control of neck and proximal arm movements (He, Dum, & Strick, 1993). Finally, CST neurons that innervate motoneurons in the lower cervical levels of the spinal cord innervate motoneurons that activate muscles involved in the performance of skilled movements of the hands and fingers. The CST is also capable of influencing reflexive actions by selectively inhibiting or exciting spinal cord motoneurons responsible for innervating muscle.

In addition to their role in controlling fine motor movements, CST neurons that originate in the somatosensory and parietal cortices and terminate in the dorsal horns of the spinal cord are also capable of modulating the flow of sensory information being conveyed by the somatosensory pathways. Likewise, the continuous sensory input that is available during movement can influence CST neurons and make it possible to adjust their motor output very rapidly in response to changes occurring in the environment as a movement is being executed.

***Medial Brainstem System.***    Three motor pathways comprise the medial brainstem system (MBS). The first of these is the vestibulospinal tract that originates in the lateral vestibular nucleus in the brainstem (see Figure 5.5b). As you will recall from our discussion in Chapter 4, this nucleus receives sensory inputs from the labyrinths of the vestibular apparatus as well as from the cerebellum. It plays an important role in equilibrium righting reactions through its excitation of alpha and gamma motoneurons that innervate the extensor, or "antigravity," muscles and through inhibition of motoneurons that inhibit the flexor muscles. The second pathway in this system is the reticulospinal tract that originates in a diffusely arranged and expansive set of nuclei known as the reticular formation. This area receives inputs from a number of areas of the brain, including the cerebellum, sensorimotor cortex, vestibular system, and the ascending somatosensory pathways. The primary function of this pathway is to activate the axial and proximal limb muscles (Porter, 1999).

The final pathway that comprises this system originates in the superior colliculus and is called the tectospinal tract. Because of its origin in the superior colliculus, the primary function of this pathway is thought to contribute to head- and neck-orienting reactions in response to visual inputs (Rothwell, 1994). According to Kuypers (1985), the collective function of the pathways that comprise the medial brainstem system is to provide the basic functions of postural control (including control of axial musculature, equilibrium righting reflexes, and head- and neck-orienting reactions) that can be further organized by cortical motor areas to produce more complex and highly differentiated movements.

***Lateral Brainstem System.***    The rubrospinal tract is the major pathway in this second brainstem system and originates in the red nucleus (see Figure 5.5b). Shortly after this pathway leaves the red nucleus, it decussates and descends to lower levels of the spinal cord. In addition, the pathway provides branches to other brain structures that include, among others, selected nuclei within the cerebellum and the vestibular nuclei. In contrast to the vestibulospinal tract, the primary role of the rubrospinal tract is to facilitate alpha motoneurons that innervate distal flexor muscles and inhibit alpha motoneurons that innervate the extensor muscles. The rubrospinal tract works in close cooperation with the CST because of its overlapping termination sites. Both tracts facilitate the same spinal reflexes and innervate the same distal flexor muscle groups (Porter, 1999).

As was the case for the ascending pathways discussed in Chapter 3, most of the descending pathways just described are also somatotopically organized. That is, the cortical neurons whose axons descend to the spinal cord and finally innervate specific muscle groups via pools of alpha motoneurons are arranged in a very orderly sequence. Moreover, as a function of the many reciprocal connections and extensive circuitry that exist between cortical and subcortical

The pathways of the medial brainstem system provide the basic functions of postural control.

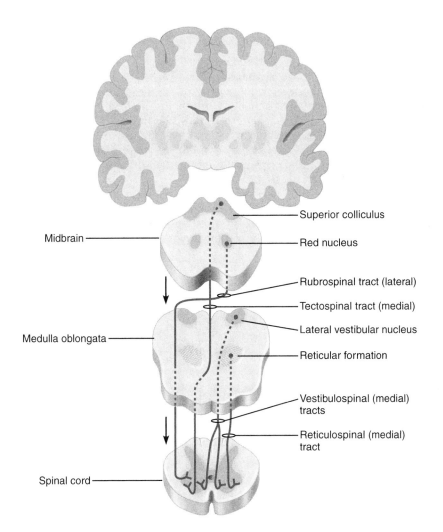

Midbrain

Superior colliculus

Red nucleus

Rubrospinal tract (lateral)

Tectospinal tract (medial)

Lateral vestibular nucleus

Medulla oblongata

Reticular formation

Vestibulospinal (medial) tracts

Reticulospinal (medial) tract

Spinal cord

**Figure 5.5b**   The medial brainstem system is comprised of three motor pathways: the vestibulospinal tract, the reticulospinal tract, and the tectospinal tract. The rubrospinal tract is the major pathway comprising the lateral brainstem system.

structures, it is most likely that parallel (as opposed to serial) processing of motor outputs occurs. Put more simply, it is not necessary that activation of a higher cortical motor area precede the activation of subcortical motor areas, as would be the case if the processing of motor signals was serial in nature.

Because of the redundancy that exists between the descending pathways due to overlapping functions (e.g., rubrospinal and corticospinal tracts), significant recovery of function is also possible following cerebral trauma. The only areas that suffer permanent loss are the hands and fingers because they receive direct projections from the motor cortex and, therefore, any injury to this cortical motor area will permanently affect the ability to perform such skilled hand and finger movements as object manipulation (Ghez & Krakauer, 2000).

## The Spinal System

Many of the final details related to the actual execution and ongoing control of movements are left to the **spinal system,** which directly regulates the timing of the various muscle activation patterns in those parts of the **musculoskeletal system** that will actually perform the desired movement. Minor adjustments to the movement pattern can also be made at this level through regulation of the firing levels of motoneurons responsible for activating the various muscle response synergies involved in the performance of the action. How the spinal system functions in the moment-to-moment control of action is the subject of the next section.

Although this description of the neuromotor processes might also suggest that information flowing through the various areas in the nervous system follows a specific and unidirectional route, this is simply not the case, particularly when one considers that the various task systems are all interconnected via an elaborate network of internal feedback loops (review Figure 5.1). These interconnections allow the CNS to make comparisons at various points in the planning process and to determine whether the movement currently being executed will effectively achieve the goal originally conceived. It is not always possible to make adjustments in the plan before the movement begins, but continuous feedback from areas both within and external to the CNS can certainly be used to modify, or even curtail, movements already in progress.

The spinal system directly regulates the timing of various activation patterns of the muscle response synergies involved in the action.

## Moment-to-Moment Control

Once the plan of action has been developed by the various subsystems within the CNS, all that remains to be done is recruitment of the appropriate muscle response synergies to execute the action plan. As the reader will recall from our discussion in Chapter 1, these groups of muscles, constrained to act as a single functional unit, enable us to reduce the number of degrees of freedom we must individually control. This has the net effect of simplifying the decision-making process for the CNS. How then does the CNS decide which muscle response synergies are actually recruited for a given action? McCrea (1992) suggests that the final decision as to which muscle groups will be activated is largely governed by two factors: the type of action produced at the joint(s) spanned by the muscle response synergy and the total number of synergies needed to generate enough force to produce a desired action. This force may be generated for the purpose of propelling an object such as a javelin or may be exerted against the ground and air as we perform the final approach run and take-off in the high jump.

It has become increasingly clear in the last two decades that the ongoing control and coordination of movement is not the sole responsibility of higher cortical structures, as early hierarchical motor programming models of motor control had assumed. Instead, coordinated movement is made possible by the interactions between multiple subsystems located at all levels of the CNS. This change in perspective has been fueled by a resurging interest among researchers in the operations performed by lower levels within the CNS (such as the spinal cord) and the musculoskeletal system with which these lower levels are ultimately interfaced.

The collective results of these many studies have prompted researchers to both modify and extend the widely held view that the spinal cord serves as a passive conduit for neural messages traveling between higher cortical levels and the skeletomuscular system. This older view has now been replaced with a considerably more dynamic view of spinal cord function. In this view, the spinal system is accorded greater responsibility for the ongoing control and coordination of a broad range of voluntary movements, and other subsystems within the CNS play a complementary rather than a dominant role. Let us begin at a neurological level by describing the different types of motoneurons found throughout the spinal cord and their respective roles in movement production and modification.

## Types of Motoneurons

*Alpha, or Skeletomotor, Neurons.*   Once the information for action has been conveyed to the spinal system, a number of neurons distributed throughout the various segments of the spinal cord are activated. One of these types of neurons assumes the responsibility of carrying the neural impulses to the appropriate muscle response synergies. This is the function of the **alpha motoneuron,** or **skeletomotor neuron,** which forms the final common pathway leading from the CNS to the peripheral musculature. These alpha motoneurons are organized into groups, or pools, within the spinal cord and are collectively responsible for the innervation of specific skeletal muscles.

The alpha motoneuron serves as the final pathway linking the CNS with the musculoskeletal system.

*Gamma, or Fusimotor, Neurons.*   The second type of motoneuron present within the spinal system is the **gamma motoneuron, or fusimotor neuron.** This second type of motoneuron is activated by the same neural impulses that activate the alpha motoneurons in a process called **alpha–gamma coactivation.** Unlike the alpha motoneurons, however, which send their impulses to the extrafusal fibers of skeletal muscle, the gamma motoneuron carries its message to intrafusal muscle fibers within **muscle spindles,** located deep within the muscle. We have already discussed the sensory function of the muscle spindle in Chapter 3; in this chapter you will learn more about the motor function of the muscle spindle.

Gamma motoneurons carry their message to the muscle spindles located within the extrafusal muscles.

*Interneurons.*   The third type of neuron located in the spinal system is the **interneuron.** The exact role played by interneurons in the ongoing control and modification of movement has yet to be elucidated, but it is clear that sophisticated networks of interneurons exist both within and between segments of the spinal cord. Advances in cell-recording technologies have provided further evidence that these networks are responsible for integrating the internally generated information arriving from other subsystems within the CNS. They are also responsible for integrating the various sensory inputs that enter the CNS at various levels of the spinal cord.

How are interneurons able to serve such a complex function? It is primarily because of their ability either to excite or to inhibit the pools of motoneurons with which they synapse. In this way, certain muscles can be inhibited while others are excited to produce coordinated movement. This process of simultaneous excitation and inhibition, or **reciprocal innervation** as it is most often called, not only permits us to make the automatic adjustments in posture necessary when we touch a hot item or step in a hole while

Coordinated action is achieved through the simultaneous activation and inhibition of motoneuron pools serving different muscle groups.

running, but also assists us in voluntarily coordinating our limbs when performing the many activities associated with daily life. We will talk more about this process a little later in this chapter. What is perhaps even more interesting is the fact that these neural circuits comprising inhibitory and excitatory interneurons appear capable of producing rhythmic movements (walking, swimming, hopping, etc.). This evidence stems from deafferentation studies (Brown, 1911; Knapp, Taub, & Berman, 1963; Rothwell, Taub, Day, Obeso, & Mersden, 1982), spinal cord isolation studies (Smith & Feldman, 1987), and spinalized animal studies (Sherrington, 1910, 1911; DeLeon, Hodgson, Roy, & Edgerton, 1998).

Although the majority of the evidence for the existence of spinal pattern generators has been based on animal studies, some recent evidence for their existence in human spinal cords has come from clinical studies conducted with patients following spinal cord injury (see highlight, Training the Spinal Cord). Current thinking is that while some type of **central pattern generator** (CPG) probably exists in the human spinal cord that is capable of generating a basic movement pattern, supraspinal centers (e.g., sensorimotor cortex, cerebellum, and basal ganglia) are responsible for turning it on as well as controlling the integrity of its operation (Muir & Steeves, 1997; Calancie et al., 1994). In addition, sensory feedback is essential for being able to respond to changes in the environment during the performance of complex locomotor activities. Nonetheless, it is argued that the existence of pattern-generating neural circuitry within the spinal cord does at least reduce the complexity of the descending motor commands from higher cortical and subcortical areas of the CNS (Field-Fote, 2000).

*Central pattern generators (CPGs) are neural circuits comprised of inhibitory and excitatory interneurons that are capable of producing rhythmic movements.*

## Muscle Activation and Force Production

*The neuromuscular junction serves as the functional connection between the motoneuron and the muscle fibers it innervates.*

As mentioned earlier in this section, the final link between the spinal and musculoskeletal subsystems is created by the alpha motoneuron synapsing with extrafusal muscle fibers at a site known as the **neuromuscular junction,** or motor end plate. This neuromuscular junction, which is spread across most or all of the muscle, serves as the functional connection between the motoneuron and the muscle fibers it innervates. At this juncture, the electrical energy conveyed by the alpha motoneuron is converted to chemical energy in the form of a transmitter called acetylcholine that binds itself to specific receptor sites on the muscle membrane, causing it to depolarize and produce a muscle action potential, which, in turn, triggers a chain of muscular events that culminate in the interaction of two very important contractile proteins (actin and myosin) within the muscle itself. This two-step process, which is called **excitation–contraction coupling,** is responsible for transforming action potentials into muscular force.

*The fundamental unit of motor control is the motor unit.*

The connection between a single alpha motoneuron and the extrafusal muscle fibers innervated by it forms the most fundamental unit of motor control, a **motor unit.** The exact size of these motor units is determined by the total number of muscle fibers innervated by one alpha motoneuron. Some alpha motoneurons (such as muscles of the leg and trunk) innervate as many as 2,000 muscle fibers; others (including muscles of the eye and fingers) innervate as few as 10 to 15 muscle fibers. These large differences in innervation ratios influence the level of motor control available in certain muscles.

# HIGHLIGHT

## Training the Spinal Cord

Evidence for the existence of central pattern generators (CPGs) has been bolstered in recent years by research studies conducted with individuals following complete or partial transection of the spinal cord (Dimitrijevic, Gerasimenko, & Pinter, 1998). Continuous electrical stimulation of the spinal cord in patients with complete spinal cord injury (SCI) has produced rhythmic and alternating locomotor-like EMG activity in the lower limbs in some studies, while in other studies analyses of EMG activity in lower limb muscles (e.g., gastrocnemius, tibialis anterior) have demonstrated the existence of locomotor-like EMG patterns that could be spatially and temporally modulated in response to changes in treadmill speed (Dietz, Nakazawa, Wirz, & Erni, 1999; Dobkin, Harkema, Requejo, & Edgerton, 1995). These findings have been attributed to the existence of a CPG in the spinal cord.

Still more recently, the plasticity of the spinal cord has been demonstrated in a small number of locomotor training studies conducted with patients with a clinically complete or severe incomplete SCI (Harkema, 2001). This new rehabilitative approach uses a body weight support and treadmill system (see figure). The goal of body weight support training (BWST) is to provide the patient with a training environment that promotes the movement of the trunk and legs while minimizing the need for maintaining postural control. Such training provides the patient with sensory cues that are specific to the patterns associated with locomotion.

Seven principles associated with locomotor training have been outlined by Behrman and Harkema (2000). They include: (1) generating walking velocities that approximate normal walking speeds; (2) providing normal load patterns to

*continues*

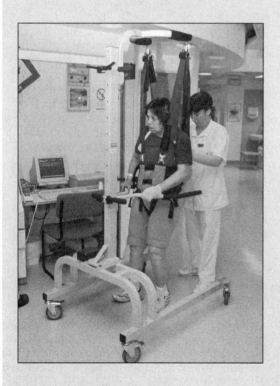

Body weight support training (BWST) is a new rehabilitative approach being used to improve locomotion in patients who have experienced spinal cord injuries.

the stance limb; (3) ensuring an upright and ex-tended trunk and head; (4) approximating ankle, knee, and hip kinematics within normal ranges; (5) synchronizing the loading and unloading of limbs during the stance phase; (6) eliminating or minimizing weight bearing on the arms so as to facilitate a reciprocal arm swing; and (7) maintain-ing symmetrical kinetics and kinematics between the limbs.

In one of the first comprehensive studies exploring the efficacy of BWST in individuals with clinically incomplete SCI, Wernig, Muller, Nanassy, and Cagol (1995) demonstrated positive func-tional changes in a majority of the patients who participated in the locomotor training. The BWST group included 44 chronic and 45 acute patients with clinically incomplete SCI. Using a functional class assessment that rated each patient's recovery of locomotion, Wernig and colleagues noted that 25 participants moved from the wheelchair-bound to the ambulatory category, and the majority of patients who were ambulatory prior to the start of the study also improved in terms of their functional classification. The improve-ments observed in the group receiving the BWST intervention were better than those obtained following conventional therapy. What was partic-ularly noteworthy about this study was that in a follow-up study, all participants had retained the functional improvements and, in some cases, even continued to improve with respect to their overground walking abilities (Wernig, Nanassy, & Muller, 1998).

What types of underlying mechanisms may account for improvements in function in the case of patients with complete or incomplete spinal cord lesions? Drawing from the large number of animal studies that have been conducted to investigate spinal cord function following spinal cord transection, as well as the promising findings emerging from recent human studies, Pearson (2001) proposed four possibilities for the improve-ments observed in locomotion. These include: (1) the regeneration of axons across the injury site and the reestablishment of descending pathways needed to initiate the locomotor pattern; (2) en-hanced effectiveness of undamaged neurons in incomplete spinal cord transections; (3) nonspe-cific facilitation of spinal reflexes and circuits that may result from transmitters being released from regenerated axons or from substances released during the locomotor training; and (4) enhanced trunk movements in proximity to the injury site that strengthen the mechanical coupling of the trunk and lower limbs via spinal reflexes.

Although the findings of a small number of studies are encouraging, many more randomized clinical trials that systematically investigate the efficacy of BWST when compared to more con-ventional therapy in both acute and chronic SCI patient populations are needed. According to Harkema (2001), there is also a need to determine if certain types of SCI are more amenable to BWST and the extent of the locomotor recovery that can be expected in these different patient groups.

Innervation ratios that are very low facilitate movements requiring fine motor control, whereas larger innervation ratios make it possible to generate the large amounts of force characteristic of more gross movements.

***Types of Motor Units.***   Three different types of motor units activate human skeletal muscles: slow-twitch, fatigue resistant motor units (SFR); fast-twitch, fatigue resistant motor units (FTR); and fast-twitch, fatiguable motor units (FTF) (Burke, 1981; Burke & Edgerton, 1975). SFR motor units are comprised of motor neurons that have small cell bodies and axons that selectively inner-vate a small number of slow-twitch or *type I muscle fibers*. As a result, the amount of force that these units are able to produce in a given muscle is quite small. In contrast, FTF motor units are comprised of motoneurons with large cell bodies and larger diameter axons that innervate large numbers of a subtype of fast-twitch muscle fibers called *type IIB muscle fibers.* These motor units are therefore able to generate large amounts of force in the muscle very quickly. One disadvantage of these motor units is that they fatigue quickly. Finally, FTR motor units are comprised of intermediate-sized motor neurons with axons that innervate a second subtype of fast-twitch muscle fibers that are more resistant to fatigue. These are referred to as *type IIA muscle fibers* and are also capable of generating large amounts of muscle force but for a longer period of time (several minutes). One can expect, then, that the level of contractile force that a muscle can generate is a function of which muscle fiber type is innervated and the number of fibers innervated by each motoneuron.

*Three types of motor units activate human skeletal muscles: slow-twitch, fatigue resistant (SFR), fast-twitch, fatigue resistant (FTR), and fast-twitch, fatiguable (FTF) motor units.*

*Motor Unit Recruitment.*     How is it that individual motor units can be activated to assist us in generating just the right amount of force necessary to produce different levels of motor control? Two mechanisms are available to the CNS to accomplish this goal. The first is related to the *order* in which the respective motor units are recruited during muscle contraction, and the second involves the *rate* at which individual motoneurons are activated. The discovery of the first of these two mechanisms can be attributed to a set of observations made by Denny-Brown and Pennybacker (1938), who reported that motor units appeared to be recruited in a very orderly sequence. Some time later, Henneman (1957, 1979) discovered that the recruitment pattern was highly correlated with the type of motoneuron (cell body size and diameter of axon) and type of muscle fiber innervated. This means that the SFR motor units will be recruited first, followed by the FTR and FTF motor units. According to Loeb and Ghez (2000), this orderly recruitment of motor units serves two functional purposes. First, by turning on the SFR units before either of the two fast-twitch motor unit subtypes, the development of fatigue is minimized during the performance of movements that do not require large amounts of force. The fast-twitch motor units are reserved for those movements requiring the application of larger amounts of contractile muscle force. Second, the orderly recruitment of motor units from the smallest to largest will ensure that the amount of force applied will be incremental and proportional to the level of force at which each individual motor unit is recruited. This second purpose allows us to perform movements smoothly and efficiently.

*The orderly recruitment of motor units from smallest to largest allows us to perform movements smoothly and efficiently.*

*The Size Principle.*     This hypothetical explanation, referred to as the size principle, is thought to apply irrespective of whether force is being increased or decreased within a given set of muscles. Not only does the orderly recruitment of motor units provide us with a mechanism for grading force production according to the type of movement being performed, but it also reduces the complexity of the decision-making process occurring within the CNS. Given this orderly recruitment of motor units, the subsystems involved in developing the action plan need only specify which muscle response synergies are to be recruited in advance of the movement. The actual selection of motor units has already been determined on the basis of the size principle.

*Rate Coding.*     In addition to recruitment of motor units via the size principle, a second mechanism for generating muscle force is available. This mechanism

Rate coding involves the firing frequency associated with individual motor units and constitutes a second mechanism for generating muscle force.

involves the firing frequency associated with individual motor units and is termed **rate coding.** It has been demonstrated that smaller motor units generate smaller action potentials at a progressively lower rate as muscle force increases. By contrast, larger motor units are capable of generating larger amounts of force because they have larger motoneurons that are capable of producing larger action potentials at rates that increase linearly as the amount of force required in a given muscle group increases.

Once all available motor units are recruited, a second component of the rate-coding mechanism can be exploited to increase the amount of force generated within the muscle. The rate at which each individual motoneuron is fired is increased by manipulating the rate at which the motoneurons send nervous impulses to the muscles being contracted. As the interval between successive firings of individual motor neurons becomes shorter, the forces generated by each impulse begin to accumulate faster than the muscle's individual twitch contraction time. This rapid summation of nerve impulses has the net effect of producing increased levels of force within the already contracting muscles.

At a practical level, the types of motor units recruited will be largely determined by the nature of the task being performed. For example, activities such as jogging that require sustained levels of muscle force will rely more on the recruitment of the smaller, fatigue resistant motor units that innervate slow-twitch muscle fibers, whereas activities requiring short bursts of muscle force as would be needed when leaping to rebound a basketball would require the recruitment of the larger, albeit more fatiguable, motor units that are capable of generating large action potentials in a very short period of time.

## Musculoskeletal Contributions to Force

As important as the many motor units are in grading the forces produced by the various muscle response synergies, other factors have also been shown to influence the level of force generated by a given muscle group. Two very important examples of these factors are the anatomical and mechanical forces acting on the body. These types of forces may be created by the way the musculoskeletal system is organized, by gravitational and reactive forces acting on the body as we stand and move in space, and by forces associated with a limb's changing moment of inertia. We will begin by describing how the anatomical position of a limb and the action to be performed influence the amount of force produced by the muscles involved.

The position of the limb and/or the relaxation of the muscle prior to innervation affect the amount of muscle force produced.

***Anatomical Limb Position.***   It has now become clear that a given level of neural innervation does not result in a fixed level of force being produced by a muscle. Nor, for that matter, does it result in a fixed movement pattern. Instead, the amount of force any given muscle is able to generate varies as a function of the limb's anatomical position and/or the degree of muscle relaxation (i.e., amount of actin–myosin overlap prior to nervous stimulation). Moreover, the velocity with which the muscle then shortens or lengthens also influences the amount of force it is capable of generating. For example, a limb that is in a slightly more flexed position can produce more force than one that is being held in an extended position. Similarly, a muscle moving at a slower velocity, whether it is shortening or lengthening, produces more force.

The additional variability that arises as a function of the limb's anatomical position and muscle relaxation prior to innervation clearly poses problems for hierarchical theories of motor control that assume that higher centers within the CNS prescribe the amount of activation for each individual muscle involved in a given movement. Turvey, Fitch, and Tuller (1982) have argued that this address-specific feature not only makes the unrealistic demand that the CNS regulate the contractile states of every muscle throughout the movement, but also ignores other sources of potential variability that emerge as a function of the changing context.

***Mechanical Properties of the Skeleton.***    In addition to the influence that anatomical limb position exerts on the level of force a muscle can produce, a second influence is mechanical in origin. One has only to look at the body's skeleton to see that the bones form a chain linked by a variety of joints permitting different types of movements. The number of movements possible at any individual joint, in turn, determines the number of degrees of freedom available to us. Although certain joints (e.g., the knee and elbow) possess as few as one functional degree of freedom, others (e.g., the shoulder and hip) provide as many as three. As the total number of joints involved in an action increases, so too does the number of degrees of freedom that must be organized for efficient movement. This factor helps explain why movements involving multilimb coordination are much more difficult to learn and/or control than single-limb movements.

Because of the way the bony skeleton is rigidly linked, we can also expect that any movement in one part of the chain will affect another, often quite distal to the joint being moved. This distal movement has the effect of generating kinetic energy that also influences the overall shape of the movement being produced. This is evident when we observe someone preparing to kick a stationary ball. As the hip joint is extended during the backswing and then flexed during the kicking phase, the lower leg and foot continue to accelerate as the kinetic energy generated by the hip's action is distributed throughout the length of the kicking leg. A similar distribution of kinetic energy is evident during the swing phase of locomotion. In this latter situation, the activation of the flexor/extensor muscles at the hip joint produces angular acceleration of the thigh, which in turn leads to greater acceleration in the more distal segments of the moving limb.

> Movement in one part of the chain of joints will affect another, often quite distal to the joint being moved.

## Subconscious Control of Movement

In addition to the many conscious modifications we are able to make to movements in progress, certain neuronal connections within the spinal system contribute to the modification of movements in progress by providing sensory information at a subconscious level. The influence of some of these reflex loops is limited to local control of muscle force, but others are capable of influencing force levels in muscle groups quite distant from those originally stimulated. These longer reflex loops are therefore capable of modifying movements to a much larger extent than the shorter reflex loops that are confined to single segments within the spinal cord. In what kinds of movement situations are we most likely to involve these different types of reflex circuits? The short reflex loops are most often called into play when minute adjustments in muscle length are needed. These adjustments are necessary when misalignment exists between intended muscle length and actual muscle length. This misalignment is most likely to occur in situations where unexpected forces are applied to the limb or the muscle begins to fatigue. Both situations can lead to an involuntary and undesirable lengthening of the muscles involved in the action. For example, when we incorrectly predict the weight of an object we are about to lift, the firing rates of the muscle spindles involved must be quickly altered. If we underestimate the weight, spindle afferent firing rates will need to be quickly increased, whereas if we overestimate the weight of the object, the firing level of the spindle afferent fibers will need to be reduced in order to avoid gross errors in performance.

### Short-Loop Reflexive Adjustments.

Now that we have a better idea of when these various reflex loops might be called on to assist us in modifying the action plan being executed, let us look more closely at how these different types of reflex loops are organized and then activated during movement control. Two important examples of short reflex loops are the spinal stretch reflex and the gamma reflex loop.

*Short-loop reflexes are limited to the local control of muscle force.*

### Spinal Stretch Reflex (SSR).

The spinal stretch reflex comprises a sensory receptor (in this case the muscle spindle), which is responsible for monitoring changes in muscle length; an afferent sensory neuron, which relays the sensory information arising in the spindle to the spinal cord; and an alpha motoneuron, which then closes the loop by acting on the incoming sensory information—specifically by causing the extrafusal muscle fibers it innervates to contract.

The SSR is triggered when the length of an extrafusal muscle is altered, causing the sensory endings within the muscle spindle to be mechanically deformed. Once deformed, these sensory endings fire, sending nerve impulses into the spinal cord via an afferent sensory neuron whose cell body, or soma, is located just outside the spinal cord. As soon as these impulses reach the spinal cord, they are transferred to alpha motoneurons that innervate the very same muscle that houses the activated muscle spindles. It is through the operation of this reflex that we are able to alter continually the tone of a muscle and/or make subtle adjustments in muscle length during movement. These latter adjustments may be in response to external factors that produce unexpected loads or forces on the moving limbs or to internal factors. For example, internal modulation of the SSR is also made possible through the influence of cortical structures and the descending pathways that are capable of altering the balance between the level of excitatory and inhibitory inputs to spinal motoneurons and interneurons. In this way, the spinal system is capable of responding to external (e.g., changing environmental events) and internal (e.g., changing task goals) influences on the movement in progress.

*The internal modulation of the spinal stretch reflex is also made possible through the influence of cortical structures and descending motor pathways.*

To illustrate how the muscle spindle contributes to the automatic regulation of muscle length in response to the external application of force, let us consider the sequence of events that occur when an SSR is activated by tapping the patellar tendon (see Figure 5.6). This is a common procedure used by clinicians to test the integrity of the SSR. When a physician or therapist taps the skin surface above the patellar tendon, a reflex chain of events results in the initially flexed leg rapidly extending. This external application of force

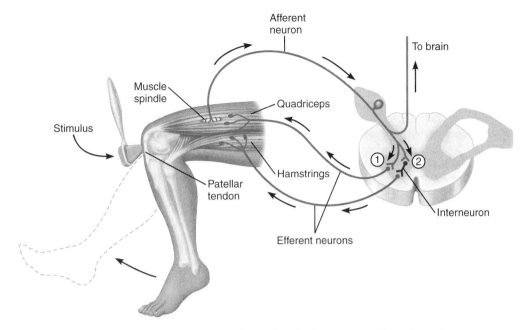

**Figure 5.6** One simple way of activating a spinal stretch reflex is to tap the skin surface above the patellar tendon. Excitation of the alpha motoneuron that innervates the lengthened muscle (quadriceps) is indicated by a ① and inhibition of the alpha moto-neuron via an inhibitory interneuron that innervates the opposing muscle group (ham-strings) is indicated by a ②.

stretches, or lengthens, the extrafusal muscle fibers of the quadriceps beyond their current resting position. The lengthening of the quadriceps muscle results in deformation of the sensory endings wrapped around the intrafusal muscle fibers of the muscle spindles contained within the muscle that has been length-ened. Physical deformation of the sensory endings causes the Ia and II affer-ents to fire and send nervous impulses to the spinal cord.

Upon entering the spinal cord, Ia and II afferents synapse with excitatory alpha motoneurons (see ① in Figure 5.6), which, in turn, send nervous impulses back to the same quadriceps muscle group that was just lengthened. The reflex loop is closed as contraction of the quadriceps muscle results in extension of the lower leg. Extension of the leg temporarily shortens, or unloads, the intrafusal fibers of the muscle spindle, leading to a cessation of firing. From a clinical perspective, triggering an SSR provides useful informa-tion about the integrity of the sensory and motor pathways involved in the SSR, as well as the level of muscle tone. Other reflexes that are typically exam-ined in clinical settings include the jaw, biceps, triceps, hamstring, and ankle.

Although we limited our discussion of the patellar tendon reflex to the chain of events involving only the alpha motoneurons that innervated the lengthened quadriceps muscle, it is important to understand that the Ia affer-ent endings leading away from the muscle spindles embedded in the extra-fusal muscle that was stretched not only directly innervate the alpha

# HIGHLIGHT

### Measuring the Spinal Stretch Reflex

Two basic experimental methods have been used to stimulate and measure the spinal stretch reflex (SSR). The first of these is via the tendon tap, and the second is via the Hoffman reflex, or H-reflex, as it is commonly called. As you may recall, tapping the tendon of the target muscle activates the sensory receptors of the muscle spindle which, in turn, activate the sensory neurons in the dorsal root ganglion that then carry the neural signals into the spinal cord, where they synapse with alpha motoneurons. In contrast to this mechanical method of activating the SSR, measurement of the reflex can also be obtained by electrically stimulating the Ia afferent nerve fibers directly.

According to Schieppati (1987), this second method of stimulating the SSR allows researchers to study the central mechanisms that influence motoneuron excitability and to do so independently of the peripheral muscle spindle receptor. Electrically stimulating the afferent pathways leading away from the muscle spindle results in the excitation of the alpha motoneurons in the spinal cord, which in turn activate the extrafusal muscle. Surface electromyography (EMG) is then used to record the level of muscle activity in the stimulated muscle. Only very low stimulation levels are needed to evoke a pure H-reflex because the sensory axons innervating the muscle spindle have much lower thresholds for stimulation than other axons.

Measuring the strength of the SSR can assist clinicians in diagnosing different medical disorders. Absent or weak SSRs are indicative of disorders affecting the sensory and/or motor components of the reflex. Activating the SSR via the tendon-tap and H-reflex methods has also provided researchers with a clearer picture of the effects of age on this important subconscious mechanism of motor control (see Myrnark & Koceja, 2001, for a more in-depth review of the age-associated changes in the SSR).

**Reciprocal innervation is the almost simultaneous process involving excitation of the agonist muscle and inhibition of the antagonist muscle.**

motoneurons that are responsible for contracting the same extrafusal muscle (the quadriceps muscle in the patellar tendon reflex), but also indirectly innervate alpha motoneurons that serve the opposing muscle (hamstrings in this example) via a special class of inhibitory interneurons referred to as Ia inhibitory interneurons (see ② in Figure 5.6). This almost simultaneous process involving excitation of agonist (quadriceps) muscles and inhibition of antagonist (hamstrings) muscles is called reciprocal innervation, a process we introduced in an earlier section of this chapter.

In addition to the important role that reciprocal innervation plays in the operation of the SSR, this same neural mechanism plays an important role in the ongoing regulation of voluntary movements. According to Pearson and Gordon (2000), inhibiting the antagonist muscles during the performance of a voluntary movement enhances the speed and efficiency of a movement. This is because the agonist, or prime moving muscles, are not working in opposition to contracting antagonist muscles. This mechanism of reciprocal innervation also acts to simplify the coordination of movements by relieving cortical areas of the need to activate the opposing muscle groups individually.

As useful as this reciprocal innervation is in the production of coordinated movements, there are other movement situations that require both the agonist and antagonist muscle groups to be activated or cocontracted. For example, there will be times when we need to stabilize a joint during the performance of a given movement that will require cocontraction of agonist and antagonist muscle groups. In these situations, descending motor signals alter the level of excitatory and inhibitory inputs acting on spinal motoneurons and interneurons so, instead of being inhibited, the antagonist muscle groups are activated just like the agonist muscle groups.

*Gamma reflex loop.*   Muscle spindles also play an important role in the ongoing control and modification of movement by virtue of their involvement in a spinal reflex loop known as the **gamma reflex loop.** Recall that the neural impulses conveyed by the two motor pathway systems discussed earlier in this chapter synapse with both alpha and gamma motoneurons once they reach the spinal cord. Whereas the alpha motoneuron sends the information it receives to the muscles involved in the pending movement, the gamma motoneuron sends the same information to the muscle spindle.

Gamma reflex loops play an important role in the control of movements by ensuring that the muscle spindles remain ready to fire if muscle length changes unexpectedly during a movement.

What could be the purpose of sending movement-related information via this second route? One early suggestion advanced by Merton (1953) was that this loop served as an alternative method of activating the muscles involved in a movement. This hypothesis has since been rejected in favor of the idea that the gamma reflex loop assists in the control of limb movements. This is made possible by the fact that the gamma motoneurons innervate the muscle spindle at its polar ends. The shortening of the intrafusal fibers at the polar ends of the muscle spindle, in turn, results in the central region of the spindle being stretched from both ends. Either the firing rate of the spindle afferent fibers increases as a result of this gamma-based activation or the afferent endings are brought closer to their threshold for firing as a result of being "loaded" again. Keeping a certain amount of stretch on the intrafusal fibers of the muscle spindle during muscle contraction is critical for ensuring that the spindle will respond quickly to any unanticipated change in muscle length during a movement and also ensuring that the muscle spindle is capable of signaling changes in muscle length across its full range. Just think how slowly we would respond to changing task demands and/or environmental events if the muscle spindle was allowed to become slack or completely "unloaded" during active muscle contraction.

The independent innervation of the muscle spindle by the gamma motoneuron is very important during muscle contraction when the intrafusal fibers of the spindle would otherwise become slack or unloaded. Gamma activation of the spindle results in the stretching of the intrafusal fibers even though the extrafusal muscle fibers are contracting. How might this gamma activity assist us during the moment-to-moment control of movement? Because it takes up the slack in the spindle caused by muscle contraction, minute changes in the length of the muscle can be detected and corrected more quickly. To illustrate how the gamma loop contributes to the rapid correction of limb position, let us consider a situation in which an additional load is added to an already loaded limb being held in a given position in space. As illustrated in Figure 5.7 on page 156, the limb is holding a book in the hand at a 90 degree angle against gravity. The muscles of the limb are contracted to a specific length, and alpha motoneurons are firing in order to maintain the desired limb position in spite of the load and gravity exerting a downward force on the limb. At the same time, gamma motoneurons are innervating the polar ends of the muscle spindle in order to keep the intrafusal muscle fibers stretched.

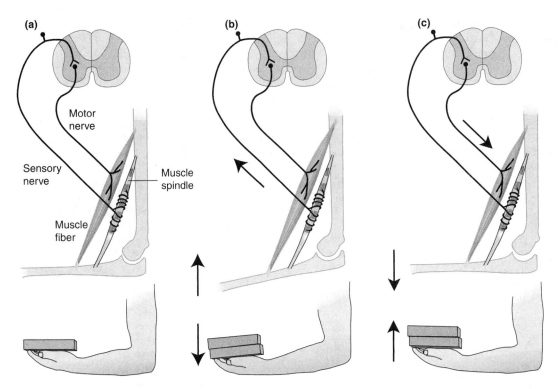

**Figure 5.7** **(a)** A muscle is under the influence of a stretch reflex when the elbow joint is flexed and maintaining a load against gravity. Gamma motoneurons (not shown) are also innervating the muscle spindle so that the intrafusal muscle fibers continue to remain stretched during muscle contraction. **(b)** A sudden increase in load lengthens the extrafusal muscle and results in muscle spindle firing and the transmission of sensory impulses to the spinal cord. **(c)** Alpha motoneurons that innervate the lengthened extra-fusal muscle are excited, sending impulses back to the muscle and causing it to contract. The elbow joint is returned to its original position.

Now an additional load is added to the end of the limb, causing the mus-cles to lengthen as the limb drops. This stretching of the extrafusal muscle fibers results in almost simultaneous stretching of the muscle spindle, which then fires and sends signals to the spinal cord and alpha motoneurons that innervate the same muscles holding the book. The firing rate of the alpha motoneurons is subsequently increased, causing the muscles in the dropping limb to be further contracted and the limb restored to its previous position. The rapid corrections would not be possible, however, if the slack was not being taken up in the muscle spindle via the gamma loop reflex.

Long-loop reflexes are used to make larger adjustments in limb and overall body position.

***Long-Loop Reflexive Adjustments.***    For larger adjustments in limb and overall body position, it is necessary to involve the longer reflex loops that extend beyond single segments within the spinal cord. The pathways involved in these neural circuits travel to the more distant subcortical and cor-tical levels of the CNS to connect with structures such as the motor cortex and cerebellum within the larger projection system. As you will recall, it is the primary responsibility of this subsystem to add the final details to the general action plan. It is perhaps not surprising, then, that certain structures within this system also play an important role in the modification of movements in progress. It has also been concluded on the basis of research studies conducted with animals and humans that two types of long-loop reflex pathways exist that appear to fulfill different functional demands. The first of these two types of long-loop pathways is mediated by the motor cortex and appears to be important in the ongoing regulation of precise movements that involve the distal musculature. Conversely, the second type of long-loop reflex pathway is more involved in the regulation of more proximal muscles that subconsciously produce movements such as maintaining balance or performing gross body movements that require much less precision, such as kicking and throwing (Pearson & Gordon, 2000). Several studies have indicated that long-loop reflexes operate to restore our limbs to their original positions in response to changes in the environment that lead to undesirable changes in muscle length. These changes may be prompted by contact with objects or other persons during many game situations, causing a momentary loss in balance or alterations in the type of surface on which we are standing or moving (Nashner, 1976). These long-loop responses can also be used to stabilize our limbs in a variety of different postures and movements.

> Two types of long-loop reflex pathways exist that appear to fulfill different functional demands.

## Solving the Motor Problem

The relationship between the brain and spinal system has been appropriately described by Turvey, Fitch, and Tuller (1982) as one wherein the two entities "relate between themselves as experts, cooperating on a problem" (p. 251). In this case, the problem to be resolved is how best to organize the many degrees of freedom available within the human system to accomplish a given movement task. As we are all too aware from our own early movement experiences, this is by no means easy. In fact, a considerable amount of practice is needed for us to learn to work with, rather than against, the many internal and external forces that act on our bodies as we move.

With repeated opportunities to experiment with different muscle activation patterns and their resulting torques, we learn to constrain and/or release available degrees of freedom, depending on the skill being practiced. In the case of learning to hit a baseball or softball, for example, we must learn to release, or free, a number of degrees of freedom, particularly in the trunk and lower body, in order to accomplish a smooth swinging action. On the other hand, to be successful in a sport such as pistol shooting, we must constrain the joints of the shooting arm to act as a single degree of freedom in order to reduce the amount of pistol movement during the aiming phase of the movement. Newell and colleagues (Newell, Kugler, van Emmerik, & McDonald, 1989) stress the importance of developing "search strategies" that can be used to explore the dynamics of an action an individual is attempting to coordinate and control. These search strategies are intended to guide the learner in the perceptual exploration of what dynamic systems theorists commonly refer to as the perceptual–motor workspace. This repeated perceptual exploration is thought to be central to the development of an appropriate solution to the motor problem at hand.

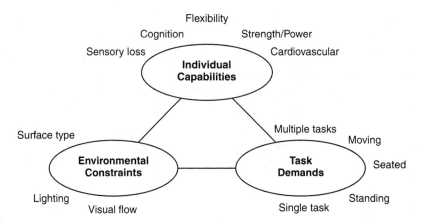

**Figure 5.8**   Three important constraints on action include the capabilities of the performer, the task being performed, and the environment in which the task is being performed.

Contrary to hierarchical theories of motor control in which the ongoing control and modification of movement is the sole responsibility of a higher cortical executive, more recent theories acknowledge the self-organizing capabilities of the CNS and the dynamic interplay of other forces external to the nervous system (the musculoskeletal system and the environment). The purpose of this section of the chapter has been to demonstrate how each of these additional forces contributes to the evolving movement pattern.

## Constraints on Action

Now that we have described how movements are planned and executed at a behavioral and neurological level of analysis, let us briefly consider three constraints that are important in shaping how movements are planned and executed. The constraints to be discussed in this final section of the chapter include those that are intrinsic to the performer, the task to be performed, and the environment in which it is to be performed (see Figure 5.8). Although only a few examples of each type of constraint will be presented in this section, it is important that the reader understand that many more constraints on action have been identified. Moreover, the degree to which each constraint described will shape the emerging action will change as the performer's experience with performing the task and its variations increases and as the performer acquires more knowledge about the performance environment itself.

### Intrinsic Capabilities of the Performer

The intrinsic capabilities or abilities that a performer brings to a movement situation will clearly shape how a movement is both planned and executed. As you have already learned in this chapter, the presence of disorders at different levels within the CNS will certainly influence how movements are planned and executed by the individual. In some cases, individuals will no longer be able to produce certain movements, while in other cases the quality of the movement will be adversely affected.

The motor abilities possessed by the performer will also influence how movements are planned and executed. The term **motor ability** is generally defined as an ability that is directly related to the performance of a motor skill. Research in the area of motor abilities has been the focus of a few scholars over the years (e.g., McCloy, 1934; Fleishman, 1972; Henry, 1961). A long-standing controversy that characterizes this research is whether individuals possess a general motor ability that will influence their performance on all movement skills (McCloy, 1934) or whether the individual possesses a large number of specific abilities that are used to perform different movement skills (Henry, 1961, 1968). Research conducted to address this controversy has provided greater support for the idea of specific motor abilities but perhaps not as many as Henry argued existed (Fleishman, 1964). In fact, on the basis of his correlational research, Fleishman grouped motor abilities into two broad categories: perceptual–motor abilities, and physical proficiency abilities. A third category related to general coordination abilities has since been added on the basis of research conducted by Keele and colleagues (Keele & Hawkins, 1982; Keele, Ivry, & Pokorny, 1987; Keele, Pokorny, Corcos, & Ivry, 1985).

At a practical level, it will be important to determine the underlying motor abilities required to perform any given movement skill and the degree to which each individual performer is able to use these abilities to perform and/or learn the required movement skill. Knowing what abilities each performer brings to a performance situation will determine where the focus of instruction will need to be in order to assist the performer in strengthening specific abilities that are weak—and therefore are undermining the performer's ability to perform the skill. The performer who is learning to pitch a baseball or softball but lacks adequate force control will require a different type of skill practice than a second performer who possesses good levels of force control but demonstrates inadequate levels of limb movement speed. Similarly, in a clinical setting, a patient may demonstrate a number of physical proficiency abilities (such as trunk strength, dynamic flexibility, gross body equilibrium) but exhibit fewer perceptual–motor abilities (such as reaction time, response orientation, multilimb coordination). Depending on the movement skill to be performed, the clinician may need to structure the practice environment very differently to maximize the patient's success and/or safety. Practitioners who know which specific abilities are well developed in a performer and which are not will better understand what types of activities the performer may be better suited to performing or the types of practice strategies that can be employed to improve or compensate for the performer's weaknesses.

> Motor abilities have been grouped into two broad categories: perceptual–motor and physical proficiency abilities.

## Task-Related Constraints

The second constraint on action is extrinsic to the performer and relates to the task to be performed. During the course of an average day we will engage in a number of different tasks that pose different levels of physical and/or cognitive demands. For example, some movements we perform will require accuracy, others will require speed, and still others will require both speed *and*

Fitts' Law has been used to explain the speed–accuracy trade-off.

accuracy. Of course, what we find is that as the speed of the movement increases, the accuracy with which it is performed declines. Although this relationship between the speed and accuracy requirements of a movement was first observed by Woodworth (1899), it was not until the work of Paul Fitts (1954) that the relationship between movement speed and accuracy was mathematically quantified. The mathematical equation describing what was to become known as the speed–accuracy trade-off is called **Fitts' Law.**

To investigate the relationship between the variables of target distance and width, Fitts instructed study participants to move a hand-held stylus continuously between two targets for 20 seconds at a time. Over the course of the experiment, the amplitude (A, or distance between the two targets) and/or the width (W) of the targets was systematically manipulated. What Fitts noted was that movement time (MT) increased as the distance between the two targets increased and as the width of the targets decreased. He subsequently developed a simple mathematical equation that beautifully described the changing relationship between speed and accuracy as a function of the changing amplitude and target width. The equation is as follows:

$$MT = a + b \left( \log_2 [2A/W] \right)$$

According to Fitts, the "$\log_2 (2A/W)$" portion of the equation equates to the **Index of Movement Difficulty (ID)** and can be used to describe how the movement times of a single performer or group of performers will be influenced as the distance between two endpoint targets increases and the width of those endpoint targets decreases. The *a* and *b* constants in the equation represent the intercept (movement time when the ID is zero) and slope (the change in movement time associated with a one-unit change in the ID), respectively.

In his multiple experiments, Fitts quantified the relationship between speed and accuracy. What his results showed was a linear increase in movement time as the ratio of 2A to W increased. Either increasing the amplitude between the targets or decreasing the width of the targets alters the ratio. Because his results further revealed that study participants were more sensitive to changes in target width as opposed to amplitude, Fitts adjusted his equation to weight target width more heavily.

At a practical level, Fitts' Law demonstrates how the temporal and/or spatial demands of the task influence how quickly and accurately the movements are performed. That is, as the accuracy requirements of a task increase, one can expect that the time to complete the movement will increase as the performer trades speed for accuracy. On the other hand, as the accuracy requirements of a task are reduced, one can expect that the performer will complete the movement more quickly. The robustness of Fitts' Law has been demonstrated repeatedly over the years, in a variety of different task settings, with different aiming movements and across different age groups (e.g., Fitts & Peterson, 1964; Kerr, 1973; Meyer, Smith, & Wright, 1982).

A second type of task demand that will shape the emerging motor control relates to its cognitive demands. We can expect that as the number of tasks that must be performed simultaneously increases, particularly those with a high cognitive load, the more likely it is that one or more of the tasks being performed will be affected in some way. We might observe a decline in the speed with which one or more of the tasks is performed or perhaps an increase in the number of errors made during the performance. In yet another situation we might see one task be curtailed while the other task is performed, particularly if the performance of both tasks exceeds the individual's attentional and/or physical capabilities. Certainly the findings of several research studies have demonstrated significant changes in motor performance when the cognitive or attentional load of one or more tasks is increased significantly (see reviews by Egeth & Yantis, 1997; Whitall, 1996).

The effect of cognitive or attentional load on motor performance is further adversely affected as a function of the aging process (Chen, Schultz, Ashton-Miller, et al., 1996; Brown, Shumway-Cook, & Woollacott, 1999) and disorders of the CNS that affect the sensory, motor, and/or cognitive systems.

## Environmental Constraints

The third and final category of constraints on action to be discussed here are those related to the environment in which the movement is to be performed. As you have already learned from your reading of Chapters 3 and 4, sensory information derived from the environment plays an important role in shaping how a movement will be planned and executed. In particular, the degree to which the environment is changing during the performance of a movement skill will significantly influence an individual's motor performance. To illustrate this point, let us try to visualize ourselves dribbling a soccer ball toward a goal on an empty field or perhaps walking through an empty corridor. Now imagine adding a number of additional players or pedestrians to each of those scenes. Will this change in the environmental context affect how we plan and ultimately control our actions? It certainly will, given that the first two movement scenes are far less complex than the latter two. The first two scenes described are examples of highly predictable and **stable environments.** This type of environment reduces the demands placed on motor control by allowing us, among other things, to proceed at a self-determined speed.

Adding more players or pedestrians to these same two movement situations renders them much less predictable and therefore creates a more **variable environment.** As a result, the level of motor control that is required increases. Our movements are now largely determined by the speed of others rather than by our own internal timing mechanisms, and we must continually adjust our movements as the constraints imposed by the environment change. Our increasing reliance on sensory feedback to guide our movements becomes evident in these variable environments. As we will see in later chapters, the characteristics of the environment in which a motor skill will ultimately be performed influence the type of instructional strategies used during the early stages of learning. It is therefore extremely important that physical educators and therapists carefully consider whether the environment in which the skill will ultimately be performed is stable or variable when they plan physical education lessons or treatment programs.

The level of motor control required varies according to whether the performance environment is stable or variable.

# Summary

The purpose of this chapter has been to provide the reader with a general understanding of both the cognitive processes involved in the planning and execution of movement and some of the neurological areas and/or structures that appear to play an important role in the planning and execution of action. For the purposes of the discussion, we assumed that a set of functional neuromotor task systems, distributed throughout the CNS, work cooperatively to produce coordinated action in response to an internally generated goal and/or to changes occurring in the environment.

The primary neuromotor task systems believed to contribute to the planning and execution of goal-directed actions were identified as the limbic system, which drives our desire to act; the association cortex, which is involved in the early development of the "best" perceived plan of action; the projection system, which provides the specific movement dynamics for the action plan; and the spinal system, which is ultimately responsible for the spatial and temporal aspects of execution.

During the planning process, communication among the various neural task systems is made possible by a rich network of feedback loops that also help the performer determine whether the action being planned or executed matches the original goal. The coordinated movements that emerge are ultimately produced by muscle response synergies that comprise groups of muscles constrained to act as functional units of action. This type of organization greatly simplifies the planning process and also provides for greater flexibility of action.

The flow of information through the CNS is strongly influenced by the nature of the environmental context in which the action is to occur. Whereas stable environments impose lower demands in terms of the level of motor control required to plan and execute the prescribed movements, acting in more unpredictable or variable environments requires greater motor control. Variable environments also lead to increased dependence on sensory feedback to guide the action.

The moment-to-moment control of movement is made possible by the activity of a variety of spinal system mechanisms that link the spinal cord with the muscles involved in the action (the spinal stretch reflex and the gamma reflex loop) and with other systems within the CNS itself (e.g., long-loop reflexes). In addition to these mechanisms, the anatomical and mechanical properties of the human system can be exploited to minimize the level of control required of the CNS. These properties determine not only the amount of force one can generate in a given movement, but also the efficiency with which it can be completed.

As learning progresses, the relationship between the performer, the task, and the environment is continually redefined until the observable behavior perfectly matches the goal of the movement and the constraints of the surrounding environment. A number of theorists aligned with the dynamical and ecological systems approaches to motor control believe that this redefining of the performer–environment relationship is achieved through repeated experimentation and exploration of the perceptual–motor workspace.

## IMPORTANT TERMINOLOGY

After completing this chapter, readers should be familiar with the following terms and concepts.

akinesia
alpha–gamma coactivation
alpha motoneuron
apraxia
association cortex
ataxia
bradykinesia
central pattern generator (CPG)
cognitive set
contralateral
corticospinal tract (pyramidal tract)
decussate
dyskinesia
excitation–contraction coupling
festinating gait
Fitts' Law
fusimotor neuron
gamma motoneuron
gamma reflex loop
hyperkinetic
hypokinetic
Hoffman reflex (H-reflex)
hypotonia
Index of Movement Difficulty (ID)
interneuron
ipsilateral
lateral brainstem system

limbic system
medial brainstem system
motor ability
motor unit
motor set
muscle spindle
musculoskeletal system
neuromuscular junction
paresis
premotor area
primary motor area
projection system
rate coding
reciprocal innervation
reticulospinal tract
rubrospinal tract
size principle
skeletomotor neuron
spinal stretch reflex (SSR)
spinal system
stable environment
supplementary motor area
tectospinal tract
tremor
variable environment
vestibulospinal tract

## SUGGESTED FURTHER READING

Krakauer, J., & Ghez, C. (2000). Voluntary movement. In E. R. Kandel, J. H. Schwartz, & T. M. Jessell (Eds.), *Principles of Neural Science* (4th ed., pp. 756–781). New York: McGraw-Hill.

MacKay-Lyons, M. (2002). Central pattern generation of locomotion: A review. *Physical Therapy, 82,* 69–83.

## TEST YOUR UNDERSTANDING

1. Identify the functional neural task system involved in each of the following cognitive processes associated with the planning and execution of action:
   a. Formulation of a general plan of action
   b. Control and regulation of movements in progress
   c. Application of movement dynamics to a general action plan
   d. Decision to act

2. Briefly describe how the cognitive processes described in question 1 are accomplished by the functional neural task systems identified.

3. Identify the specific functions that the basal ganglia and cerebellum appear to serve in the planning and execution of action.

4. Identify the specific function(s) of the three motor cortical areas in the planning and/or control of movements.

5. Briefly describe the two-step process known as excitation–contraction coupling.

6. Explain how the muscle spindle is involved in the automatic regulation of muscle length. Provide a real-world example to illustrate your response.

7. Describe the two mechanisms used to generate the appropriate amount of force in a muscle.

8. Briefly describe the musculoskeletal contributions to muscle force.

9. Describe the role(s) played by the gamma reflex loop in the subconscious control of movement. Provide a real-world example to explain how this loop operates.

10. Identify the three variables that are known to constrain how an action is produced. Provide a real-world example that illustrates how each variable can influence the type of action produced.

11. Briefly describe how neurological disorders in the following structures or areas within the CNS are likely to affect an individual's motor control:
    a. Basal ganglia
    b. Cerebellum
    c. Primary motor area
    d. Premotor area
    e. Descending motor pathways

12. Identify the major pathways responsible for transmitting the dynamics of movement to the spinal system. How do the functions of these cortical and subcortical pathways differ?

13. Describe two ways in which the decision-making process is simplified.

## PRACTICAL ACTIVITIES

1.  In order to better understand how certain features of a task influence motor performance, we have constructed a small experiment for you to try that is based on Fitts' Law. First, you will need to draw each of the three sets of targets illustrated below on a sheet of paper with the following specifications:

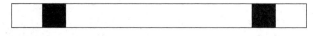

Target size: 2" diameter          Distance  between targets: 6"

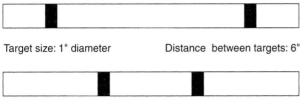

Target size: 1" diameter          Distance between targets: 6"

Target size: 1" diameter          Distance between targets: 3"

Second, on the basis of your knowledge of Fitts' Law, try to predict on which set of targets you will be able to complete the most and least taps within a 20-second time period. Write down your predictions on a piece of paper and put it aside.

Now that you have made your predictions, let's begin the actual experiment. Using a pen or pencil, begin tapping each target in a back and forth motion, continuously alternating between right and left targets for 20 seconds without stopping. (A partner can time you using a stopwatch for the duration of the trial.) Count the number of target taps you complete within the 20 seconds, and divide the number into 20 seconds to obtain your average movement time. For example, if you were able to complete 26 taps in 20 seconds then your average movement time would be $26 \div 20 = 1.3$ taps per second. After you complete your 20-second trial, switch with your partner so that he or she can be the study participant and you the timer. This will allow you to rest between trials and also to observe each other's performance on the different pairs of targets.

When you have each completed all three 20-second trials, compare your actual movement times across the three sets of targets to the predictions you made prior to the start of the experiment. On the basis of what knowledge did you make your predictions? Were your predictions correct? A quick review of our earlier discussion of Fitts' Law may help you make better predictions.

2.  Now that you have learned how the different sensory systems and the motor system contribute to the planning and execution of action, let's see if you can put it all together by describing what happens at a neurological level in the following movement scenarios:
    a. Standing upright against gravity with the eyes open
    b. Walking along a busy street

    Write your thoughts down on paper, and compare them with other students in a small group. Don't forget to consider how the sensory *and* motor systems contribute to the action you are describing.

# 6

# INTRODUCTION
# TO MOTOR LEARNING

*Motor learning is a process that depends on the movement skill to be learned,*
*the conditions under which it is to be learned, and the learner.*

## CHAPTER OBJECTIVES

After studying this chapter, you should be able to:

- Define and explain what is meant by the term *motor learning*.

- Explain the motor learning–motor performance distinction and why the former must be inferred from the latter.

- Provide examples of motor performance changes that do and do not qualify as evidence that motor learning occurred.

- Explain closed-loop, schema, and ecological theories of motor learning.

- Describe what happens as learners go through the stages of motor learning.

- Explain how developmental level, learning style, and motivation influence the readiness to learn.

Do you ever find yourself wondering how expert performers are able to control their body movements so effortlessly? Whether they are leaping across a stage, dribbling a basketball down court, or twisting and turning through a set of uneven parallel bars, these performers appear to direct very little attention to the mechanics of the performance. Their seemingly automatic behavior is in stark contrast to that of novice performers who are learning their first dance routine or the fundamental ballhandling skills necessary to play basketball. The movements of novice performers usually demand a considerable amount of physical and mental effort as they attempt to discover how the skill should be performed to achieve a certain movement goal.

Many thousands of hours of instruction and skill-specific practice separate novice and expert performers as they learn to "solve" the motor problem at hand. In observing the learning process one is often struck by the variety of solutions that are found to achieve a particular movement goal. Despite the fact that a group of learners often observe the same model perform the skill, receive the same type of instruction, and are provided with similar opportunities to practice, very few of these individuals appear to learn and/or perform the skill in the same way. This is not surprising when one considers the differences in the performers. They vary physically in height, weight, limb length, muscle strength, and flexibility, as well as in their cognitive and perceptual abilities.

The combined influence of the many performer-related differences that are evident, coupled with the changing constraints of the environment in which a given skill is first learned, ensures that the learning process remains challenging for both learner and instructor. We will begin exploring the many facets of the learning process by considering a number of theories that have been advanced to explain *how* the learning of motor skills is accomplished. Starting with this theory-based discussion will help us better understand *why* certain instructional strategies are used to foster learning in applied settings and why the learning environment is manipulated differently throughout the learning process. This discussion of the various learning-related theories will be followed by an account of *what* changes we can expect to observe in the learner at various points along the learning continuum. We can then use the knowledge gleaned from these descriptions to determine *when* to apply certain instructional strategies or, perhaps, alter the learning environment to enhance the learning process.

## Defining Motor Learning

Definitions of **motor learning** vary among scholars, but most agree that motor learning is a function of (a) the movement skill to be learned, (b) the learner, and (c) the conditions under which the learning takes place. Motor learning depends on the nature of the movement skill to be learned, including its meaningfulness and difficulty level. Motor learning also is a function of the learner's personal qualities, such as his or her emotional, physical, and intellectual developmental level; background of prior experiences, including previously learned knowledge and skills; motivation to learn; and learning style. Lastly, motor learning depends on the conditions under which the learning is to occur. These conditions include factors such as who is doing the teaching, how the teaching and practice is carried out, how emotionally supportive and constructive the atmosphere is for learning, how well the learner relates to and interacts with the practitioner directing the learning, and how conducive the equipment and facilities are for learning.

In spite of the differences in definition, today's scholars also agree that motor learning not only involves motor processes, but also perception-cognition-action processes. Whether trying to learn a new motor skill or reacquire one lost through injury (recovery of function), the learner actually searches for a solution by exploring the task to be learned and the environmental constraints or conditions under which the learning must take place. The task solution that emerges involves the reorganization of both the perception and action systems in relation to the task and conditions of learning. Indeed, the task solution that emerges is a new strategy for perceiving and acting (Newell, 1991).

Regardless of the differences among definitions, most of them attempt to distinguish between the types of movement performance changes with their associated antecedents (a) that *do* qualify as evidence for motor learning, and (b) that *do not* qualify as evidence for motor learning. Most definitions of motor learning attempt to distinguish between types of movement changes because not all changes in movement performance reflect learning. The following definition is offered as an example of how to distinguish between the types of changes and their correlated antecedents that *do* and *do not* qualify as motor learning:

*Motor learning is a process by which the capability for producing movement performance and the actual movement performance are reliably changed through instruction, practice, and/or experience.*

As with other definitions, this definition is provisional and not formally satisfactory due to the number of terms that are not operationally defined. However, it will serve as a basis for elaborating on exactly what we mean by the term *motor learning*.

## Motor Learning Is Inferred from Performance

It is important to understand that motor learning is a process that takes place within the learner and therefore cannot be directly observed. We cannot readily see the process by which the capability for producing movement performance is reliably changed. The process that takes place to change the capability for producing movement performance lies *within* the learner. Moreover, although numerous changes occur within the nervous system infrastructure as a result of learning (for example, level of neuronal activation, synaptic efficiency, cortical reorganization), ordinarily we cannot easily see these changes taking place in humans either. What can be directly observed are reliable changes in the actual movement performance that result from learning. Thus, **movement performance** (the act of executing or performing a movement skill) can be directly and easily observed—motor learning cannot. Consequently, whether motor learning has occurred or the extent to which it has occurred is inferred based on the extent of change that is directly observed in the learner's movement performance. This is the approach teachers of motor skills and physical therapists use most often to determine whether a particular instructional, rehabilitation, or training program or procedure has been successful in producing learning. These observable changes in movement performance can be documented over time and used to determine how far along the continuum a learner has progressed. As we will see later in this chapter (page 171), several theoretical models have been developed that eloquently describe the changes in the perception-cognition-action processes that occur with learning.

## Performance Is Not a Perfect Index of Motor Learning

Since motor learning must be inferred from changes in motor performance, they are not the same. Although changes in motor performance are our best indicator of the extent to which motor learning has taken place, it is not a perfect index of motor learning. The fact is that all observable changes in motor performance during or following acquisition in which instruction, practice, or training take place do not reflect motor learning. For example, suppose a learner is taught a handstand in gymnastics for the very first time and through practice is eventually able to perform it, albeit with questionable form and balance. It would be reasonable to infer that some learning took place because there was a change in the learner's movement performance, which in this case was an improvement in handstand performance. If the learner gradually improved his or her form and balance with continued practice, it would be reasonable to infer that further learning occurred because there were further changes or improvements in his or her movement performance. Thus, in this example the performance changes observed could be used as evidence to infer that learning had occurred.

> Motor performance is our best indicator of motor learning, but it is not perfect.

Another situation in which motor performance can be less than a perfect indicator of motor learning is when there is an absence of observable changes in motor performance during or following acquisition. For example, what if a learner is unable to perform the handstand that was taught and practiced during acquisition or was able to execute a crude version of the handstand following instruction and some initial practice but showed absolutely no improvement in handstand performance with continued practice? Indeed, it is possible that some learning took place but not enough to result in an observable change (improvement) in handstand performance. It is possible that the learner was engaged in a trial-and-error process during which different strategies for performing the handstand were being tried and, when found ineffective, they were eliminated. Thus, the learner was finding out that these strategies were ineffective in helping him or her perform the handstand, but such learning did not result in an observable improvement in performance. In this case it would be safer to conclude that if learning had occurred, there was no evidence of it in the movement performance that was observed. You see it is very easy to be mistaken when making an inference about whether learning has or has not occurred. Before we infer that little or no learning has occurred, we must be certain to take into account those variables that affect performance but do not affect learning.

> The motor learning process is not readily observable and therefore must be inferred from repeated observations of performance.

## Motor Learning Produces Reliable Performance Changes

Also very important to consider when making inferences about motor learning is how reliable or dependable the changes are as a result of instruction, practice, training, or experience. Changes in movement performance that are inconsistent or temporary (they don't persist over time on repeated attempts to execute the movement skill) would not be reliable and hence would not be evidence that motor learning had occurred. For changes in movement performance to qualify as evidence to infer that motor learning has occurred, the changes must be the result of practice or experience or instruction (antecedents) *and* be consistently demonstrated on repeated attempts to perform the motor skill. If the changes in performance are consistently repeated time after time, they would be considered highly reliable and serve as evidence to infer that what was learned was well learned. If the changes in performance are repeated less consistently on future attempts to perform the skill, they

> Motor learning produces durable changes in performance.

would be less reliable and suggest that, although some learning took place, it was not well learned. Thus, how well a movement is learned can be inferred by assessing the extent to which the movement performance changes are reliable and can be consistently repeated on future attempts to perform the skill.

So, at the behavioral level, reliable changes in motor performance emanate from motor learning, and these changes can be directly observed. Underlying these behavioral level changes are changes that take place at a neurological level. For example, there is evidence that through learning (a) the brain's chemistry is altered (for a review see Dunn, 1980), (b) the cortical representations of body parts involved in the learning are changed (Pascual-Leone, Grafman, & Hallet, 1994), and (c) morphological (structural) changes in the central nervous system occur (Glickstein & Yeo, 1989). These changes include increased dendritic branching, an increase in the number of synaptic connections between neurons, and structural alterations to pathways entering and leaving certain areas and/or structures within the nervous system. In addition to these structural changes, a number of functional changes can also be observed within the nervous system. These may lead to changes in the nature or prominence of the roles played by certain neurological subsystems as control strategies used to coordinate movement are altered (Brooks, 1986). Research also suggests that certain reflexive pathways are altered as a function of learning (Fournier & Pierrot-Deseilligny, 1989; Wolpaw & Carp, 1990). Although much more research is needed to fully identify and understand all of the changes that take place at the neurological level as one learns, it is clear that they form the basis for the reliable changes we readily observe at the behavioral level.

## Motor Learning May Not Lead to Performance Improvement

Motor learning can lead to improvement or deterioration in performance.

We expect the reliable changes in performance to be in the form of consistent improvements in movement technique or outcome, but it is important to understand that the changes could be consistent errors in movement technique or outcome. When learning a motor skill, we can learn incorrect movement techniques as well as correct movement techniques because learning is indifferent with regard to correctness. If we are taught and/or practice incorrect movement techniques we will learn them just as well as correct movement techniques. How often have you heard a learner say, "the more I practice the worse I seem to get" or "I've practiced and played this game for years, and I don't seem to get any better—in fact, I think I'm getting worse!" How often have you heard a teacher or coach say that someone is getting worse instead of better? These individuals are learning, but they are learning the wrong things. The process of learning does not select only the correct things to acquire and automatically filter out the incorrect things that should not be acquired. Such filtering is usually done by a teacher, coach, trainer, or physical therapist who is responsible for directing the learning. That is why we often see individuals who taught themselves new motor skills (such as those found in sport) seeking instruction from teachers later on in an attempt to relearn those skills the correct way. If we want learning to lead to improvement we must be taught the correct way and practice or train the correct way.

## Motor Learning and Instruction, Practice, and/or Experience

To qualify as evidence that motor learning occurred, the reliable movement performance changes observed must be the result of antecedents such as instruction, practice, and/or experience. These changes cannot be the result of maturation or temporary states of the learner that are caused by variables such as fatigue, motivation, or drugs. Clearly, developmental, motivational, and fitness training antecedents promote movement performance changes, but such changes do not qualify as evidence for learning. The reliable movement performance changes we see when a child develops the capability to crawl, walk, skip, and jump cannot be solely attributed to motor learning because developmental readiness factors also significantly contributed to these changes. No amount of instruction, practice, or experience in teaching a child to walk will get him or her to learn to walk until the neuromuscular infrastructure has developed properly. More will be said about developmental readiness for motor learning later in this chapter. Motivation, fitness training, and drug-related changes in movement performance are usually temporary and unreliable and therefore would not qualify as evidence that motor learning has taken place.

> Motor learning occurs as a function of instruction, practice, and/or experience.

For example, if an individual completes a two-month fitness program designed to improve cardiovascular endurance, muscle strength, and overall flexibility, we expect to see discernible changes in performance. However, if this individual does not continue to maintain or increase his or her level of training, then performance can be expected to decline. This deterioration does not occur when a skill has been learned.

It will become clear in Chapter 9, when we discuss how best to organize the practice environment, that it is not only the amount of practice that determines how well a skill is learned, but also how that practice is varied by the instructor or therapist. In general, practice influences such things as the type and quality of decisions made by the performer, the dynamics of the emerging coordination pattern, and how well the performer is able to exploit the performance environment.

## Theories of Motor Learning

A fundamental assumption associated with traditional motor learning theories is that learning is characterized by the development of an appropriate memory representation of the acquired skill. These representations are then used to guide performance, the specific movement parameters being prescribed according to the goal of the movement. Two theories that foster this assumption are the **closed-loop theory** of motor learning developed by Adams (1971) and Schmidt's (1975) **schema theory.** Indeed, a considerable amount of research conducted in the area of motor learning has been devoted to testing the predictions set forth in each of these theoretical frameworks.

The assumption that the development of some sort of representation is the end product of learning runs counter, however, to another approach that has emerged. This alternative view of motor learning, known as the ecological theory of perception and action (Gibson, 1966, 1979; Turvey, 1974, 1977; Fowler & Turvey, 1978), dismisses the need for discrete representations of action and focuses on the changing relationship between the learner and the environment in which the learning takes place. Let's examine the basic tenets of each of these theories as they are related to the acquisition of skills within the motor domain. Their respective contributions to our present level of understanding of motor skill learning will also be discussed.

## Adams' Closed-Loop Theory

Adams' closed-loop theory relied heavily on feedback to guide learning.

Perhaps the first contemporary theory developed to describe how simple movements are learned was advanced by Adams (1971). In an attempt to overcome what he perceived to be the shortcomings of earlier, open-loop accounts of motor behavior, Adams set about developing a theory of motor learning that relied heavily on the availability of feedback to guide the learning of a motor skill. Contrary to the assumptions of open-loop theories, Adams argued that feedback was necessary to guide each performance attempt during the early stages of learning and that it also served as an important source for the detection and correction of errors in performance. Adams' closed-loop theory was predicated on the complementary operations of two distinct memory states. The first of these, called the **memory trace,** was responsible for selecting and initiating a given plan of action. The **perceptual trace** then served as a comparator mechanism, comparing the movement in progress with a correct memory of the movement. Adams considered the strengthening of these two distinct memory states central to the learning of a given motor skill.

Adams' theory stimulated a number of research investigations designed to test his two-state memory system (Adams & Goetz, 1973; Christina & Anson, 1981; Christina & Merriman, 1977; Newell, 1974; Schmidt & White, 1972). Although a number of these studies provided support for the theory, its value as a comprehensive theory of learning was considered limited. This perceived shortcoming was based on the overuse of slow, linear-positioning movements to test the various predictions associated with the theory. These slower movements were not considered sufficiently representative of the full range of movements possible.

The results of a number of deafferentation studies (Lashley, 1917; Taub & Berman, 1968) also proved difficult to reconcile by using Adams' theory. As you will recall from our earlier discussions of the various motor control theories in Chapter 1, animals and humans deprived of all sensory feedback are still able to accomplish a variety of movements. Given the central role played by feedback, Adams' closed-loop theory cannot account for this ability to perform movements in its absence.

## Schmidt's Schema Theory

In addition to the troublesome empirical findings outlined in the preceding discussion, Schmidt (1975) identified two further theoretical problems associated with Adams' closed-loop theory of motor learning. The first of these problems was related to storage. That is, how is it possible to store a mental representation for every movement ever performed? Surely we would exceed the capacity of human memory at some point. The second problem was related to an individual's ability to perform quite accurately what appear to be novel skills: movements not previously observed or physically attempted. Adams' theory provides no mechanism to explain how skills not previously experienced could be initially performed. These apparent shortcomings of Adams' theory inspired Schmidt to develop an alternative theory of learning. This new theory of motor learning came to be known as schema theory (see Figure 6.1 on page 174).

Although schema theory retained the need for two independent memory states, the *recall* and *response recognition* schemas proposed by Schmidt were less rigidly conceived and therefore better able to account for a learner's ability to acquire a broad range of movement skills. Like Adams' memory trace, Schmidt's **recall schema** was involved in producing a movement by being responsible for selection of the parameter values that specified that particular movement. Examples of these movements are throwing a ball using an overarm as opposed to underarm pattern or climbing a flight of stairs with different stair riser heights. Once these values were selected and the movement executed, it became the responsibility of the **response recognition schema** to evaluate the correctness of the completed movement in terms of both the amount and the direction of errors. Schmidt further hypothesized that as the learner continued to practice and receive feedback from his or her own sensory mechanisms and other external sources, the strength of both schemas would be enhanced.

In addition to the two schemas, a core feature of Schmidt's theory was the **generalized motor program (GMP),** an abstract memory structure that could be prepared in advance of a movement. This mechanism provided the means by which a specific movement was executed. It was thought to contain the temporal and spatial patterns of muscle activity needed to accomplish a given movement. Thus, the GMP played a particularly important role in the execution of ballistic movements, where the opportunity to use feedback to guide the movement was limited or nonexistent. Although Adams argued that his memory trace was, in essence, a form of motor program, it operated only long enough to initiate the movement (e.g., a few milliseconds). In contrast, Schmidt's generalized motor program was capable of operating much longer (e.g., one or more seconds) and therefore was not dependent on feedback or on the response recognition schema to complete certain movements.

How were the recall and response recognition schemas thought to be developed? According to schema theory, their development was contingent on the learner's ability to extract four important pieces of information from every performance. These were the initial conditions associated with the movement (such as body position, characteristics of the object being thrown or held), the specific movement parameters or response specifications chosen (for example, force, velocity), the sensory consequences emerging from the actual performance of the movement (such as how the movement felt), and the movement's outcome.

Once each individual piece of the movement puzzle was extracted from the performance, the learner would begin to put the pieces together, relating certain individual pieces to others. For example, the relationship between the initial conditions and the particular movement parameters selected was thought to contribute to the development of the recall schema, whereas the response recognition schema's development was assumed to be based more on

The GMP is thought to contain the spatial and temporal patterns of muscle activity needed to perform a given movement.

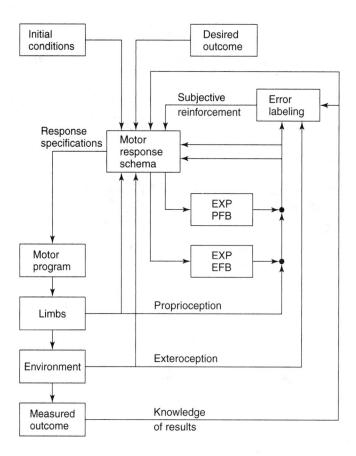

**Figure 6.1**   Schmidt's schema theory of discrete motor learning. The motor response schema (recall and recognition schemas are combined for clarity) is shown in relation to events occurring within a movement trial.

Abbreviations: EXP PFB = expected proprioceptive feedback; EXP EFB = expected exteroceptive feedback.

*Source:* Schmidt, R. A. (1975). A schema theory of discrete motor skill learning. *Psychological Review, 82,* 225–260.

the relationships among the initial conditions, the movement's outcome, and the sensory consequences generated (Schmidt, 1982b, 1988b). Once these relationships were abstracted, certain rules or principles of operation could be formulated and used to guide selection of the appropriate motor program for action.

Although interest in schema theory as an all-encompassing account of motor skill acquisition has largely waned, certain theoretical constructs emerging from the theory have endured. These constructs continue to be extensively studied by a number of motor learning researchers. Two of the more often investigated aspects of schema theory are the generalized motor program (Magill & Hall, 1990) and the variability-of-practice hypothesis (Bird & Rikli, 1983; Gabriele, Hall, & Buckholz, 1987). Schmidt argued that learning was not only dependent on how much a skill was practiced, but also how the skill being practiced was varied. The variability-of-practice hypothesis has received a considerable amount of research attention in the past 20 years. At this time, however, the predictions associated with the hypothesis have yet to be unequivocally supported. See Van Rossum (1990) for a comprehensive review of research on the variability of practice.

## Ecological Theories of Perception and Action

The beginnings of an ecological approach to perception and action emerged with an influential set of papers written by Turvey and colleagues (Turvey, 1974; Turvey & Carello, 1988; Fowler & Turvey, 1978). In these studies, the authors outlined a new theory of motor learning that not only incorporated the major concepts described in Gibson's ecological theory of direct perception (Gibson, 1979), but also extended Bernstein's work (1967) in the area of movement coordination to the learning of motor skills. You may recall that Gibson and Bernstein provided the impetus for development of the dynamic systems framework of motor control that we described in Chapter 1. These two theories share a common theme: interaction between the performer and the dynamics of the environment in which she or he is moving. The ecological approach has therefore extended the ideas embodied within the dynamic systems approach to a perceptual level of analysis.

In contrast to the more traditional motor learning theories developed by Adams and Schmidt, which describe the products of learning in terms of schemas or memory traces, the ecological theory of perception and action dismisses such memory-based explanations of learning. Central to the ecological approach to perception and action is the idea that the learner seeks to discover the lawful properties or invariant relationships between, among other things, the physical features of objects in the environment that make it possible to learn certain motor skills. Having discovered these properties, the learner becomes better able to generate a solution for any given movement problem that is encountered. Just as the dynamic systems approach focused on the interaction between performer and environment in the control of movement, the ecological approach emphasizes the changing relationship between the perceptions of the performer and the action environment in which the learning takes place.

In a review article contrasting the various theories of motor learning, Newell (1991) identifies two major weaknesses associated with the more traditional theories of motor learning. The first is their inability to explain how new patterns of coordination are learned. At best, schema-based accounts can only describe how modifications to existing patterns of movement are accomplished. The second weakness identified by Newell is the inability of traditional theories to account for the spontaneous compensations made in response to perturbations, or changes, that occur in the environment while a movement is in progress. Ecological approaches to motor learning appear better able to address this ability without resorting to elaborate cognitive processing or the

*Ecological theories emphasize the changing relationship between a performer's perceptions and the action environment.*

need for a preexisting reference of movement correctness (such as a memory trace or motor program).

Traditional motor learning theorists have countered the claims made by ecological theorists by pointing out certain perceived weaknesses of their own. Schmidt (1988a), the originator of schema theory and of the generalized motor program concept, argues that the role of the GMP has been misinterpreted by advocates of the ecological approach and that it is considerably more flexible and nonspecific in its function than ecological theorists imply. A second criticism of the ecological approach is that it places relatively little importance on the role of cognition during learning. In a review article addressing the controversy, Colley (1989) describes a number of movement scenarios in which some form of cognitive processing or mental representation is needed to guide the action. Certainly, it is difficult to imagine how we are capable of performing the appropriate actions in a variety of rule-based sports settings without resorting to a mental representation of some kind. For example, how does one know how to interact with an approaching soccer ball unless the conditional rules are already stored in memory? As we noted in Chapter 5, simply seeing the approaching soccer ball is insufficient to define the nature of the interaction.

Even though the basic tenets of the ecological approach have only just begun to be systematically applied to the acquisition of movement skills, a growing base of support for this new theoretical approach is building among the scientific community. At the very least, the emergence of this alternative approach to studying skill acquisition has renewed interest among researchers in better understanding how novel motor skills are learned. As was the case in our earlier discussion of the various theories advanced to explain how movements are controlled, it is unlikely that a single, all-encompassing theory of motor learning will emerge.

## How Does Motor Learning Really Occur?

In 2003, Schmidt reevaluated his schema theory and concluded that it has provided some useful insights into several aspects of movement skill learning. However, he also was quick to point out that schema theory has a number of deficiencies. Consequently, he called for the development of a new theory which would include many of the aspects of schema theory that are still viable and exclude or modify many of the other aspects to reflect new research evidence and thinking.

In another critical review of schema theory, Sherwood and Lee (2003) identified several of the deficiencies. Essentially, they found schema theory to be inconsistent with the research evidence in the areas of mental practice and observational learning (especially the evidence showing motor learning in the absence of movement), augmented feedback presentation, and variability and order of practice. Further, they provided a strong rationale for the importance of cognitive processes in motor skill learning. They argued that schema theory failed to adequately explain the role of cognitive processes and cognitive effort in motor learning. For instance, it did not explain how motor learning can be advanced without movement as has been demonstrated in the mental practice and observational learning literature.

In yet another critical review of schema theory, Newell (2003) contrasted schema theory with the ecological theories of perception and action, especially the muscle response synergies (coordinative structure) and dynamic systems perspectives. He pointed out that a major limitation of theories of motor learning such as closed-loop and schema theories is that they have tended to undervalue the importance of change in movement behavior over time in favor of the study of the amount of some averaged change in behavioral outcome. He argued that the muscle response synergies and dynamic systems approach to motor learning overcome this limitation because it directly relates to the problem of change in behavior over time. This approach holds that the change(s) in movement behavior and outcome that occur in action are actually manifestations of multiple time scales of change in a dynamical system. Thus, he envisions the time scales of change as being central to the development of a new theory of motor learning.

So how does motor skill learning really occur? Does it occur as proposed by Adams (1971) in his closed-loop theory or by Schmidt (1975), who developed the schema theory of motor learning? Alternatively, does Gibson's (1979) ecological theory of direct perception better explain the observable changes in movement performance as a motor skill is learned? More specifically, do learners always have to cognitively process information in elaborate ways and develop cognitive representations (e.g., generalized motor programs) when they learn to execute movement skills? Is the execution of these skills dependent on cognitive representations that are controlled by brain centers at the top of the central nervous system hierarchy that direct lower centers to carry out the execution? Conversely, is it possible for people to learn to directly perceive the relevant information in the environment without the need for elaborate cognitive processing because it is immediately meaningful for the planning involved in executing movement skills? Does the execution of these skills depend on the availability of a particular motor program, or does it depend on the interaction of multiple subsystems (neurological, biological, musculoskeletal) with no one subsystem being capable of planning and controlling the movement's execution or having priority over another subsystem? The answers to these questions are still a matter of some uncertainty and will be the target of much debate among scholars for some years to come. Certainly, further research will be needed before the validity of the answers proposed by the different theories of motor learning can be ascertained.

However, if we were to speculate at this time based on the available evidence we would say that both motor programming and ecological models can operate at different times or in different situations when people are learning to perform movement skills. Clearly, there is sufficient evidence available to suggest that this is the case. What needs to be determined is when or in what context each one operates. For instance, it would be helpful for practitioners to know which environmental situations or types of skills demand elaborate cognitive processing of information and which ones allow for direct perception to operate. It also would be useful to know if the learner's developmental level and the stage of learning play a role in determining the extent to which elaborate cognitive processing and direct perception is used. By knowing this information, practitioners could construct conditions of learning that would be more appropriate for allowing elaborate cognitive processing of

Motor programming and dynamic systems models may operate at different times or in different contexts during motor learning.

information to operate and other conditions that would be more suitable for allowing direct perception to function.

Unfortunately, we do not know enough at this time about when or in what context each proposed theory of motor learning operates. This being the case, practitioners have little choice but to strive to provide instructional and practice conditions that allow learners the possibility to learn to perform movement skills by both elaborate cognitive processing of information and direct perception. In spite of this limitation of knowledge, both theories still provide us with very useful conceptualizations of how people learn to execute movement skills, which clearly enhance our understanding of the motor skill learning process. Each of these alternative theoretical accounts of how the learning of motor skills occurs will be discussed in more detail in a later section of this chapter.

## Stages of Motor Learning

Despite the fact that considerable controversy exists about which theory of motor learning best describes how motor skills are acquired, existing theories offer practitioners much help in understanding the nature of the learning process. One aspect of applying what we know about motor learning is of great practical significance: being able to describe the nature of the behavioral changes we can expect to see during various stages of the learning process. Fortunately, a number of useful models have been developed that eloquently describe the behavioral changes that accompany learning. We will consider three such models.

### Fitts' Three Stages of Learning

**The learner attempts to understand how to perform the movement skill during the cognitive phase.**

As early as 1964, a prominent researcher by the name of Paul Fitts identified three major stages of motor skill acquisition. The first, which Fitts called the **cognitive stage of learning,** is thought to be characterized by a learner's attempt to understand the nature of a particular motor skill using information from a variety of different sources. This information may be derived from watching a peer or instructor perform the skill, receiving verbal feedback from a coach who observes the learner practice the skill, or from attending to the learner's own sensory feedback generated through physical practice. Numerous errors that are quite gross in nature typically accompany performance during this stage, and learners can often be seen talking to themselves as they attempt to produce an appropriate movement pattern. Through a trial-and-error process, novice performers are beginning to discover both the kinematic (form) and the kinetic (force) properties that define the skill being learned.

As they enter the second stage of the learning process, learners begin to find it easier not only to detect errors in performance, but also to prescribe the appropriate solutions. Although the movement pattern is still not flawlessly reproduced, the learner who has entered the **intermediate,** or **associative stage,** is beginning to understand how the various components of the skill are interrelated. The learner also begins to modify and/or adapt the movement pattern as the movement situation demands. These abilities may be observed in the young tennis player who is able to direct her forehand stroke to different areas of the court because she better understands how the position of her body and the movement of her feet prior to ball contact can be altered to produce a different outcome. Similarly, a patient entering this phase of relearning during rehabilitation is capable of detecting errors and solving problems, independent of the therapist. Thus the use of facilitation techniques and/or manual guidance is counterproductive after the patient enters this second stage of learning.

The learner begins to modify and/or adopt the movement pattern as needed during the intermediate stage.

Once the learner has reached the **autonomous stage** of learning, the focus is on automatizing the movement pattern so that attention can be directed to other aspects of the performance. These aspects might include the position of other players on the court or the development of movement strategies that can be used to guide subsequent movements. Learners in this stage are now able to perform the necessary set of movements consistently in a variety of different movement situations. Errors become much less frequent during performance, and learning begins to slow during this stage, as the subtle changes necessary to improve performance become more difficult to master.

During the autonomous phase, movement execution becomes more automatic, and attention can be directed elsewhere.

It is also argued that the cognitive aspects of the performance are no longer accessible to the learner, who has largely given over control of the movement to other subsystems at lower levels within the central nervous system. The clinician should now be able to introduce distracters during the patient's treatment session. Ongoing conversations should be possible while the patient is performing a well-practiced task. The introduction of multiple tasks should also be possible if the patient has reached this level of learning. As O'Sullivan (1994) warns, however, many patients who have experienced traumatic head injuries affecting motor control will never reach this level of performance. They may perform consistently in very structured or stable environments, but any change that renders the environment more unstable or unpredictable often results in a dramatic deterioration in performance.

Although it remains difficult to know exactly when a learner is entering each of these **learning stages,** Fitts' description nicely illustrates how motor behavior changes as a function of instruction and/or practice. Thus it provides the teacher of motor skills with valuable observational clues from which to develop appropriate instructional strategies. This description of learning continues to appear in various instructional textbooks and literature read by instructors and therapists alike (Magill, 2001; Christina & Corcos, 1988; O'Sullivan & Schmitz, 1994).

## A Neo-Bernsteinian Perspective

A different view of the learning process has emerged in the writings of ecological theorists (Vereijken, van Emmerik, Whiting, & Newell, 1992). For want of a better label, we will call it the neo-Bernsteinian perspective. This perspective can be traced back to the writings of Bernstein (1967) in which he described the learning process in terms of "mastering redundant degrees of freedom" (p. 127). According to Bernstein, the learning of a motor skill can be likened to the solving of a problem, the problem being how best to harness the many degrees of freedom available in the human motor system (see Figure 6.2).

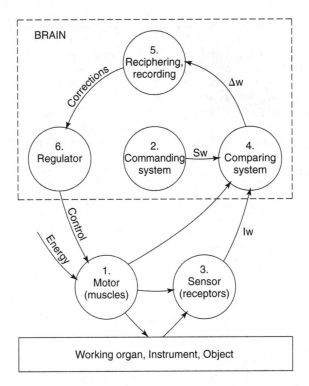

**Figure 6.2**  The simplest block diagram of an apparatus for the control of movements. (1) **Effector** (motor) activity, which is to be regulated along the given parameter; (2) a **control element,** which conveys to the system in one way or another the *required value* (Sw) of the parameter which is to be regulated; (3) a **receptor** that perceives the *factual course of the value(s)* of the parameter and signals it by some means to (4) a **comparator device,** which perceives the discrepancy between the *factual* and *required* values (Δw) with its magnitude and sign; (5) an **apparatus** that encodes the data provided by the comparator device into correctional impulses that are transmitted by feedback linkages to (6) a **regulator,** which controls the function of the *effector* along the given parameter.

During the novice stage, the learner simplifies the movement problem by "freezing out" some of the available degrees of freedom.

Combining the intuitive logic of Bernstein's early writings and the ideas embodied within an ecological framework, Vereijken (1991) proposed a three-stage model of learning that describes how the learner attempts to manipulate the dynamics of a movement in order to "solve" a given movement problem. During the **novice stage,** the learner simplifies the movement problem by "freezing out" a portion of the degrees of freedom. This reduction in the number of degrees of freedom is thought to be accomplished in two ways. The first involves keeping all joint angles in the body rigidly fixed throughout the movement, and the second involves temporarily constraining, or coupling, multiple joints so that they are forced to move almost in unison. Unfortunately, either solution results in a performance that is rigidly executed and unresponsive to changes in the action environment. One has only to observe the rigidly constrained swinging action of a novice batter attempting to hit a pitched ball to see how counterproductive these types of freezing out strategies are. See the highlight, How the Available Degrees of Freedom Are Manipulated and Influenced by the Goals of the Skill Being Learned, on page 183.

As learners move into the **advanced stage** however, they begin to reinstate degrees of freedom and/or release additional degrees of freedom. These released joints are now incorporated into larger functional units of action or, to use dynamic systems terminology, coordinative structures or muscle response synergies. During this advanced stage of learning, the dynamics of the action are becoming more apparent to learners as they begin to alter the kinematics associated with the movement. The relationship among the joints and their associated muscle synergies is altered, permitting some joints to continue to move in synchrony while others move independently of each other. The result is a more fluent performance that can be readily adapted to changes occurring in the action environment.

> During the advanced stage, the learner begins to reinstate and/or to release additional degrees of freedom.

Finally, Vereijken hypothesized that during the **expert stage** of learning, the learner continues to release additional degrees of freedom and reorganize others until all the degrees of freedom needed to accomplish the goal of the task have been manipulated in the most economical fashion. What differentiates this stage of learning from the previous one is the learner's ability not only to manipulate his or her own degrees of freedom, but also to exploit additional passive forces (such as inertia and friction) that are external to the learner but inherent in the movement situation. Thus the relationship between the learner's perception of what is required to solve the movement problem and the emerging dynamics of the resulting action is permanently redefined.

> The performer's ability to exploit additional passive forces that are external to him or her is evident during the expert stage.

## Gentile's Two-Stage Model

A third description of the learning process that warrants discussion was developed by Gentile (1972). Her description was originally intended to provide teachers of motor skills with a more cohesive account of motor skill acquisition than appeared in many of the motor learning textbooks available at that time. Gentile not only considers how the nature of the movement environment in which the task is to be performed influences the nature of the information a learner must acquire, but also provides a number of instructional strategies that a teacher can implement to facilitate a learner's progress through each stage. Our discussion in this chapter will be largely theoretical, but many of the practical strategies she describes in her working model will be incorporated in our discussions of practice and feedback in later chapters.

According to Gentile's model (see Figure 6.3 on page 182), the learner's goal during the first of two stages of learning is **getting the idea of the movement**—that is, discovering how the movement must be organized to accomplish a particular goal within the constraints of the movement environment. In order to accomplish this goal, however, the learner must identify and selectively attend to those aspects of the skill and environment that are directly relevant to the performance. Gentile referred to these relevant aspects as the **regulatory conditions** associated with the learning environment. In the case of a child attempting to catch a fly ball, for example, the regulatory conditions

> During the first stage, the learner must learn to identify and selectively attend to the regulatory conditions related to the movement.

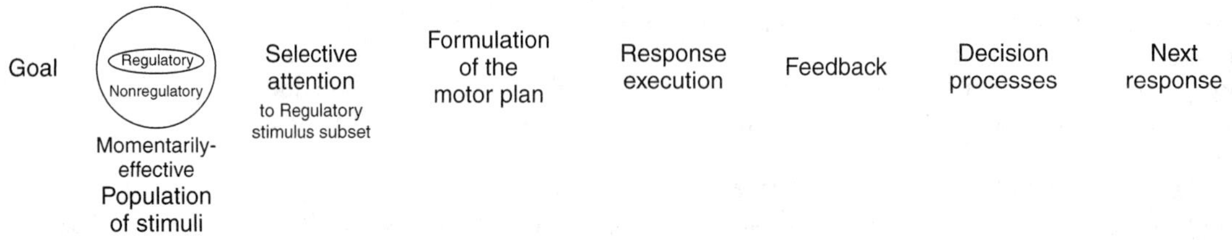

Goal ( Regulatory / Nonregulatory )    Selective attention to Regulatory stimulus subset    Formulation of the motor plan    Response execution    Feedback    Decision processes    Next response

Momentarily-effective Population of stimuli

**Figure 6.3**   The initial stage of Gentile's working model of skill acquisition. Motor learning involves at least two stages: the initial stage ("getting the idea of the movement") and the later stage ("fixation/diversification"). The initial stage is similar to Fitts' (1964) cognitive stage, and the later stage incorporates Fitts' associative and autonomous stages.

include the ball and its trajectory as it moves through space. These two characteristics determine how the performer organizes his or her movement pattern to reach the desired position in space at the appropriate time to interact successfully with the ball. How the performer then spatially orients the catching limb to position the glove hand to intercept the ball constitutes a second set of regulatory conditions to which the learner must selectively attend.

Getting the idea of the movement is often made more difficult for the learner by the fact that nonrelevant aspects of the environment often distract the performer from the task at hand. In order to accomplish the goal of the movement, the learner must ignore these nonrelevant or **nonregulatory conditions.** As we know from the developmental literature, however, this task is not an easy one for young children, who tend to be easily distracted from the goal by nonrelevant aspects (Thomas, 1984).

As the learner reaches the second stage of learning, described by Gentile (1972) as the **fixation/diversification stage,** the objective becomes matching the newly acquired movement pattern to the environment in which it is to be performed. If the environment is generally stable, the emphasis falls on making the movement pattern as consistent as possible on each successive attempt. For example, a performer attempting to learn a new dive from the tower and a gymnast learning a new floor routine are both operating in a stable environment and are therefore more concerned with developing a movement pattern that can be performed consistently on every attempt.

On the other hand, if the skill being learned is to be performed in a variable and often unpredictable environment, the primary goal for the learner is to learn to diversify the movement pattern so that it permits flexibility of action. This is certainly the goal for a soccer player, who must be able to pass the ball to other team members from stationary and moving positions and at a variety of different angles. Developing a flexible locomotor pattern is also the goal for a patient who is learning to walk again. After completing the initial stage of gait training using parallel bars and/or assistive devices, patients must learn to alter their gait pattern to accommodate changes in terrain, surface, and a number of obstacles or people moving along a crowded corridor or street. Although Gentile's working model was originally developed and

During the second stage, the learner attempts to match the newly acquired movement pattern to the performance environment.

## HIGHLIGHT

### How the Available Degrees of Freedom Are Manipulated and Influenced by the Goals of the Skill Being Learned

As you will recall from our discussion of the different stages of learning models on pages 178 to 181, the three-stage model of motor learning described by Vereijken (1991) proposes that learners in the novice stage attempt to simplify a movement problem by "freezing out" a portion of the degrees of freedom (e.g., joints, muscles). As the learners enter the advanced stage of learning, however, they begin to reinstate the frozen degrees of freedom and even release additional degrees of freedom. Finally, in the expert stage, learners continue to release and reorganize the degrees of freedom while also learning to exploit additional external forces (such as inertia and surface friction) that are inherent in the learning environment.

In recent years, researchers have begun to challenge this single-path view of motor learning, largely because of its failure to adequately consider how the goals of the skill to be learned might influence the learning process. Ko, Challis, and Newell (2003) recently tested the neo-Bernsteinian perspective by having young adults learn how to maintain upright balance on a force platform that was moving sinusoidally in a forward and backward direction. The authors speculated that an alternative pattern of change as it related to controlling the available degrees of freedom would occur due to the nature of the skill to be learned and the environment in which it was to be learned (in this case, a moving support surface).

As the authors predicted, the results of their experiment were not in agreement with Bernstein's (1967) original ideas related to how the degrees of freedom would be manipulated in each of the three stages of learning. Instead, Ko and colleagues found that the way in which the learners manipulated the available degrees of freedom was actually reversed in the first two stages. In contrast to Bernstein's predictions, their subjects actually released degrees of freedom in the early stage of learning while suppressing previously released degrees of freedom as learning progressed. Moreover, the authors also discovered, at least for their dynamic balance task, that the process of exploiting or utilizing external forces began much earlier in the learning process than previously described. The subjects in this study were learning to exploit the reactive forces related to the moving support surface at the same time they were learning to manipulate the available degrees of freedom.

The findings of this study serve to remind us that the pathway to skill acquisition may not always follow the same route but instead may take many different routes based on the characteristics of the learner (e.g., age, previous movement experiences, motor abilities), the goal(s) of the skill to be learned, and the environment in which the skill is to be learned.

applied to the teaching of motor skills in physical education settings, she has extended many of the ideas embodied in this early model to the physical therapy domain (Gentile, 1987).

## Benefits of the Three Models of Motor Learning

The three descriptions of learning that we have just discussed enhance our knowledge of the learning process in a number of ways. Whereas Fitts helps us better understand the nature of the cognitive and behavioral processes that characterize a learner's progression through the various stages of learning, Vereijken explores the changing relationship between the learner's perception and the dynamics of the action environment that contribute to the learning process. In so doing, she links the learner to the environment in which the learning is taking place. Gentile adopts a similar approach in her working model of skill acquisition by also considering how the nature of the environment in which the skill is ultimately to be performed influences the goals to be achieved by the learner. This is particularly evident in her description of the second stage of learning. Gentile's application of the model's theoretical constructs to the development of instructional strategies for use in applied settings also distinguishes her model from those developed by Fitts and Vereijken.

In addition to offering insights into the learning process from a theoretical standpoint, these three different models provide the practitioner with a multilevel perspective on the learning process. They illuminate the changing nature of the cognitive processes used by the learner and also address the dynamics of action we can expect to see at various points in the learning process. Vereijken and Gentile, in particular, stress the important role played by the environment in which the skill is to be learned. Only by considering the individual in the context of the learning environment can we truly understand *all* the variables that contribute to learning. Armed with this knowledge, the practitioner can begin to manipulate the learning environment in a way that fosters optimal learning.

# Readiness for Motor Learning

How ready people are to learn different motor skills and the rate at which they will learn them greatly depends on how developed their various unique personal qualities are at the time of learning. Some of the more important qualities include the following:

- *Emotions*—the ability to direct and control one's feelings so that they are appropriate for learning the skill.
- *Intelligence*—the ability to appropriately analyze, problem solve, and make appropriate decisions in learning the skill.
- *Capabilities*—the prerequisite abilities, skills, and knowledge that must be in place in order to learn the skill.
- *Previous Experiences*—the extent and quality of prior experiences that can be used to enhance the learning of the skill.
- *Physical Characteristics*—strength, speed, endurance, physical condition, flexibility, body build, and any physical limitations that can affect learning the skill.

Although conditions can be identified that will affect many learners in a similar way, there is a need to understand those personal qualities that differ from learner to learner and that are of major importance in determining motor skill learning. In this section we will learn about some of these personal qualities and how they can influence motor learning. These personal qualities are discussed under the headings of developmental qualities (that is, those found in growing children), learning styles, and motivational qualities.

# Developmental Qualities

Readiness to learn a motor skill largely depends on the child's level of development. The level a child reaches at a particular chronological age depends on the combined influences of heredity and environment. Heredity provides the basic potential for the learner's development, but the appropriate experiences are needed for that potential to be realized. A child's level of development mainly depends on three factors:

1.  prior experiences, including his or her background of previously learned knowledge and skills;
2.  the traits with which he or she is hereditarily endowed; and
3.  the rate at which these traits unfold, which is his or her maturation rate.

**Developmental readiness** for learning various motor skills does not occur simply because a child gets older. Nor does it occur without appropriate accompanying experiences. It results from an interaction between a child's heredity potential and life experiences. According to a position statement of the National Association for Sport and Physical Education (1995), the age-related developmental changes we see in children as they learn have the following seven characteristics:

1.  *Change is quantitative.* The amount of change in performance is measurable. For example, children tend to throw farther, run faster, and jump higher as they get older, and these performance changes can be measured.
2.  *Change is qualitative.* Inherent in the performance change is a degree of skillfulness or excellence. For example, children tend to perform skill movement patterns more proficiently as they get older.
3.  *Change is sequential.* Movement skills develop in an orderly sequence from simple to complex. For example, children walk before they run.
4.  *Change is cumulative.* Previously acquired movement patterns, experiences, or skills form the foundation for later emerging skills. For example, walking forms the foundation for running.
5.  *Change is directional.* Children's motor skill performance tends to progress toward some goal such as greater proficiency or adaptability. However, it also can regress and become less proficient or adaptable. In either case, there is directionality to the performance change.
6.  *Change is multivariable.* Performance change is the result of many variables acting together. For instance, a child can perform a one-footed hop when he or she has the strength, balance, perceptual capabilities, and motivation to do so. Its emergence is not the result of any one of these personal qualities but emanates from interactions among all of them. Also the rate of performance change may be constrained by a lack of progress in one or more of these qualities.
7.  *Change is individual.* Although the rate of change differs among children, the general sequence of change is the same for everyone. For example, many children have acquired the developmental sequence of galloping, hopping, and skipping by five years of age, but other children may be six years old before acquiring skipping, which is the last locomotor skill

Readiness to learn a motor skill largely depends on a child's level of development, which is influenced by heredity and environment.

in the sequence. Change emerges from many different personal qualities that come together in various ways at various times for different children, who themselves are changing in very special ways.

All children will tend to follow a predictable pattern of motor development that progressively proceeds from the simple to the complex. However, the rate of development will differ considerably among children, which is one reason why all children are not ready to learn the same motor skill at the same age. Some children demonstrate successes in learning and performing motor skills sooner than others. However, early learning and performance successes do not necessarily provide a valid index for predicting later successes. As children grow and develop, their bodies change with respect to size and shape. These changes are accompanied by unpredictable changes in ability. Some children who excel in motor skill learning and performance early on do not excel much as they get older. Conversely, some children who do not excel early do excel more as they get older. For instance, it is not uncommon for a child who experiences learning and performance difficulties early on, but who remains deeply interested in a sport, to later blossom into a skillful athlete.

## Learning Styles

Two major theories were advanced in the twentieth century in an attempt to interpret human differences and design educational models to accommodate these differences. Learning-style theory has its roots in the psychoanalytic community, whereas multiple intelligences theory emanated from cognitive science. Essentially, learning styles are concerned more with differences in the process of learning, and multiple intelligences focus more on the content and products of learning. Learning-style theory began with Carl Jung (1927) who noted major differences in the way people perceived, the way they made decisions, and how active or reflective they were while interacting. Subsequently, scholars have concluded that people have different learning styles, which can affect their readiness for learning.

**Learning styles** may be defined as the various ways that people would set about to learn new motor skills or knowledge if "they were in charge" of the learning. People can learn in different ways, but they prefer to learn in certain ways. Each person develops a relatively unique learning style that has certain advantages and disadvantages. By trying to understand a person's learning style, a teacher or therapist is in a better position to individualize his or her instruction or therapy program and make learning effective and efficient for that person.

Over the years, experts in the field of education have identified various student learning styles. Although these learning styles differ somewhat, there are commonalities among them. It is beyond the scope of this book to examine all of the different learning styles that have been identified, but it would be useful to examine a couple of them to provide examples. Reissman (1977), for instance, proposed three principal styles of learning: *visual (watching), aural (listening),* and *physical (performing).* Although all students will use all three styles at various times when learning new knowledge or motor skills, they appear to rely more on one style, especially early in learning a new skill or perhaps when first trying to make corrections in a previously acquired skill.

---

*All children follow a predictable pattern of motor development, but the rate of development differs among them.*

*People can learn in different ways, but they prefer to learn in certain ways.*

For example, some students seem to learn best by spending more time watching demonstrations of how a new skill or correction should be performed and perhaps visually imaging what they saw. Others prefer to concentrate more on the verbal description/discussion of how the new skill or correction should be performed, often making use of auditory cues or figurative explanations. Still others appear to learn most effectively by focusing more on trying to physically perform the new skill or correction immediately from the outset.

McCarthy (1987) described four learner styles:

- *Dynamic.* They prefer to learn by trial and error and by self-discovery. They prefer to experience variety and flexibility when learning. They tend to be risk-takers, ignore authority, are at ease with others, adventurous, intuitive or insightful thinkers, and synthesizers of information.
- *Innovative.* They prefer to learn through social interaction, discussion, and personal involvement. They tend to be divergent thinkers, idea people, innovative, imaginative, cooperative, and sociable.
- *Common sense.* They prefer security when learning and tend to learn by doing and having hands-on experience. They enjoy solving problems, knowing how things work, and having or making real-life applications. They tend to be prudent and judicious thinkers.
- *Analytic.* They prefer to learn in traditional instructional environments and desire recognition. They tend to be logical and intellectual rather than emotional thinkers and place emphasis on personal control. They tend to seek facts, collect data, separate entities into their component parts or constituent elements, and be systematic when learning.

When these four learning styles are combined with Kolb's (1985) cycle of learning (see Figure 6.4 on page 188) we find that both dynamic and common sense learners tend to rely on active experimentation (doing). However, dynamic learners prefer concrete experience (feeling) and common sense learners prefer abstract conceptualization (thinking). Both innovative and analytic learners prefer to use reflective observation (watching); but innovative learners prefer concrete experience, whereas analytic learners prefer abstract conceptualization (thinking).

Although learning-style theorists interpret the personality in various ways, most models have two things in common. First, learning-style models tend to concern themselves with the process of learning, especially in terms of how people absorb and think about information and evaluate the results. Second, learning-style theorists generally believe that learning is the result of a personal, individualized act of thought and feeling. Most theorists appear to have agreed upon the following four basic learning styles (Silver, Strong, & Perini, 1997):

- **Mastery style learner.** This style learner takes in information concretely, processes it sequentially in a step-by-step fashion, and evaluates the value of learning in terms of clarity and practicality.
- **Understanding style learner.** This style learner focuses more on ideas and abstractions; learns through a process of questioning, reasoning, and testing; and judges the value of learning by standards of logic and use of evidence.

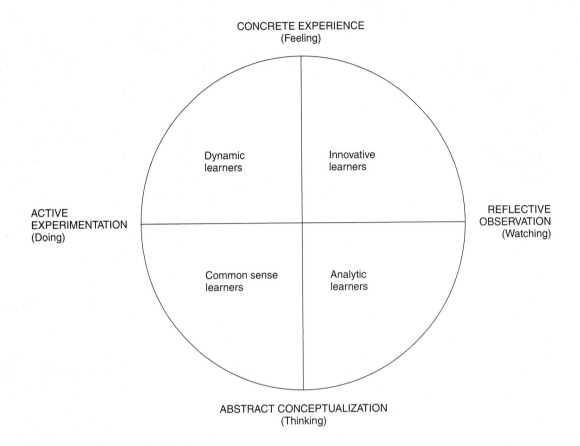

**Figure 6.4**  McCarthy's (1987) four styles of learning combined with Kolb's (1985) cycle of learning. Both **dynamic** and **common sense learners** tend to rely on active experimentation, but **dynamic learners** prefer concrete experiences whereas **common sense learners** prefer abstract conceptualization. Both **innovative** and **analytic learners** tend to use reflective observation, but **innovative learners** prefer concrete experience whereas **analytic learners** prefer abstract conceptualization.

■  **Self-expressive style learner.** This style learner looks for images implied in learning, uses feelings and emotions to construct new ideas and products, and judges the value of learning in terms of its originality, aesthetics, and capacity to surprise or delight.

■  **Interpersonal style learner.** This style learner is similar to the mastery-style learner in the sense that he or she focuses more on concrete, palpable information. However, this learner prefers to learn socially and judges the value of learning in terms of its potential use in helping others.

Although some learners will fit nicely into one of the learning styles previously described, others will seem to use some combination of these styles. It would be incorrect to say that one style is better than the others, but it would be correct to say that each learner has a certain preference for one style over the others.

Learning styles are not fixed throughout life but are modified as a person learns and develops. Many theorists agree that all people develop and experience a mixture of styles as they live and learn. Often these styles flex and adapt to various contexts, though to differing extents. Many people seek a sense of wholeness by practicing all four styles to some extent. One implication for practitioners is that they should strive to help learners discover their unique profiles, as well as a balance of styles that is most appropriate for facilitating their learning.

## Motivational Qualities

Readiness for learning motor skills depends not only on a person's developmental level and learning style, but also on his or her motivation (Atkinson & Birch, 1978; Maslow, 1970; McClelland, 1965; Nicholls, 1979; Piaget, 1972). For this reason, teachers, coaches, and physical therapists regularly strive to understand their students' or patients' various motivations and search for appropriate ways to motivate them to learn, perform, and behave as desired. What they soon discover is that motivation is the result of a complex interaction of different attitudes, aspirations, environments, and self-concepts. They also discover that there is no one simple method that will motivate all learners in the same way or to the same degree. Instead, they come to understand that what motivates some learners can be the very thing that fails to motivate others and that the same learner can be motivated by different things at different times.

*What Is Motivation?* **Motivation** may be thought of as the "GO" of a learner's personality, and it is a powerful variable for achieving his or her goals. It may be defined as the mechanisms within learners that arouse and direct their performance. It involves both the availability of energy for them to use and the direction of their action to achieve some goal. Motives are needs or desires that cause learners to act and, hence, feel motivated. **Motives** energize, direct, and help learners select behaviors or performances that are most appropriate for achieving their goals. Thus, the feeling of being motivated that learners experience is actually a psychological state of mind that results from the activation their motives.

Clearly, motivation is a dynamic, ongoing process in which learners become motivated in different ways, at different times, and for different reasons. Learners are continuously motivated to maintain and enhance their personal feelings of self-worth. For instance, at the most basic level, a learner's motivation appears to begin with the need for an acceptable degree of self-satisfaction, which may be interpreted as the need to do something for and with oneself—that is, to be somebody.

*Motivation Is Inferred from Performance.* Like learning, motivation is a process that cannot be directly observed and therefore must be inferred from the learner's behavior and motor performance. For instance, direct observation of a learner's behavior and motor performance (or absence of it) denotes what he or she *can* do or is *able* to do. Based on this direct observation of

Readiness for motor learning depends not only on a person's developmental level and learning style, but also on his or her motivation.

The mechanisms within learners that arouse and direct their performance are referred to as motivation.

Motivation is a dynamic, ongoing process in which learners become motivated in different ways, at different times, and for different reasons.

behavior and performance, we make our inference about the extent to which the learner is motivated. In other words, we make our inference about what the learner *wants* to do. As with learning, our inferences about motivation must be made very carefully because it is easy to be mistaken—motivation and performance/behavior are *not* the same. Although performance/behavior is our best indicator of the extent to which someone is motivated to learn, it is not a perfect indicator. For example, poor motor skill performance may not be so much a reflection of low motivation as it is a lack of ability to perform the skill, a lack of understanding of how to perform the skill, or perhaps even that the skill is developmentally inappropriate for the learner. Before we infer that the poor skill performance is the result of poor motivation, we must rule out variables such as these that affect performance but do not reflect motivation. The more we are aware of the operation of such performance variables, the more likely we are able to make accurate inferences about the extent to which learners are motivated and want to do what we want them to do.

Intrinsic motivation comes from within the learner, while extrinsic motivation comes from outside the learner.

***Intrinsic and Extrinsic Motivation.***    There are two kinds of motivation: intrinsic and extrinsic (Franken, 1982). **Intrinsic motivation** is the drive within learners that propels them forward and onward with energy provided by their own curiosity and interest. For example, if learners work hard in practice to acquire and refine their motor skills because they enjoy the sport and really want to learn it to perform their very best, their motivation is intrinsic because the reason for working hard resides within them. Conversely, if learners work hard to gain their coach's favor, receive praise from others, or earn awards or trophies, their motivation is **extrinsic** because the reasons lie outside of themselves. Both extrinsic and intrinsic motivation are important to understand in motor learning. While intrinsic motivation can sustain learning itself, extrinsic motivators such as praise, rewards, and criticism get learners to begin learning when the interest is lacking. The ultimate goal for practitioners (e.g., teachers, coaches, therapists) is to get learners who are extrinsically motivated to become intrinsically motivated.

## Summary

Motor learning is a process that depends on the movement skill to be learned, the conditions under which it is to be learned, and the learner. It is a process by which movement performance is reliably changed through instruction, practice, and/or experience. Since motor learning cannot be directly observed, it is inferred from our direct observations of motor performance. Although changes in motor performance are our best indicator of the extent to which motor learning has occurred, it is not a perfect indicator of motor learning because not all performance changes reflect learning. Some changes can be attributed to maturation or to temporary states of the learner such as fatigue and motivation. Both the structure and function of the central nervous system are altered in numerous ways as learning proceeds. For example, dendrites experience significant branching, pathways are altered structurally, the level of neuronal activation changes, and cortical representations of body parts are altered. Motor learning is indifferent with regard to correctness. People can learn incorrect movements as well as they can learn correct ones, which is one reason why practice does not always lead to improvement in performance.

Several theories have been advanced to explain how the learning of motor skills is accomplished. Whereas closed-loop and schema theories of motor learning emphasize the development of memory-based representations of action, the ecological theory of perception and action emphasizes the changing relationship between the performer and the movement environment. According to the ecological perspective, rather than broadening their repertoire of memory-based representations, learners discover and exploit the lawful properties of the environment that define the type of action most appropriate for solving a given movement problem.

We discussed three models that describe the performer-related changes evident during various stages of the learning process. Fitts' (1964) three-stage model describes the cognitive and behavioral changes that occur at each stage, whereas Vereijken's (1991) three-stage description of learning is focused at the level of the action itself. According to this second model, the learning process is characterized by the "freezing" and subsequent "releasing" of the degrees of freedom available within the motor system. The antecedents of this model are evident in the writings of Bernstein (1967). A third model of motor skill acquisition, developed by Gentile (1972), considers how the regulatory and non-regulatory conditions associated with a given motor skill influence the movement goals to be accomplished by a learner at each stage of the learning process.

Practical implications were discussed in relation to the various theories and models of motor learning that were discussed. One implication was that practitioners strive to provide instructional and practice conditions that allow learners the possibility to learn to perform movement skills by both elaborate cognitive processing of information and direct perception. Another was that the models and theories presented enhance our understanding of how people learn to perform movement skills. Such understanding provides a very important basis for determining the most appropriate instructional and practice conditions for individuals to learn movement skills.

Readiness for learning depends on a number of personal qualities of the learner. Readiness to learn largely depends on an individual's level of development, style of learning, and motivation. Each child's level of development depends on three factors: (a) his or her background of prior experiences, including previously learned knowledge and skills; (b) the traits with which he or she is hereditarily endowed; and (c) the rate at which these traits unfold, which is his or her maturation rate. People have different learning styles, which can affect their readiness for learning. Learning styles are the various ways that people would set about learning new motor skills or knowledge if they were in charge of their own learning. Motivation is the impetus behind a learner's personality, and it is a powerful variable for achieving his or her goals. It is the mechanism within a learner that arouses and directs his or her performance. Motives are the needs or desires that cause learners to act and, hence, feel motivated. The feeling of being motivated that learners experience is actually a psychological state of mind that results from the activation of their motives.

Practical implications were also discussed for readiness for learning in relation to developmental level, learning styles, and motivation. What we know about developmental readiness for learning suggests that instruction should be individualized as much as possible. Although children should not be expected to learn a sport or sport skill before they are developmentally ready, many sports and skills can be safely introduced by modifying such things as the rules of the game and/or the equipment and/or facilities or playing fields. This will enable children to learn some basic knowledge and skills of a sport that have the potential to transfer to the learning of the nonmodified sport and skills at a later stage of development. Once we know the preferred learning styles of the people we teach, we are in a position to adapt our teaching, coaching, and practice or treatment sessions in relation to how they prefer to learn. Learners become motivated in different ways, at different times, and for different reasons. The ultimate goal is to get learners who are extrinsically motivated to become intrinsically motivated.

## IMPORTANT TERMINOLOGY

After completing this chapter, readers should be familiar with the following terms and concepts.

advanced stage of learning
autonomous stage of learning
closed-loop theory
cognitive stage of learning
developmental readiness
ecological theory of perception and
    action
expert stage of learning
extrinsic motivation
fixation/diversification stage
generalized motor program (GMP)
getting the idea of the movement
intermediate, or associative, stage
    of learning
interpersonal style learner
intrinsic motivation
learning stages

learning styles
mastery style learner
memory trace
motivation
motives
motor learning
movement performance
nonregulatory conditions
novice stage of learning
perceptual trace
recall schema
regulatory conditions
response recognition schema
schema theory
self-expressive style learner
understanding style learner

## SUGGESTED FURTHER READING

Christina, R. W. (1997). Concerns and issues in studying and assessing motor learning. *Measurement in Physical Education and Exercise Science, 1,* 19–38.

Gentile, A. M. (1987). Skill acquisition: Action, movement, and neuromotor processes. In J. Carr, R. Shephard, J. Gordon, A. M. Gentile, & J. Held (Eds.), *Movement science foundations for physical therapy* (pp. 93–130). Rockville, MD: Aspen.

Newell, K. M. (2003). Schema theory (1975): Retrospectives and prospectives. *Research Quarterly for Exercise and Sport, 74,* 383–388.

Schmidt, R. A. (1992). Motor learning principles for physical therapy. In *Contemporary management of motor problems* (Proceedings of the II STEP Conference, pp. 65–76). Alexandria, VA: Foundation for Physical Therapy, Inc.

Schmidt, R. A. (2003). Motor schema theory after 27 years: Reflections and implications for a new theory. *Research Quarterly for Exercise and Sport, 74,* 366–375.

Sherwood, D. E., & Lee, T. D. (2003). Schema theory: Critical review and implications for the role of cognition in a new theory of motor learning. *Research Quarterly for Exercise and Sport, 74,* 376–382.

## TEST YOUR UNDERSTANDING

1. Define the term *motor learning.* Identify the various factors that influence learning.

2. Cite the kinds of neurological changes that occur as the individual learns a new motor skill or movement pattern.

3. List the fundamental assumptions of the closed-loop and schema theories of motor learning. How do the fundamental assumptions associated with these two theories differ from those that characterize ecological theories of perception and action?

4. Briefly identify the major empirical and theoretical weaknesses associated with the theory of motor learning developed by Adams (1971).

5. Identify the major theoretical weaknesses associated with traditional theories of motor learning.

6. Compare and contrast the various models that describe the performer-related changes occurring during each stage of learning.

7. According to Gentile (1972), how do the regulatory and nonregulatory conditions associated with the learning of different types of motor skills influence the nature of the movement goals to be accomplished by the learner?

8. Identify and explain the personal qualities that contribute to the readiness for learning motor skills.

9. How can developmental level, learning style, and motivation influence readiness to learn motor skills? What are the practical implications for teaching motor skills?

# 7

# HOW MOTOR LEARNING IS STUDIED

*We study motor learning, not only because we are curious about how people come to learn the movement skills they can perform, but also because of the practical benefits to be gained.*

## CHAPTER OBJECTIVES

After studying this chapter, you should be able to:

■ Distinguish among the different approaches to the study of motor learning.

■ Explain why inferences about motor learning should be based on both acquisition and post-acquisition performance measures.

■ Explain the various ways in which motor learning is assessed in acquisition and post-acquisition.

■ Become familiar with the various ways to distinguish temporary performance changes

from the durable changes produced by learning.

■ Become familiar with the various measurement techniques used not only to discover the types of abilities that distinguish experts from novice performers, but also to quantify the learning-related changes in perception and cognition.

■ Become familiar with the types of measurement techniques used to quantify the learning-related changes in how the pattern of coordination is controlled.

How does the learning of different motor skills take place? What are the mechanisms underlying the learning of movement skills, and how do they operate? What variables determine how rapidly we learn motor skills? What variables determine how long we remember the motor skills we have learned? These are but a few of the kinds of questions to which basic research in motor learning has been seeking answers. This type of research is motivated by the need to secure scientific understanding of the processes and mechanisms of motor learning with no requirement to demonstrate practical value or relevance. Ultimately, basic research seeks to develop a body of theory-based knowledge that will enable us to explain how and why the learning of motor skills occurs as it does and what variables influence that learning. Once such knowledge is developed, we will be able to manipulate conditions that optimize the acquisition of motor skills and have the power to make predictions about motor learning.

This need to develop theory-based knowledge in order to further our scientific understanding is not the only reason for wanting to study motor learning. Quite often we also are driven by practical needs. There are many professionals who need to help performers find immediate solutions to specific learning problems that occur in real-world settings such as those found in physical rehabilitation, physical education, and sports. We think immediately of practitioners such as physical and occupational therapists, teachers, and coaches who are constantly searching for (a) more effective ways to convey how to perform a motor skill during the early stages of acquisition, (b) better methods of diagnosing performance errors and of determining appropriate corrections or treatment plans, and (c) more effective ways of structuring practice environments or providing information feedback to their learners. Essentially, these practitioners are looking to construct the best learning conditions and methods to enhance motor learning and thereby optimize performance. Thus, we study motor learning, not only because we are curious about how people came to learn the movement skills they can perform, but also because of the practical benefits to be gained. This chapter focuses on the approaches, methods, and measures most commonly used to scientifically study motor learning.

> The development of theory–based motor learning knowledge is needed to further the scientific understanding that can help people find solutions to learning problems in practical settings.

## Approaches to the Study of Motor Learning

There are a number of approaches to studying motor learning. This section examines five of these approaches: the traditional approach, method-oriented approach, problem-oriented approach, doctrine of disproof approach, and cooperative approach.

### Traditional Approach

The **traditional approach** is based on the "scientific method." It has been and continues to be widely used to study motor learning. Essentially, it consists of the following five steps; the example provided after each step is based on a motor learning study that was conducted by Dunham (1976):

> The five steps that comprise the traditional approach are based on the "scientific method" and how motor learning is defined.

1. Identify the motor learning problem to be studied.

   *Example:* The problem of Dunham's research was to study the learning of a novel, gross motor task as a function of practice distribution.
2. Define a dependent variable (e.g., a movement performance) that can be reliably observed and that is appropriate for studying the problem.

   *Example:* Dunham defined his dependent variable as the number of rungs climbed per practice trial on a Bachman ladder, which is a novel gross motor ladder climbing task that relies heavily on dynamic balance for success.

3. Develop the experimental design, procedures, and learning opportunities in which the defined movement performance (dependent variable) occurs under the conditions specified by the independent variable.

   *Example:* A double transfer design was used in which groups 1 and 2 experienced distributed practice and groups 3 and 4 experienced massed practice during the acquisition phase. The distributed practice groups had sixteen, 30-second practice trials in acquisition with 30-second rests between trials followed by a 4-minute rest. The massed practice groups had 8 minutes of continuous practice followed by a 4-minute rest. In the transfer phase, group 1 continued with distributed practice; group 2 shifted to massed practice; group 3 continued with massed practice; and group 4 shifted to distributed practice. Participants performed six 30-second practice trials in the transfer phase.

   The experimental design and procedures also must exclude changes in the defined movement performance that are a function of nonlearning factors such as maturation or temporary states of the learners that may be caused by motivation, fatigue, or drugs.

   *Example:* The experimental design and procedures Dunham used excluded all nonlearning factors as possible explanations for the observed performance changes (see Figure 7.1). The only variable that caused a temporary effect on the dependent variable was massed practice, which led to a decrement in performance in acquisition and in transfer for the two groups that experienced it. However, the fact that the group (group 4) that transferred from massed to distributed practice performed as well as the group (group 1) that had distributed practice in acquisition and transfer may be interpreted as evidence that the decrement caused by massed practice was temporary and did not affect learning.

4. Observe, record, and analyze changes in the defined movement performance.

   *Example:* In addition to statistically analyzing the data, Dunham plotted the changes observed, and the performance curves are shown in Figure 7.1.

5. Make one or more inferences about motor learning as a function of the independent variable being manipulated, provided that the change in the defined movement performance is reliable and the result of instruction and/or practice.

   *Example:* One inference that can be made based on Dunham's findings is that distributed practice produced superior performance and massed practice led to a decrement in performance, but not motor learning.

These five steps are based on the well-known scientific method and on how motor learning is defined. It is relatively easy to recognize how the major elements of most definitions of motor learning, including the one we offered in Chapter 6, manifest themselves in the five steps.

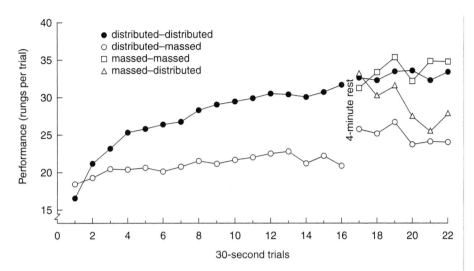

**Figure 7.1** Performance curves for distributed and massed practice on the Bachman ladder climb task.

*Source:* Distribution of practice as a factor affecting learning and/or performance, by P. Dunham, 1976, *Journal of Motor Behavior, 8,* 305–307.

## Method- versus Problem-Oriented Approach

Scholars who have studied motor learning have used both method-oriented and problem-oriented approaches. The **method-oriented approach** restricts the study of motor learning problems to one particular method (whether it be a certain experimental design, statistical analysis, or measurement technique). This limits the scope of the problems that can be studied, however. Some scholars are restricted to conducting motor learning research on problems that can only be studied by their particular method. One consequence is that many important motor learning problems that fall outside the boundaries of their method are not studied. Another consequence is that problems that need to be studied using more than one method (disciplinary or interdisciplinary) are studied with a single method, and thus provide only limited information about the solutions. Although scholars who use the method-oriented approach have generated valuable findings, this approach is not recommended because it is too limited to thoroughly study the many motor learning problems that exist. Moreover, frequent use of this approach by a majority of scholars in the future will likely impede the further development of our motor learning knowledge and its applications.

How we approach the study of motor learning, first and foremost, should be a function of the problem to be solved. This is the **problem-oriented approach.** It requires scholars to put aside their favorite method and learn the methods that are most appropriate for thoroughly studying the problem. It also requires that they join forces with scholars in other subdisciplines of kinesiology (e.g., biomechanics, sport psychology, exercise physiology) or

The problem-oriented approach requires scholars to learn the methods that are most appropriate for thoroughly studying a particular motor learning problem.

disciplines outside of kinesiology (e.g., gerontology, education, biology) who are already familiar with these methods. The resulting effect is a team of scholars who, armed with more than one method, are equipped to thoroughly study a motor learning problem. As members of such a team, scholars are able to go beyond the boundaries of any single favorite method of study and address motor learning problems that are the most important to study—and also to investigate them more thoroughly. Increased use of the problem-oriented approach by more scholars in the future could substantially advance the development of motor learning knowledge and its applications.

## Doctrine of Disproof Approach

The study of some motor learning problems will demand descriptive methods because they are applied or atheoretical in nature. Other problems will require the inferential methods that are characteristic of hypothesis and theory testing in science. When inferential methods are used, scholars should adhere to the **doctrine of disproof,** which holds that science advances only through disproof (Kuhn, 1962; Popper, 1959). If motor learning is to advance appreciably as a field of science, this doctrine must be consistently and rigorously applied in our research, especially our basic research. The doctrine demands systematic application of the **method of inductive inference** to every motor learning problem studied by using the following four steps that were described by Platt (1964):

1. Formulate alternative hypotheses (that is, solutions or answers).
2. Design one or more decisive experiments with alternative outcomes, each of which will exclude at least one hypothesis.
3. Conduct each experiment so as to obtain an unambiguous result.
4. Repeat steps 1 to 3 to refine the remaining possibilities. (Continue repeating steps 1 to 4 as needed.)

*The doctrine of disproof approach demands the systematic application of the method of inductive inference to every motor learning problem studied.*

The field of motor learning can do much better at systematically applying the four steps of the method of inductive inference. Scholars unfamiliar with these steps can begin by learning them. They can then become proficient at using them by rigorously applying them to every motor learning problem they study. Once they have learned the steps and can effectively apply them, they should teach them to others in the field. Scholars who already know the steps but who have been inconsistent or less than rigorous in applying them simply need to change how they do business. They must become more consistent and rigorous in applying them not only to the motor learning problems that they study, but to problems studied by others as well.

One very simple strategy that can be used to effectively apply the steps of the method of inductive inference is what Platt (1964) termed "The Question." He suggested that each time you hear someone propose a hypothesis, you should ask the question: *What experiment could disprove this hypothesis?* Each time you hear someone describe an experiment, you should ask the question: *What hypothesis does this experiment disprove?* "The Question" goes straight to the heart of whether we are effectively applying the four steps of the method of inductive inference and adhering to the doctrine of disproof. It directs us to concentrate on whether we are or are not taking a testable scientific step forward.

**Table 7.1**
Levels of Relevance of Motor Learning Research for Finding Solutions to Practical Problems

| Level 1:<br>Least Direct Relevance | Level 2:<br>Moderate Direct Relevance | Level 3:<br>Most Direct Relevance |
|---|---|---|
| **Basic Research** | **Applied Research** | **Applied Research** |
| *Ultimate goal:* Develop theory-based knowledge appropriate for understanding motor learning in general with no requirement to demonstrate its relevance for solving practical problems. | *Ultimate goal:* Develop theory-based knowledge appropriate for understanding the learning of practical skills in practical settings with no requirement to find immediate solutions to practical learning problems. | *Ultimate goal:* Find immediate solutions to practical learning problems in practical settings with no requirement to develop theory-based knowledge at either level 1 or level 2. |
| *Main approach:* Test hypotheses in a laboratory setting using experimenter-designed motor tasks. | *Main approach:* Test hypotheses in a practical setting or in a laboratory setting similar to it using practical skills or motor tasks that have the properties of those skills. | *Main approach:* Test solutions to practical learning problems in settings described under applied research at level 2. |

## Cooperative Approach between Basic and Applied Research

From about the 1970s to the early 1990s, there was less than a cooperative approach between basic and applied research in the field of motor learning. Applied research was seen as subordinate to and almost completely dependent on basic research and therefore was considered mainly an extension of it. This view led to the argument that a major systematic effort to conduct applied research before the fundamental knowledge from basic research on motor learning was sufficiently developed was a highly questionable endeavor and should be discouraged. Christina (1987, 1989) strongly disagreed with this view and argued that it would be more productive to adopt a **cooperative approach** between basic and applied research. He envisioned this approach as consisting of three research levels as shown in Table 7.1. These levels ranged from the most basic to the most applied research of human motor learning and were divided based on their relevance for providing solutions to practical problems.

The cooperative approach encourages scholars to think of all three levels as independent but cooperating endeavors that have a synergistic relation. The cooperative approach not only acknowledges that research at levels 2 and 3 can be an extension of basic research, but also recognizes that applied research can take place independently of basic research. Moreover, it holds that research at levels 2 and 3 can contribute to the ultimate goal of basic research just as basic research can contribute to the ultimate goal of research at levels 2 and 3.

In areas in which theory-based knowledge from basic research is sufficiently developed, scholars can determine the appropriateness of applying that knowledge to practical settings through research at levels 2 and 3.

The cooperative approach views basic and applied research as independent but cooperative endeavors that have a synergistic relation.

However, many scholars fail to realize that specialized knowledge can be developed solely by level 2 research in areas in which the theory-based knowledge of basic research at level 1 is not adequately advanced. Likewise, there is no reason why immediate solutions to practical problems cannot be found solely by level 2 research when theory-based knowledge of basic research at level 1 (or even the specialized knowledge of level 2 research) is not sufficiently developed.

If a new idea or hypothesis is developed, or some new information emanates from either level 2 or 3 research, the contribution to fundamental motor learning knowledge can be evaluated by subjecting the development or discovery to the rigor of controlled laboratory testing of basic research at level 1. In this way, applied research at levels 2 and 3 can contribute to basic research at level 1. Thus, it is clear that when scholars view research at levels 1, 2, and 3 as independent but cooperating endeavors, the three levels have the potential to contribute to one another. This is a much more viable and promising approach to adopt to guide future research efforts than the view that holds that applied research at levels 2 and 3 is an extension to basic research. It appears that since the early 1990s an increasing number of scholars in the field of motor learning have accepted and are adopting the cooperative approach.

## Assessing Motor Learning in Acquisition

### Performance Curves

A performance curve is a plot of an individual's or a group's performance on some dependent measure as a function of practice trials in acquisition.

Perhaps the most common way of examining motor learning in acquisition is to plot what has traditionally been referred to as a **learning curve** but which we will refer to as a **performance curve** to maintain the distinction between learning and performance. A performance curve is a plot of an individual's or a group's performance on some dependent measure (dependent measures were discussed in Chapter 2) as a function of practice trials in acquisition. The performance curve tells us something relatively special about performance changes in the dependent measure under the conditions defined by the independent variable from which an inference about learning can be made. However, before an inference is justified, two conditions must be met. First, one must rule out all explanations that would attribute the performance changes observed in the curve to variables that do not qualify as motor learning (e.g., maturation or temporary states of the individual caused by factors such as motivation, fatigue, and drugs). Second, one must be able to advance the explanation that the changes were reliable and a function of instruction, experience, or practice.

The shape of a performance curve is largely dependent on the nature of the task to be learned, the learner(s), the conditions under which the task is learned, and how the performance is measured.

*Shape of a Performance Curve.*    The shape of a performance curve is largely dependent on the nature of the task to be learned, the learner(s), the conditions under which the task is learned, and how performance is measured. Although many different types of performance curves are possible, quite often they display substantial improvement during early practice trials followed by a more gradual improvement as practice continues. This improvement is displayed either as a steep rise or fall in the slope of the curve as a function

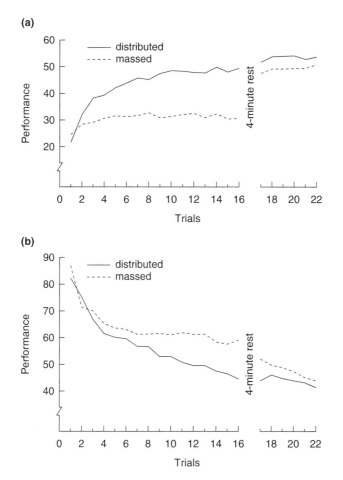

**Figure 7.2**   (a) The performance curves for distributed and massed practice groups on the Bachman ladder; scores were determined by the total number of rungs climbed in a 30-second trial. **(b)** The performance curves for the distributed and massed groups on the stabilometer; scores represented total amount of board movement as measured by a work ladder per 30-second trial, with one movement unit equal to 12 degrees of board movement.

of the early practice trials. If the dependent measure (e.g., number of correct responses made or time on target) is a measure that increases as one improves with practice, the curve will reveal a rise in the slope over the early trials as shown in Figure 7.2a. If the dependent measure (e.g., number of errors made or time off target) is a measure that is likely to decrease as one improves with practice, the curve will display a fall in the slope over the early trials as shown in Figure 7.2b.

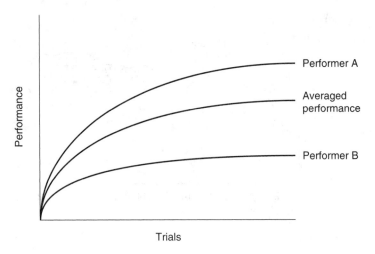

**Figure 7.3**  Hypothetical performance curves for two learners and a curve representing the average of their performances.

Further, the method of measurement determines the smoothness of a performance curve regardless of whether it is a curve for one learner or a group of learners. The more performance measures are averaged together over practice trials, the smoother the curve becomes. However, it is important to keep in mind that a substantial amount of information can be lost about individual or group learning when data are averaged. With an individual performance curve (a curve for a single learner), there is one measure per practice trial; whereas with a group performance curve, data are averaged across learners in the group for each trial. Group performance curves are useful for summarizing information, testing hypotheses or theories, and for making theoretical inferences about learning. However, inferences about learning based on a group performance curve should not be applied to an individual curve (Estes, 1956). The risks in making generalizations about learning from a group curve to an individual curve are substantial, especially in terms of experimental and statistical violations. Moreover, the shape of a group curve does not determine the shapes of the curves of the individuals within the group (see Figure 7.3). Indeed, the group curve is insensitive to the variability in performance between the individuals in the group. Lastly, much information about individual learning is lost when data are averaged to form group performance curves. For instance, within-person variability (the variability in performance that each individual in the group displays over practice trials) is lost. This is a serious loss of information because when people learn, often their performance not only gets more accurate with practice, but also becomes less variable or, conversely, more consistent. Newell (1991) contends that if one really wants to know how a learner solves any given motor problem, then "the change in performance with practice needs to be examined on an individual-subject basis over individual practice trials" (p. 223).

***Scoring Sensitivity.***    The shape of any performance curve (individual or group curve) also can be affected by the **scoring sensitivity** of the dependent measure used to plot the curve. The problem is that a curve may be misinterpreted at different stages of practice, and effects attributed to the independent variable actually can be *artifacts* produced by the scoring sensitivity of the dependent measure that was arbitrarily selected by the experimenter. A study by Howland and Noble (1953) serves as an example to illustrate this problem. Howland and Noble attempted to evaluate the independent variable effects of control loading (manipulating different types of resistance on a control device used to track a target) on tracking performance and used time-on-target (TOT) scores as their dependent measure. The resulting performance curves in acquisition displayed an increasing separation with practice, which led them to conclude that the differential effects of control loading upon tracking performance increase as practice progresses. Bahrick, Fitts, and Briggs (1957) plotted these curves again for a larger target-scoring area and found that this increasing separation among the performance curves disappeared. Indeed, the increasing separation of the curves was an artifact of the gradually increasing sensitivity of the target area rather than the result of different control loadings. In other words, the arbitrary choice of target size by Howland and Noble produced dependent measure scoring artifacts that they mistakenly attributed as effects of the independent variable. Essentially, TOT scores used alone are of limited value, particularly if performance on different manipulations of the independent variable at different stages of acquisition varies over a wide range and the scores are either very low or very high for some of the distributions (Bahrick & Noble, 1966).

> Scoring sensitivity of the dependent measure used to plot the performance curve can affect its shape.

***Ceiling and Floor Effects.***    The shape of a performance curve also can be affected by *ceiling and floor effects.* When tasks are relatively easy to learn, and/or the range of potential improvement is somewhat restricted or insensitive because of the scoring method, **ceiling effects** as evidenced by asymptotes in performance curves are reached quickly. Let's consider the following example. Suppose ten normal functioning adults were given 50 practice trials to learn to make a two-foot putt. The dependent measure, or scoring method, is the number of putts made. The task is very easy to learn, and the scoring method is insensitive to measuring putts that miss the hole. We may see a few putts missed on the early practice trials, but very few, if any, missed on the remaining trials. Indeed, some of the participants may have made 50 out of 50 putts because the task was so easy. The group performance curve that results probably would reveal a sharp rise on the initial trials and a leveling off (asymptote) on the remaining trials. This leveling off would represent a ceiling effect.

> Ceiling effects occur when the task to be learned is too easy, while floor effects occur when the task is too difficult to learn.

If these adults were given 50 practice trials to learn to make a ten-foot putt instead of a two-foot putt, the shape of the curve would be quite different because the task is more difficult. It is unlikely that any of the participants could have made all 50 putts. We would probably see more missed putts on the early practice trials and some improvement over the remaining trials. The group performance curve that results would probably show a rise on the initial trials and some gradual increases on the remaining trials, with an asymptote or ceiling not being reached. Another way to change the shape of the curve is to make the dependent measure a more sensitive measure of putting performance by measuring the distance (in centimeters) of the putts that were missed and assigning a zero score to the putts made (no error). By doing this we have increased the scoring sensitivity so that the dependent measure is now a more sensitive measure of putting performance.

Conversely, **floor effects** result when the task is too difficult to learn and/or the range of potential improvement is restricted or insensitive because of the scoring method. For instance, if we change the task to be learned in the above example to a 30-foot putt instead of a 2-foot putt and measured performance as the number of putts made, we would observe floor effects in the curve. We would expect very few, if any, putts to be made by the ten participants over the 50 trials. The performance curve that results would probably asymptote along the x-axis and show no improvement in performance as a function of practice.

Ceiling and floor effects are often observed in clinical instruments also because the test is either too easy or too difficult for the patient population being assessed or is insensitive to performance changes over time because the range of possible scores is very limited. For example, functional performance scales with ordinal scales that range from zero to one or two (e.g., Tinetti, 1994) will not be as sensitive to performance changes over time when compared to other functional performance scales (Berg, Wade, & Greer, 1989; Rose & Lucchese, 2003) with ordinal scales that range from zero to four.

A learning plateau represents a leveling off in performance.

*Learning Plateaus.*   Have you noticed that learners improve performance up to a certain level and then seem unable to improve with continued practice? This leveling off in performance is known as a **learning plateau,** which can be readily seen when the dependent measure is plotted over practice trials. A learning plateau represents a leveling off in performance preceded and sometimes followed by accelerated performance increments. It is a phenomenon that has not been found to occur in many learning studies that have used laboratory tasks. Indeed, it has been argued that learning plateaus may not actually exist (Keller, 1958). However, a classic example of a plateau was found by Bryan and Harter (1897) who used a task that had participants learn to receive telegraphic signals in American Morse code. These two researchers found that positive improvements in performance speed (letters transmitted per minute) occurred during the first twenty weeks of practice but then ceased improving for the next six weeks, suggesting that learning had reached a plateau. Somewhat surprisingly, performance began improving steadily again during the last six weeks of practice. These results would seem to indicate that the plateau was not reflecting that learning had ceased, but rather that the learning that was continuing to occur was not being reflected in the overt performance of the telegraphers.

At least four hypotheses have been proposed to explain why learning plateaus occur. One hypothesis suggests that plateaus occur because learners are in transition between performance strategies. They may be trying different strategies of executing the skill in an effort to perform it better. While trying these strategies, which are often ineffective at improving the performance of the skill, performance levels off. However, once the appropriate strategy is found, performance begins to improve again. A second hypothesis proposes that plateaus occur because of the hierarchy of subskills or prerequisite skills that have to be acquired while attempting to learn a complex motor skill. For example, a prerequisite skill might be the acquisition of a fundamental basketball skill such as dribbling with the preferred hand while standing in one place. Once acquired, the next step in the hierarchy might be to learn to dribble while moving down the court alone. The last step might be to learn to dribble down the court in the presence of one or more defenders similar to a game context. It is possible, depending on the way in which the complex skill of basketball dribbling is taught and how the learner is engaged, that a performance plateau could occur during any one of these transitional periods.

A third hypothesis holds that plateaus are the due to psychological factors such as (a) the learner's inability to control his or her arousal level (level of anxiety) to perform well enough to show improvement, (b) the learner's lack of motivation (boredom) to learn to improve his or her performance, (c) the learner's personal problems (loss of a friend or failing grades) distracting him or her from learning to improve his or her performance, and/or (d) fear of failure.

A fourth hypothesis proposes that plateaus are due to physical factors such as a deficiency in physical fitness (e.g., lack of strength, flexibility, or endurance), a physical injury of some sort, or a lack of physical readiness. Other hypotheses include (a) the learner focusing on the wrong cues during learning, (b) a lack of understanding of the instructions provided, and (c) setting learning goals that are too low. Indeed, if plateaus do occur in the learning of motor skills in the real world (although not clearly demonstrated using laboratory tasks), more than one of these hypotheses or factors may be operating.

### Limitations of Performance Curves.

Performance curves were once used as the primary source of evidence from which to draw inferences about motor learning. This is a mistake, however, because performance curves developed over the course of an acquisition phase can really only inform us about the specific performance changes observed in the dependent variable under the experimental conditions in which it was studied. They should not, therefore, be used to make inferences about learning in general.

Performance curves should not be used as the main source of information on which to base inferences about motor learning for two main reasons. First, these curves, by themselves, do not provide sufficient evidence that the observed changes in performance resulting from practice are reliable or durable. To determine if the performance changes are reliable, post-acquisition measures also have to be used. (These measures will be discussed later in the section "Assessing Motor Learning in Post-Acquisition" on page 209. Second, by themselves, these curves do not provide sufficient evidence to rule out the possibility that the observed changes in performance as a function of practice were due to variables that do not qualify as evidence for motor learning (e.g., maturation or temporary states of the learner caused by variables such as motivation, fatigue, drugs). Other sources of information must be used as evidence to rule out this possibility. Thus, while performance curves can help us to understand and make certain inferences about motor learning, they must be used in conjunction with other sources of information (e.g., post-acquisition measures, retention and/or transfer designs, specific experimental procedures) to determine the extent to which the performance changes observed are reliable and durable and, therefore, a true reflection of motor learning.

> Performance curves should not be used as the main or sole source of information on which to base inferences about motor learning.

## Setting a Criterion of Mastery

Motor learning is considered complete in acquisition when some arbitrarily defined criterion of mastery is achieved.

Important to the assessment of motor learning in the acquisition phase is determining when practice (that is, learning) is complete. Usually, it is considered complete when some arbitrarily defined **criterion of mastery** (an arbitrarily defined level of performance) is achieved. Although historically in the literature it has been common to refer to the best level of performance reached in acquisition as the **level of original learning,** we prefer to use the expression **level of performance** achieved in acquisition because it preserves the distinction between learning and performance. How the level of performance or criterion of mastery is selected (how it is defined and assessed in terms of when it is satisfactorily achieved) is quite arbitrary. The level or criterion is usually measured in terms of trials needed, time required, or frequency of errors made until it has been achieved. In most published studies reviewed, however, the criterion has been established either at a minimal level of mastery (e.g., the first trial performed without an error) or at a slightly more than minimal level (e.g., three successive trials performed without an error). Minimal criterion levels such as these do not provide very convincing evidence that the skill being practiced has been mastered reliably if only correctly demonstrated in as few as one to three practice trials. Achieving a criterion of mastery set at a level demanding somewhat stable or consistent performance over many more practice trials (e.g., ten successive trials without an error) would provide more convincing evidence that the skill being practiced had been reliably mastered. In addition to setting an arbitrary criterion of mastery, the slope of the curve in acquisition could be used to determine when performance has stabilized at or above the predetermined criterion level (Jones, 1985). When the slope has begun to plateau at or above the criterion level of mastery, practice may be considered complete and learning evident.

Clearly, the arbitrary nature of the criterion of mastery makes it difficult to perform certain comparisons across studies because the criterion varies from study to study. It depends on how the criterion of mastery in acquisition is defined and how it is quantified in terms of when learning is judged to be complete. These complications notwithstanding, the criterion of mastery continues to be used to study learning in the acquisition phase. Moreover, if the same criterion was used consistently across studies investigating the same motor-learning problem, it would be possible to conduct meaningful comparisons across studies. Of course, temporary performance effects caused by the selected independent variables (e.g., knowledge of results, distribution of practice, or variability of practice) could contaminate the use of any performance measure obtained in acquisition such that the measure might not reflect learning. If temporary performance-effect contamination is suspected in the planning of the study, it must be dealt with in a reasonable way, which typically involves using an experimental design and procedures that allow for the assessment of performance in post-acquisition using retention or transfer tests. More will be said about this issue in the section entitled "Assessing Motor Learning in Post-Acquisition" on page 209.

# Over-Learning

Regardless of the criterion of mastery selected to determine when learning is complete in acquisition (level of original learning), one way to enhance retention is to provide supplementary practice on a task after the criterion has been reached. For example, a teacher could have his or her beginning basketball players continue to practice free throw shooting even though they achieved the mastery criterion of making 25 out of their first 50 shots. This method may be interpreted as post-mastery learning and is usually referred to as **over-learning.** The level of over-learning is usually expressed as simply the number of practice trials that learners complete after the criterion of mastery has been achieved in acquisition. Alternatively, it is expressed in percentage terms, for example, 50% over-learning means that the learners completed half again the number of trials that they required to achieve the established criterion of mastery in acquisition. The arbitrary nature of mastery and over-learning criteria can make it difficult to compare findings across studies. That is because a trial that is part of mastery in acquisition for one study can be part of over-learning for another study. It depends on how one defines *when* the original learning is complete, how one quantifies the level of original learning or mastery, and how one defines the level of over-learning. Nonetheless, it is clear that retention is better for over-learned tasks (e.g., Loftus, 1985; Schendel & Hagman, 1982; Slamecka & McElree, 1983). The timing of when to introduce the supplementary trials does not appear to be a critical factor for enhancing retention; the level of over-learning is far more important than the time at which the supplementary practice trials are introduced (Schendel & Hagman, 1982). The literature also reveals, however, that providing over-learning trials reaches a point of diminishing returns (e.g., Bell, 1950; McGeoch & Irion, 1952; Melnick, 1971). In other words, increasing the number of over-learning trials may not produce proportionate increases in retention. Thus, although 100% over-learning may result in better retention than 50%, the additional gain that occurs may not be worth the additional time and practice.

> One way to enhance the retention of a motor skill is to provide supplementary practice on the skill after the criterion has been reached.

# Level of Automaticity

Another way to assess the level of performance achieved or mastered in acquisition *(level of original learning)* is by using a dual-task paradigm to determine the degree of automaticity of performance. Using this paradigm, a second task, in addition to the one already being practiced, is introduced to learners to sample their spare cognitive capacity while they are performing the primary task (Shiffrin & Schneider, 1977; Schneider & Shiffrin, 1977; Schneider, Dumais, & Shiffrin, 1984). The point at which neither of the tasks causes a performance decrement on the other is considered an acceptable degree of automaticity and, hence, the level of performance achieved or mastered in acquisition. Although the dual-task paradigm can be an effective way of assessing the **degree of automaticity,** it is not without its critics (see, for example, Fendrich et al., 1988; Jonides, Naveh-Benjamin, & Palmer, 1985). Theoretically, skills that require only a minimum amount of attention and cognitive capacity to perform are either completely or partly automatic, whereas skills that require

> A dual-task test is often used to determine the level of automaticity that has been achieved in the performance of a motor skill.

cognitive resources and effort involve controlled processes. Schneider et al. (1984) defined an automatic process as one that does not make use of general cognitive resources. Thus, capacity reductions do not influence automatic processing because an automatic process is not subject to conscious control and can be executed in response to relevant external stimuli to which little attention is paid.

The more automatic the skill is, the greater the chance that it will be retained during periods that it is not practiced.

Whether a skill is classified as automatic or controlled depends largely on the level of original learning. Many skills require controlled processes early in learning, but the processes become automatic with extensive practice and more so if that practice contains a high degree of consistency. *Practice consistency* means that a learner makes the same response each time a certain event occurs (e.g., defender in basketball attempting to block offensive player's movement toward the basket). The proposed explanation for this phenomenon is that retention of a skill depends heavily on the degree to which a skill is automatic or can be performed without conscious awareness. The more automatic the skill is, the greater the chance that it will be retained over nonuse periods. However, automated skills that are acquired through practice (e.g., speed of soldering joint) can be expected to deteriorate more during nonuse periods than automated skills that are less dependent on practice (e.g., encoding of temporal or spatial information). The implication for designing a skill maintenance program is that more emphasis should be placed on the automated skills that were acquired through practice.

## Limitations of Assessing Motor Learning in Acquisition

One major challenge for those who attempt to assess motor learning in acquisition is that the performance changes observed may or may not reflect learning, and the absence of any performance changes may or may not be evidence that learning has occurred. Some practice and training procedures known to enhance performance during acquisition might or might not enhance learning. Conversely, other procedures that make the practice environment more difficult for the learner (e.g., contextual interference) and that impair performance during acquisition might in fact foster learning (Christina & Bjork, 1991; Schmidt & Bjork, 1992). Thus, assessing performance in acquisition has some limitations for making inferences about motor learning, especially in determining the extent to which the performance observed is durable.

What is observed in acquisition is performance localized in a given place and time that may or may not reflect learning.

Based on the current definition presented in Chapter 6, motor learning is optimized when there is some durable change in the learner's capacity for performing a movement. Moreover, learning must be inferred from a reliable change in performance that was caused by learning variables such as instruction, practice, or training. What is observed during acquisition is performance localized in a given place and time. At a later time, in another place, the learner might perform quite differently, in some cases at an inferior level compared to the level achieved in acquisition and in other cases at a superior level of performance. The performance observed during acquisition might be mediated by instruction or practice variables that produce a temporary effect that either enhances or depresses it rather than a reliable or durable effect that is indicative of learning. Since the level of performance or criterion of mastery achieved in acquisition may or may not be an accurate indicator of the extent to which motor learning has occurred, it also is necessary to assess performance in post-acquisition with retention and/or transfer tests.

# Assessing Motor Learning in Post-Acquisition

## Retention Tests

Motor learning is assessed in post-acquisition using a retention design and test mainly to determine the extent to which the level of performance achieved in acquisition or original learning can be reproduced after some time period of disuse (no experience or practice on the task), which is referred to as a **retention interval.** If the level of performance achieved in acquisition was due to learning, it will be reliable (durable) and should be able to be reproduced after the retention interval on the **retention test.** However, if the level of performance achieved in acquisition was due to variables that produced temporary effects that do not qualify as motor learning, it will not be reliable and should not be able to be reproduced after the retention interval on the retention test.

When studying retention, traditionally a distinction is made between the acquisition and retention phases of the study. The acquisition phase involves the time or trials required to achieve a certain level of task proficiency (e.g., criterion of mastery). The retention phase follows the acquisition phase and consists of a retention interval (time period of nonuse or no practice) that might vary from being very short (e.g., seconds, minutes, or hours) to long (e.g., weeks, months, or years) and a retention test. The retention test usually consists of a test to determine how much of the task proficiency gained during the acquisition was retained or, alternatively, how many trials were saved in relearning the task that was learned in the acquisition phase. Thus, it is common to use the term *retention* when performance on the task practiced during the acquisition phase is assessed in the retention phase under conditions that are essentially the same as those that existed in the acquisition phase. In contrast, the term *transfer* is used when the task and/or conditions present in the retention phase differ from those that existed in the acquisition phase.

For the purposes of this book, the common usage of these two terms is followed, but it is important to understand the concept that retention so defined is actually a special case of transfer. Retention and transfer are related in the sense that the post-acquisition context can differ from the acquisition along the dimensions of time and overall similarity. These dimensions are related in that, with the passage of time during a retention interval, the acquisition and post-acquisition contexts tend to become less similar because the mechanisms that affect the emotional, physical, and cognitive states of the learner are operating. For example, the mechanisms that produce forgetting or alter one's motivation to perform a skill are operating during the retention interval. In this sense, a retention test can be interpreted as a test of transfer of learning to a context that appears to match the context of the acquisition phase.

Although retention designs, tests, and measures used to assess the reliability of motor learning are very effective, they should be used in conjunction with performance measures recorded during acquisition (e.g., an acquisition

The term *retention* is used when performance on the task practiced during the acquisition phase is assessed in the retention phase under conditions that are essentially the same as those that existed in the acquisition phase.

The term *transfer* is used when the task and/or conditions present in the retention phase differ from those that existed in the acquisition phase.

performance curve). Acquisition measures provide us with information about the level of performance achieved in acquisition, whereas retention test measures provide us with information about the durability of the level of performance achieved in acquisition. Each of these measures tells us something different about performance, and the information they provide should be used in relation to each other to draw inferences about motor learning. When used conjointly the different types of information generated by the different measures complement each other and fit together like pieces of a puzzle to provide a more complete picture about the durability of motor learning.

## Maintaining the Learning–Retention Distinction

When we measure motor performance in acquisition we are studying the learning of a defined performance. However, when we measure motor performance in retention we are studying the persistence of the acquired defined performance over time. It is important to maintain this **learning–retention distinction** because they are not the same. It's easy to make the mistake of thinking that retention performance measures are measures of learning when in fact they are measures of the retention of learning. Performance measures in acquisition are used to make inferences about mechanisms, processes, and outcomes of learning, whereas performance measures in retention are used to make inferences about memory mechanisms and forgetting processes that operate during the retention interval to affect what was learned in acquisition.

When we use a retention test to assess the durability of the motor learning that occurred in acquisition, care must be taken through our design and procedures to control or account for the effects due to factors such as warm-up, motivation, and forgetting that could operate during the retention interval to contaminate measures taken on the retention test. For example, longer retention intervals would allow for more of the massed practice schedule effects that temporarily depress performance in acquisition to dissipate and thus, make the retention measures less contaminated by these effects. At the same time, however, longer retention intervals could increase the decrement in performance measured on the retention test caused by forgetting or by not warming up, or they could produce an increment in performance due to increased motivation. The use of retention tests to assess the durability of motor learning could confound the amount learned in acquisition with these factors if they operate over the retention interval and if our experimental design and procedures do not control or account for their effects (Christina & Shea, 1988, 1993).

> Performance measures in acquisition are used to make inferences about learning, whereas performance measures in retention are used to make inferences about memory and forgetting.

## Transfer Tests

Motor learning is assessed in post-acquisition with a transfer design and test mainly to determine:

1. if the performance changes observed in acquisition are temporary and due to variables that do not qualify as learning, or if they are reliable and the result of variables (e.g., instruction, practice) that do qualify as evidence for learning

2. the direction of transfer; that is, if the training in acquisition produced learning that enhances (which is a positive transfer), impedes (negative transfer), or has no effect (neutral transfer) on performance in the post-acquisition context
3. the generalization of transfer; that is, the extent to which training in acquisition produced a level of motor learning that prepares people to perform in a post-acquisition context that differs from the acquisition context or to perform a new but similar motor skill to the one presented during acquisition (e.g., the skating technique in cross-country skiing after first learning to in-line skate on Rollerblades)

Transfer designs, tests, and measures to assess motor learning are very helpful, but they should be used wisely and in conjunction with performance measures recorded in acquisition.

One common way to determine if the level of performance achieved in acquisition is temporary or durable is to use an experimental design that allows for the assessment of performance in post-acquisition using a **transfer test.** The ideal way to accomplish this is to use a complete transfer design (double transfer design) in which all of the tests and necessary control and experimental groups are included in both the acquisition and transfer phases. An example of a study that used a double transfer design was conducted by Dunham (1976), and discussed on page 196 (see also Figure 7.1). In the acquisition phase of a practice distribution experiment, for instance, two groups (groups 1 and 2) practice according to a distributed practice schedule, and two groups (groups 3 and 4) practice according to a massed practice schedule. In the transfer phase, group 1 continues in the distributed practice schedule, group 2 shifts to a massed practice schedule, group 3 continues in the massed practice schedule, and group 4 shifts to a distributed practice schedule.

Compared to an incomplete transfer design, a double transfer design puts us in a better position to make an inference about the effect of massed and distributed practice on motor learning. The double transfer design enables us to separate durable performance changes that we attribute to learning from temporary changes caused by variables that do not qualify as evidence for learning (the effect of switching conditions and massed practice). In spite of the great value of a double transfer design, often, incomplete designs are used (e.g., see Figure 7.2 a, b) because they "cost" less in terms of the number of participants and the amount of time needed to conduct the research. However, what we save in terms of this cost might not be worth what we lose in terms of scientific benefit. Conversely, this cost might not be worth what we gain in terms of scientific benefit. Whenever faced with a decision about whether to use a complete design or an incomplete design, we would be wise to ask whether the design we have selected adheres to the doctrine of disproof that was discussed earlier in this chapter. If we think it does, we should be able to answer "The Question"—What hypothesis does this experimental design disprove?

Like the measurement of retention effects, the measurement of transfer effects has been plagued by several problems. Different methods of measuring transfer effects, like those to measure retention effects, have problems associated with them that can influence the validity of the conclusions that are reached not only within a given study, but across studies as well. We will discuss this problem in more detail in Chapter 12.

One way to determine if the level of performance achieved in acquisition is temporary or durable is to use a double transfer design.

# Measuring Learning-Related Changes in Perception and Cognition

In addition to the information provided by the use of retention and/or transfer tests, the practitioner and researcher alike are also interested in discovering the types of abilities that distinguish expert from novice performers and the nature of the perceptual and cognitive changes that can be attributed to learning. Fortunately, several measurement techniques and methods of analyzing experimental data have been developed to assist us in this endeavor. We will begin with a discussion of the most common techniques and methods used to make comparisons between expert and novice performers and also to measure the learning-related changes in perception and cognition.

## Expert–Novice Comparisons

The expert–novice approach has been used primarily to compare the perceptual–cognitive characteristics that appear to differentiate elite from subelite and/or novice performers.

A common experimental approach used to describe the characteristics of motor performance at various points along the learning continuum involves the comparison of expert and novice performance across a broad range of cognitive and motor skills. The **expert–novice approach** has been used primarily to compare the perceptual–cognitive characteristics that appear to differentiate elite from subelite and/or novice performers. This approach has been successfully applied to a number of cognitive and motor skills, including chess playing (Chase & Simon, 1973), physics problems (Chi, Feltovich, & Glaser, 1981), dinosaur knowledge (Chi & Koeske, 1983), basketball (French & Thomas, 1987), tennis (McPherson & Thomas, 1989), and baseball (McPherson, 1993).

In general, such studies have identified significant perceptual differences between expert and novice performers. These differences have specifically involved how a given visual display is searched, the speed at which it is searched (Bard & Fleury, 1981), what elements of the display are selectively attended to (Allard & Starkes, 1980), and how quickly the important information is extracted from the visual display prior to movement (Abernethy & Russell, 1984, 1987b). Expert performers search a visual display more quickly than novice performers, but they are also able to locate objects quickly and extract only those elements of the display that are relevant to the forthcoming response (see highlight, Do Experts See Things Differently in a Field of Play?). In addition to these perceptual inequalities, cognitive differences are also readily apparent. For example, expert performers are better able to interpret and organize skill-related information in memory so as to facilitate superior recall of that knowledge (Allard, Graham, & Paarsalu, 1980; Borgeaud & Abernethy, 1987).

The research tools used to identify the perceptual and cognitive differences that differentiate expert from novice performers typically include visual occlusion techniques, eye movement recordings, and memory recall tests. A discussion of each technique and how it has been used in various experimental settings follows.

# HIGHLIGHT

### Do Experts See Things Differently in a Field of Play?

Williams and colleagues (1994) demonstrated that in contrast to an inexperienced group of soccer players who tend to watch the ball and the player who is passing it (Box), expert players focus on the more peripheral aspects of a game, such as the positions and movements of players "off the ball." These systematic differences in visual search strategies are evident in the graph below, which shows how long experienced and inexperienced players fixated on certain areas of the playing scene.

To demonstrate these contrasting visual search strategy patterns, Williams et al. used an eye movement recording system capable of monitoring the eye movements of a group of inexperienced and experienced soccer players as they watched a series of soccer action sequences on a large projection screen. In order to determine how the different visual search strategies might influence the decisions made by players, the researchers also measured how quickly and accurately each player decided where on the field the ball would be passed. They did this by asking the player to announce aloud the grid number corresponding to the selected pass destination on the field. Not surprisingly, the experienced players demonstrated significantly faster response times than their inexperienced counterparts. The experienced players were clearly anticipating the ball's

destination even before the ball was kicked, an outcome that underscores their ability to make better use of advance information.

Perhaps one of the most interesting findings of this study was that the experienced players tended to fixate on many more field locations and to alternate their fixation locations more frequently during each trial. The faster scan rates observed by Williams et al. were in contrast, however, to those recorded in previous studies (Helsen & Pauwels, 1990). The authors attributed these differences to the fact that they had created a more complex open-play situation by representing more players in each of the filmed sequences.

According to the authors, research findings such as these emphasize the need for coaches to help inexperienced players develop more appropriate visual search strategies that not only encompass the passing player and the ball being passed, but also acknowledge the importance of the positions and movements of players in the immediate vicinity of the unfolding play. The authors conclude their discussion by suggesting a number of soccer-related training activities that coaches might use to help players develop more effective visual search strategies. These include using activities such as "one touch" and "silent" play lead-up games.

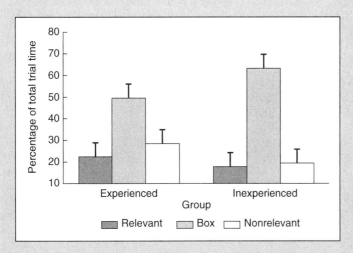

The experienced soccer players tended to fixate on many more field locations and to alternate their fixations more frequently than inexperienced players.

## Visual Occlusion Techniques

**Visual occlusion** has been used in a series of studies designed to investigate whether expert and novice performers attend to and extract the same types of visual cues from a visual display (Abernethy & Russell, 1987b; Starkes & Deakin, 1984). Vision of the movements of a videotaped or filmed performer is blocked at certain points during the action sequence, and the observer is asked to make certain predictions about the outcome of the movement. This same technique has been used to occlude certain body parts of a performer during execution of a movement. By doing this, researchers can begin to identify what aspects of the performer's movement appear to provide the most meaningful information for the forthcoming response.

Visual occlusion techniques are used to investigate whether expert and novice performers attend to and extract the same types of visual cues from a display.

Abernethy and Russell (1987b, experiment 1) used the visual occlusion technique to demonstrate that expert badminton players were significantly better than novice performers at predicting the landing location of an approaching badminton shot when the film was stopped at the exact moment of racquet-shuttlecock contact or as early as 83 ms before contact. The researchers demonstrated that the expert performers were extracting meaningful information from the display much more quickly than the novice performers. In a second experiment conducted by the same authors, certain body parts of the filmed performer were occluded during the performance. During one sequence, the racquet and arm of the performer were eliminated; the lower body, face and head, or racquet only were occluded during other sequences. The results indicated that novice performers attended primarily to the movements of the racquet in order to anticipate where the shuttlecock would travel. In contrast, the expert performers made their predictions by watching the movements of the arm and the racquet held by the performer. Monitoring the location of the arm controlling the racquet was clearly providing the expert performer with information about the direction of the shot much earlier than watching the racquet alone.

Although such visual occlusion techniques have advanced our knowledge concerning the aspects of visual information that appear to be important to skilled performance, the limitations of the methodology have prohibited its use as a perceptual training and assessment tool in actual play situations. As a result of recent advancements in technology, however, visual occlusion techniques may become an extremely useful perceptual training tool in the years to come. Starkes and colleagues (Starkes, Edwards, Dissanayake, & Dunn, 1995) recently completed the first field test using a new technology known as liquid crystal visual occlusion spectacles (Milgram, 1987). The lenses of these spectacles can be manipulated to provide full or occluded vision by means of an electrical pulse manually delivered to the glasses.

Using the visual occlusion spectacles, Starkes and colleagues were able to manipulate the visual fields of a group of volleyball players during various stages of a live serve. Following the serve, each player was required to place a marker on the court where she thought the ball had landed and then rate how confident she felt about her decision. The results of this study were similar to those of previous studies using more traditional visual occlusion approaches, which suggests that the new technology may eventually assist researchers in conducting studies in more realistic sports situations than has ever been possible.

## Eye Movement Recordings

An alternative method of determining exactly what aspects of a visual display performers are attending to while they are watching a movement or play situation unfold involves the use of more sophisticated devices to record eye movement. This computer-based technique is designed to track the movements of the observer's eyes while also providing information about gaze fixation time (the length of time the eyes are fixed on a given area of the display). Bard and Fleury (1981) have successfully used this technique to demonstrate that expert ice hockey goal tenders fixate for a longer period of time on the stick of the shooter, whereas novice goal tenders fixate more on the puck. As was the case in the badminton study conducted by Abernethy and Russell (1987b, experiment 2), watching the arm and implement being controlled, instead of the object being contacted, gives expert performers more time to anticipate what type of shot will be performed and therefore enables them to initiate a response more quickly. Eye movement recordings have also been used to identify differences among expert and novice performers in tennis (Goulet, Bard, & Fleury, 1989), soccer (Helsen & Pauwels, 1990), and gymnastics (Vickers, 1988).

Certain problems with the use of eye movement recordings to compare the perceptual abilities of expert and novice performers have been identified. First, the device itself has not yet been refined to the point where it can be worn in the actual movement setting. In order for the recordings to yield accurate eye movement data, the observer must be stationary and must generally be seated in a chair. The ecological validity associated with the use of this technique remains questionable as a result. Second, Adams (1966) correctly points out that the recording of eye movements identifies only what the observer is looking at, not what she or he is actually seeing. Thus eye movement recordings do not necessarily indicate what cues are being extracted for the purposes of making a response. One final criticism involves the device's inability to monitor peripheral vision as well as focal vision. We already know from our discussions on the role of vision in motor control that peripheral vision can provide the performer with important information on which to formulate a response.

*Eye movement recordings track the movements of the fovea and also provide information about gaze fixation time.*

## Pattern Recognition and Memory Recall Tests

The method most often used to investigate the cognitive processes that appear to form the basis of expertise has been the **pattern recognition** and **memory recall tests.** These tests have been used to demonstrate that expert performers not only take in very large quantities of information from a visual display in a very short period of time, but also organize it in a form that facilitates superior recall of that information. This organization of the information is thought to involve the **"chunking"** of individual pieces into larger units in memory. We will discuss this memory process in more detail in Chapter 8.

DeGroot (1966) and Chase and Simon (1973) were among the first researchers to use this type of test successfully to study cognitively based skills such as playing chess, writing computer programs, and solving mathematical

*Pattern recognition and memory recall tests have shown that experts are able to extract large amounts of information quickly from a visual display and that they organize it in a form that promotes superior recall.*

problems. In using the test to compare expert and novice chess players, Chase and Simon (1973) found that expert players were able to recall the exact location of a significantly higher number of chess pieces immediately following a 5-second look at a game board. Less skilled players were able to recall the locations of significantly fewer chess pieces. What is most interesting about their findings, however, is that experts demonstrated superior recall only when the locations of the chess pieces conformed to an actual game setup. On those trials where the pieces were randomly located, there were no differences found in recall ability among the various skill levels. This suggests that the expert performer's ability to chunk information is dependent on his or her familiarity and experience within the specific skill environment rather than on a preexisting ability to store more information in memory.

Pattern recognition and memory recall tests have since been used to study open sport skills that are primarily performed in variable environments. Unlike closed skills, open skills test a performer's ability to extract large amounts of information from a continuously changing visual display. (See highlight, The Classification of Motor Skills) In one such study, Allard, Graham, and Paarsalu (1980) presented several slides of basketball play situations to varsity- and intramural-level basketball players. Half of the slides depicted players in structured game positions; the remaining half showed random game positions such as scrambling for a loose ball. Following a 4-second viewing of the slide, players were asked to recall the position of as many players as possible by placing magnets on a game board provided. As was the case in Chase and Simon's study, the varsity players exhibited superior recall when compared to intramural players but only for those slides that depicted structured play situations. These findings have since been replicated using other sports, such as field hockey (Starkes & Deakin, 1984) and volleyball (Borgeaud & Abernethy, 1987).

### *Limitations of the Tests.*

As effective as the use of pattern recognition and recall tests appears to be in differentiating between expert and novice performers in their perceptual abilities, it is not without limitations. These limitations were highlighted in an article by Abernethy and colleagues (Abernethy, Burgess-Limerick, & Parks, 1994), who share the concerns expressed by advocates of direct theories of perception (see Chapter 5). They also suggest that the use of static "snapshots" of action may not adequately capture the dynamic nature of perception in a real sports environment. It is clear that this method of exploring perceptual differences between expert and novice performers is based on an indirect/computational view of perception. Recall that researchers aligned with this more traditional view of perception assume that the visual image received at the level of the retina is both static and impoverished—and therefore in need of considerable elaboration before the observer can perceive it as meaningful. A second concern raised by Abernethy et al. involves the erroneous conclusion that the superior perceptual abilities demonstrated by experts are the sole cause of differences in the quality of performance observed. They argue that improved perceptual abilities may simply be by-products of other factors, such as task experience and familiarity, that might contribute more to the differences observed in performance.

# HIGHLIGHT

## The Classification of Motor Skills

It has been a common practice in research on motor skill learning to categorize motor skills according to different criteria. One classification system that has been referred to extensively in the motor learning literature categorizes skills into two general classes according to the type of environment in which they are performed. The two classes of skills are closed and open (Poulton, 1957). Let us briefly contrast the defining characteristics of these different types of motor skills.

*Open skills* have customarily been described as those skills that are performed in variable environments and therefore must be repeatedly adapted to the changing demands of the environment. Given that a changing environment rarely permits the use of the same movement response on two successive attempts, it is important that the performer be able to execute many subtle variations of the skill. Examples of open skills can be found in soccer, basketball, football, and ice and field hockey.

*Closed skills* are performed in stable, unchanging environments. The goal for the learner in these types of movement situations is the development of a consistent movement pattern that can be performed in exactly the same way from trial to trial. Examples of these types of skills include springboard and platform diving, figure skating, and gymnastics.

Unfortunately, this method of classifying skills has created as much confusion as clarity for the reader of motor skills research. This is because many skills are really neither open skills nor closed skills. Consider, for example, golf and pole vault. Although both skills are performed in relatively stable environments, subtle changes are occurring from trial to trial. Wind direction and velocity may change between golf strokes, and the height of the bar to be jumped in the sport of pole vault is raised repeatedly throughout a competition. Couple this problem with the fact that many open skills have components that can be classified as closed skills (e.g., free throw shooting in basketball), and the dichotomous classification of skills becomes still more imperfect.

Writers such as Magill (1993b) have suggested that much of the confusion can be avoided if we consider these two very different types of skills to represent the two opposite extremes of the motor skill continuum. Thus there is room between the "poles" to place a number of motor skills that are more like one than the other type of skill.

# Development of a Knowledge Base

Although comparisons between expert and novice performances have provided us with knowledge about the attention and cognitive abilities that appear to differentiate novice from expert performers, this methodology has contributed little insight into *how* a novice performer actually learns to become an expert. This major shortcoming of the expert–novice paradigm was first identified by Thomas, French, and Humphries (1985), who called for a more systematic approach to the study of motor skill acquisition—one that better elucidates the processes underlying the acquisition of what the authors referred to as a domain-specific knowledge base. Thomas and colleagues (French & Thomas, 1987; McPherson & Thomas, 1989; McPherson, 1993) have since developed a comprehensive **knowledge-based paradigm** and successfully applied it to a variety of sport-related settings.

The paradigm developed by Thomas et al. involves the administration of appropriate knowledge tests and skill-specific tests to children at different levels of learning: extensive verbal interviews designed to test the children's knowledge of a game's rules (declarative knowledge) and their understanding of when to apply certain game-specific strategies (procedural knowledge). Each of these tests is supplemented with the videotape coding of game performances. These videotape recordings are then used to evaluate the learning-related changes in the level of skill exhibited, in the quality of decision making during match play, and in the performer's ability to execute the decisions successfully.

As a consequence of their efforts to explore all these relationships simultaneously, Thomas and colleagues have been able to show that expert performers possess a larger, more complex, and better organized knowledge base than novice performers in certain sports settings. The authors further speculate that this major difference in knowledge base lies in the expert performer's tendency to develop IF-THEN-DO productions with incorporation of the DO portion being the defining element of expertise (see McPherson & Thomas, 1989, for a more detailed review).

> The difference in knowledge base lies in the expert's ability to incorporate the DO portion into the IF-THEN-DO productions.

## Measuring Learning-Related Changes in the Dynamics of Action

In addition to the many perceptual–cognitive changes that occur in connection with learning, it is clear that many subtle and not-so-subtle changes are also taking place in the pattern of coordination at various points along the learning continuum. Although the practitioner with acute observational skills is able to observe directly many of the not-so-subtle changes in the dynamics of the action that evolve with practice, more sophisticated technology and methods of analysis are necessary if the more subtle changes in behavior are to be identified.

We will discuss two types of measurement in this section: physiological and mechanical measures of efficiency. Both of these measurement techniques have been successfully used to quantify the more subtle learning-related changes that occur in the dynamics of the action.

### Measures of Metabolic and Mechanical Efficiency

If, indeed, one of the defining characteristics of skilled performance is movement efficiency, then research directed at studying how this component changes as a function of practice would seem worthwhile. Sparrow and colleagues (Sparrow, 1983; Sparrow & Irizarry-Lopez, 1987) have shown particular interest in this aspect of performance and have employed physiological and mechanical indices of efficiency to explore the relationships among practice, mechanical work rate, and metabolic energy expenditure.

In one such study, Sparrow and Irizarry-Lopez (1987) examined the changes in the amounts of metabolic energy expended and mechanical work accomplished by the legs and arms of adults who repeatedly practiced a crawling movement on a motor-driven treadmill over the course of ten days. The authors hypothesized that changes in these two aspects of performance would be closely related to any modifications being made to the movement pattern during practice. This initial hypothesis was generally supported when the various physiological and mechanical parameters measured were correlated. The authors found that as subjects "optimized" their pattern of interlimb coordination, the amount of energy expended decreased. And although the improvement was not statistically significant, the level of mechanical efficiency demonstrated by the subjects had also improved as much as 13.7% by the last day of practice.

Considerably more research is necessary to examine fully the relationship between movement kinematics and mechanical efficiency, but the results of this study suggest that this will be a fruitful area of research. Research in this area may also yield important practical information for rehabilitation therapists concerned with helping patients learn functional movement patterns. The development of a movement pattern that minimizes the amount of energy expended and the mechanical work involved is an important goal for the patient.

> The level of metabolic and mechanical efficiency has been shown to increase as a movement skill is learned.

## Identifying the Learning-Related Changes in Performance

It is clear that the use of the many experimental methods and techniques described in this chapter has contributed much to our understanding of the perceptual, cognitive, and mechanical processes that form the basis of skilled performance. More research is needed to delineate exactly how a performer progresses along the skill-learning continuum, but we can identify a number of performer characteristics that are directly influenced by learning.

- *The focus of attention.* As learning progresses, performers allocate attention to different types of salient cues and become able to extract meaning from a visual display with greater speed and precision.
- *Knowledge base.* Both the breadth and the structure of the knowledge base can be expected to change as a function of learning. Expertise appears to be accompanied by knowledge not only of what to do but also of when to do it.
- *Dynamics of the action.* The learner begins to manipulate more appropriately the degrees of freedom available within the motor system to accomplish the goal of the movement. Changes in the temporal and spatial patterning of musculature are also evident as the learner searches for the optimal solution to the motor problem at hand.
- *Metabolic and mechanical efficiency.* There is some evidence to suggest that modifications in the kinematics of movement associated with learning are strongly related to reductions in the amount of physiological and mechanical energy expended.

# Summary

In this chapter, four approaches to studying motor learning were discussed. The traditional approach is based on the "scientific method" and on how we define motor learning. A problem-oriented rather than method-oriented approach was recommended because it enables researchers to go beyond the boundaries of any one method. Also recommended was the doctrine of disproof, which holds that science advances only through disproof. Lastly, the approach that views basic and applied research as independent but cooperating endeavors, rather than applied research solely as an extension of basic research, was recommended if motor learning is to develop a body of knowledge that is enriched with relevance.

Additionally, in this chapter, we discussed how we assess motor learning in acquisition, especially in terms of performance curves; the factors that affect performance curves and the study of motor learning (such as scoring sensitivity, ceiling and floor effects, and plateaus); and the ways of assessing motor learning by means of setting a criterion of mastery or measuring the degree of automaticity to determine when learning is complete in acquisition and how the criterion of mastery relates to over-learning were discussed. Because performance measures taken in acquisition may or may not be an accurate indicator of motor learning, it is necessary to combine them with post-acquisition performance measures taken on retention or transfer tests. These tests help us determine the durability of the level of performance achieved in acquisition and the direction and generalization of transfer.

Differences in perceptual abilities between novice and expert performers have been demonstrated by using two related research methods: visual occlusion techniques and eye movement recordings. As a consequence of attending to different salient cues in a visual display, expert performers are able to extract more meaningful information more quickly than novice performers. These perceptual differences ensure that the expert performer is able to respond more quickly and appropriately in game situations.

The use of memory recall tests has revealed differences in cognitive abilities between expert and novice performers. In general, expert performers have learned to organize, or "chunk," large amounts of information into larger memory units that can then be retrieved with greater speed and ease of recall.

The relationships among development of a knowledge base, skill performance, and decision-making abilities is currently being systematically explored in a number of different sports contexts. Current research findings suggest that as the learning of a sport proceeds, the learner develops more and more IF-THEN productions, which are then linked to a number of DO productions. The successful linking between these two sets of productions may herald the arrival of expertise in a given sport.

The changing dynamics of action that accompany learning are being quantified using a variety of measurement and analytical techniques, which include measures of physiological and mechanical efficiency. Research conducted using these techniques has provided evidence that as individuals optimize their pattern of interlimb coordination, the amount of energy expended decreases and mechanical efficiency improves.

## IMPORTANT TERMINOLOGY

After completing this chapter, readers should be familiar with the following terms and concepts.

ceiling effects
chunking
cooperative approach
criterion of mastery
degree of automaticity
doctrine of disproof
expert–novice approach
floor effects
knowledge-based paradigm
learning curve
learning plateau
learning-retention distinction
level of original learning
level of performance

memory recall test
method of inductive inference
method-oriented approach
over-learning
pattern recognition test
performance curve
problem-oriented approach
retention interval
retention test
scoring sensitivity
traditional approach
transfer test
visual occlusion

## SUGGESTED FURTHER READING

Christina, R. W. (1997). Concerns and issues in studying and assessing motor learning. *Measurement in Physical Education and Exercise Science, 1,* 19–38.

Snyder, C. W. Jr., & Abernethy, B. (1992). *Understanding human action through experimentation.* Champaign, IL: Human Kinetics.

McPherson, S. L. (1994). The development of sport expertise. Mapping the tactical domain. *Quest, 46,* 223–240.

## TEST YOUR UNDERSTANDING

1. Distinguish among the following approaches to the study of motor learning: traditional, method-oriented, problem-oriented, doctrine of disproof, and cooperative.

2. Explain how the shape of a performance curve can be affected by each of the following: method of measurement, scoring sensitivity, and ceiling and floor effects.

3. Why is it inappropriate to make inferences about an individual's motor learning based on a group performance curve?

4. What is a plateau in a performance curve, and why does it occur?

5. What are the limitations of using performance curves to assess motor learning?

6. Explain how one can determine when learning is complete in acquisition by setting a criterion of mastery and using a degree of automaticity.

7. Why are retention and transfer tests used to assess motor learning?

8. Describe two experimental methods used to identify the perceptual characteristics that differentiate novice from expert performers. Explain the nature of the perceptual differences revealed by these two methods.

9. How have memory recall tests been used to identify differences between experts and novices in cognitive abilities? Describe the major research findings that have emerged from the use of such tests.

10. Briefly describe a research paradigm that has been used to study how the novice performer learns to become an expert. How does the expert's knowledge base appear to differ from that of a novice performer?

11. Describe two methods that have been used to investigate how the dynamics of action change as a function of learning. Outline the major findings that each method has yielded.

# 8

# SETTING THE STAGE FOR MOTOR LEARNING

*How a movement skill is presented to learners sets the stage for understanding*
*how to perform it as well as how effectively it is learned.*

## CHAPTER OBJECTIVES

After studying this chapter, you should be able to:

- Explain the role of motivation in motor learning and how goal setting, praise, criticism, success, failure, self-esteem, competition, and cooperation can operate to motivate people to learn.

- Describe the key elements to consider when introducing and explaining a new movement skill to learners.

- Identify and explain the variables that have been shown to influence the effectiveness of using a model when learning movement skills.

- Identify practical strategies and techniques that can be used to enhance the effectiveness of a model in a variety of learning situations.

- Explain the two primary theoretical positions that account for the effectiveness of modeling in the learning of movement skills.

- Explain the alternative technique called discovery learning for teaching a new movement skill or pattern of coordination.

- Identify ways in which the environment can be structured to promote discovery learning of movement skills or patterns of coordination.

A recurring issue for teachers and clinicians alike is the construction of an environment in which the learning or relearning of movement-based skills is optimized. Although it is important for the learning environment not to overwhelm the learner with its complexity, it should progressively challenge the individual and eventually mirror the environment in which the skill to be acquired will be performed. For example, during the course of a rehabilitation program in which a patient is learning to regain function following a cerebrovascular accident, the learning environment should resemble the place where the skills will ultimately be performed. To achieve this end, many rehabilitation facilities construct elaborate complexes complete with full-scale kitchens, grocery aisles stocked with items to be selected and carried, and modified motor vehicles designed to train the patient in advanced transfer skills.

In motor skills settings, a similar approach is desirable. Once the fundamental skills of a sport have been introduced, further practice should take place in a learning environment that mirrors the game situation. Undesirable complexity can be controlled by limiting the skills needed in modified game situations or the number of players participating. In this way, the learning environment is progressively shaped to reproduce that of the game.

Numerous factors must be considered when setting the stage to optimize motor learning. Some of the more important ones include how to effectively motivate learners and help them set learning goals, as well as how to introduce, explain, and demonstrate the motor skill to be learned. Of course, central to the implementation of effective demonstrations is understanding how observational learning and modeling works. This chapter also discusses an alternative instructional approach referred to as *discovery learning*. Let's examine these factors more closely and determine how practitioners can manipulate them to effectively set the stage to optimize motor learning.

## Motivating People to Learn Motor Skills

Being appropriately motivated to learn is a prerequisite for optimizing learning.

Being appropriately motivated to learn a motor skill is a prerequisite for optimizing learning. Essentially, people get out of their learning experience what they put into it. If they are not motivated to learn a movement skill, the stage is set for little or no learning to take place. If they are moderately motivated to learn a movement skill, the stage is set to learn some, but not all, that is necessary to optimize performance. And, if they are highly motivated, the stage is set to learn all that is needed to optimize motor skill performance. Consider, for example, your own handwriting. How many years have you been practicing your handwriting? Has the proficiency of your handwriting continued to improve, improved to a certain level and then stayed about the same, or become worse over the years? If it has stayed the same or become worse, you can probably attribute either of these results to your lack of motivation to improve it. Essentially, you were practicing your handwriting without the intent to improve it. When you practice a movement skill without the motivation to improve it, the amount and conditions of practice are likely to have little or no effect on improving performance.

Motivating people to learn when setting the stage for practice can create a momentum of interest and excitement in acquiring the new movement skill that is likely to carry into the actual practice session. If they are motivated to learn the new movement skill after it has been introduced, explained, and demonstrated, they will be motivated to learn it during the initial stage of practice. Thus, it is important that appropriate motivators be not only interwoven into the introduction, explanation, and demonstration of the skill to be learned, but also inserted immediately before practice begins if necessary. Of course, motivation can wane as practice continues, so learners must keep their motivation at the appropriate level when acquiring a new movement skill. Motivation (extrinsic and intrinsic), motives, and needs were introduced in Chapter 6 and will not be repeated here. Instead, the focus is on the roles of goal setting, praise, criticism, success, failure, self-esteem, competition, and cooperation in motivating people to learn.

# Goal Setting

**Goal setting** motivates people to get the most out of their learning. This process involves establishing challenging but realistic learning goals before practice or training to learn the movement skill begins. This motivational approach has been studied in industrial settings (for reviews see Locke & Latham, 1985; Tubbs, 1986) and in exercise and sport situations (for reviews see Burton, 1993; Locke, 1991; Weinberg, 1994). At least in industrial environments, setting well-defined and challenging goals results in better performance than either no goals or vague goals such as "do your best" or "give it 100%" (Locke & Latham, 1985). Well-defined and challenging goals are ones that (a) focus specifically on what activities have to be done, (b) assist in managing the effort given to these activities, (c) help to sustain watchfulness in striving to achieve the goals, and (d) function as a referent against which the performance achieved can be compared.

The findings from research on goal setting in exercise and sport have not consistently supported those emanating from research in industrial environments. This may be due to the inherent difficulty of manipulating external goals in exercise and sport environments because quite often performers are intrinsically motivated (Burton, 1993; Locke, 1991; Weinberg, 1994). Consequently, when they are instructed in a study to set external goals, regardless of whether the goals are vague or specific, they may be secretively setting intrinsic goals that are, in fact, well-defined and very challenging. Indeed, if this is happening, they will attend to their intrinsic goal setting more than the researcher's manipulations of external goal setting, which makes it difficult to determine the actual effects of goal setting in exercise and sport. In spite of this difficulty, Kyllo and Landers (1995) reported from their meta-analysis of the research literature that explicit, well-defined goals that are moderately challenging to achieve were beneficial to exercise and sport performance. Further, they indicated that short-term goals and short-term goals combined with long-term goals were more effective than only long-term goals.

Much of the research on goal setting has studied its effect on performance, which raises a question about its effect on learning. Boyce (1992) attempted to answer this question. She studied three groups of participants who established various goals before they learned to shoot at a target with a rifle. One group was instructed to "do your best" (instructor sets general goal); the second group was instructed to set their own specific goals (learner sets specific goals); and a third group was given explicit, well-defined goals that were made gradually more challenging on each day of practice (instructor sets specific goals). Following a target shooting pretest, the three groups of learners completed five days of practice over three weeks in which they trained using the goal-setting strategy to which they were randomly assigned. A retention test was given one week after the last day of practice. The findings, shown in Figure 8.1 on page 226, reveal that except for the first day of practice, shooting performance was better in acquisition and retention for the two groups in which specific goals were set by the learners and by the instructor than it was for the group in which the instructor set the general goal to "do your best." This finding supports

*Explicit, well-defined goals that are moderately challenging to achieve are effective.*

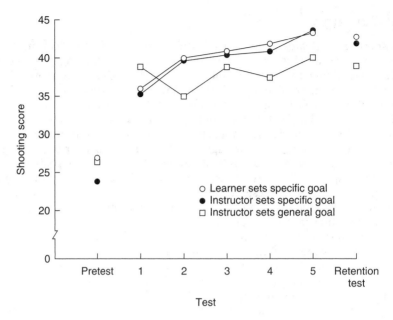

**Figure 8.1**   Influence of goal setting on the learning and retention of shooting at a target with a rifle.

the hypothesis that specific, well-defined goals are more beneficial for motor learning and its retention than a general goal to "do your best."

## Praise and Criticism

Usually praise is more powerful in motivating learners than criticism.

Not all people are motivated before they begin learning, but this does not mean that they cannot become motivated as they engage in learning. The judicious and appropriate use of praise and criticism can be very helpful in motivating people to learn (Brophy, 1981). Usually, **praise** is more powerful in motivating learners than criticism, but at times even **criticism** can be better than receiving no recognition at all. As a general rule, praise is best to use with learners who have introverted personalities. Some learners with extroverted personalities tend to respond best to criticism. In order for praise and criticism to have their greatest positive effect on the motivation to learn, learners must perceive that (a) praise and criticism are not given automatically and unconditionally, (b) not everyone receives praise and criticism all the time, and (c) praise and criticism fit the situation and the learner. How criticism is given makes a difference. **Constructive criticism** given in a friendly, positive way and in the spirit of helpfulness is much more effective than destructive criticism that focuses on put-downs that are hurled at learners out of frustration and anger. Constructive criticism is essential for enhancing learning, but destructive criticism, which makes learners feel like their self-esteem is under attack, can be quite detrimental to learning.

# Success and Failure

Generally, learners who experience frequent **success** in learning and performing motor skills tend to feel more adequate, confident, and self-enhanced. Learners who experience frequent **failure** tend to feel anxious, less adequate, less confident, and less able to set realistic goals for themselves. Essentially, success tends to enhance learning and, to an even greater extent, failure tends to impair it (Lantz, 1945; Rhine, 1957; Steigman & Stevenson, 1960). Moreover, repeated failure tends to depress self-confidence and motivation for further learning.

Success tends to enhance learning to a greater extent, and failure tends to impair it.

When teaching people who are highly motivated to achieve, providing them with learning experiences that offer opportunities for a blend of successes and failures are most likely to sustain their high level of motivation (Weiner, 1972). When teaching people who have a low level of motivation to achieve, providing them with learning and practice experiences that offer opportunities mainly for successes are more likely to sustain their motivation level. When teaching people who have experienced many more failures than successes, try to help them feel worthwhile, adequate, and successful during the numerous interactions that you have with them. A friendly smile, positive comment, or a pat on the back when deserved are examples of ways of communicating the idea that they are "worthwhile" and "successful" as human beings. Find desirable behaviors (e.g., their effort) and successful performances (even if only a part of the skill was performed correctly) to praise, but be certain the praise given is deserved. Also, don't hesitate to give constructive criticism when appropriate. Lastly, design learning experiences in which difficulty levels are adjusted appropriately in relation to the different capabilities of the learners.

# Self-Esteem

Learners' **self-esteem** refers to how they view themselves as individuals (Lynch, Norem-Hebeisen, & Gergen, 1981; Rosenberg, 1979). Self-esteem is important to consider when trying to understand how and why success and failure experiences motivate different learners in different ways. Usually, learners strive to behave in a manner that tends to be consistent with their self-esteem. Generally, high self-esteem learners develop "success-type" personalities and search for ways to succeed while low self-esteem learners develop "failure-type" personalities and may actually seek ways to fail (Covington & Berry, 1976; Hamachek, 1978; Lowin & Epstein, 1965).

High self-esteem learners who are confident in their self-appraisal tend to accept their successful experiences regardless of whether the successes were self-determined or a result of external circumstances. High self-esteem learners who are not confident also tend to welcome their successful experiences regardless of the source of successes. Low self-esteem learners who are confident in their self-appraisal tend to reject their successful experiences to be consistent with their failure image; however, they are inclined to be motivated by successes they perceive as resulting from luck or fate. Lastly, low self-esteem learners who are not confident tend to accept their successful experiences regardless of whether their successes were self-determined or a result of external circumstances.

High self-esteem learners tend to develop "success-type" personalities and search for ways to succeed.

## Competition and Cooperation

Some people prefer competitive conditions, whereas others prefer cooperative conditions in which to learn movement skills.

Competition and cooperation can function as motivators to enhance learning (Johnson & Johnson, 1975; Michaels, 1977; Okun & DiVesta, 1975; Sharon, 1980; Slavin, 1980). **Competition** is a contest between rivals who are striving for some objective, such as victory, whereas **cooperation** is an association with two or more for a mutual benefit. For example, competition can be seen between opposing teams playing games such as basketball, baseball, or soccer and between two individuals playing a game such as tennis or golf. Cooperation is evident in sport when players on a team work together to execute plays and function successfully as a unit on offense or defense. The question for practitioners directing learning is what works best to motivate people to learn movement skills—competitive or cooperative conditions? Actually, it appears that some learners prefer competitive conditions more often to learn to perform their best, whereas other learners prefer cooperative conditions more often to enhance their learning.

There are at least two recommended guidelines for manipulating competitive conditions appropriately to meet the different needs and desires of learners and to minimize the impact of losing without compromising the positive benefits of competition. First, although learners compete against others to determine the outcome, each person should be encouraged to do his or her personal best and to compete against him- or herself. Second, strive to arrange competitive situations in which learners with different skill levels and capabilities can have a chance for success and be acknowledged for their best efforts. If learners know for certain that there are some skills they can perform reasonably well and that this performance is appreciated, the skills they cannot perform as well are likely to be kept in perspective and not likely to be as disappointing.

# Introducing and Explaining Movement Skills

The first step in setting the stage for practice and learning involves **introducing** the movement skill to be learned. The next step involves **explaining** and **demonstrating** how to perform it. How you introduce, explain, and demonstrate the new skill should not only help learners understand how to perform it, but also motivate them to want to learn it.

## Setting the Stage for the Introduction

The introduction should tell the learners what they will be learning and why it is important.

The introduction should enthusiastically inform learners what they are about to learn and why it is important to learn it. Further, it should prepare them for the explanation and demonstration that follows. If learners are to obtain the greatest benefit from the introduction of a new movement skill, the instructor must first make sure that he or she captures their attention, and then organizes them into a formation that is appropriate for everyone to hear what is said and see what is about to be demonstrated. The background the learners see behind the instructor should be free from visual distractions, and the area selected should have minimum background noise.

## Delivering the Introduction

Once the learners are properly arranged it is time to deliver the introduction. Be enthusiastic and make it *brief, simple, accurate,* and *direct* (Landin, 1994; Siedentop, 1991). It should cognitively prepare the students for learning the skill that is about to be explained and demonstrated. As mentioned, it should tell them what they are going to learn and why they need to learn it. Avoid introductions that are too detailed, elaborate, or abstract, and use language that is easy to understand and appropriate for the age level of the learners. Lastly, use part of the introduction to motivate the learners to acquire the new skill not only by explaining how they will benefit, but also by identifying others (to whom they can relate) who have been successful in learning and using it. The more students are convinced of the relevance and importance of the new skill being introduced and how they will benefit, the more motivated they will be to learn it.

## Delivering the Explanation

Like the introduction, the explanation should be enthusiastically presented, appropriate for the age level of the learners, and consist of language that they can easily understand. The explanation should be *brief, simple, accurate,* and *direct* (Conrad, 1962; Landin, 1994; Siedentop, 1991; Waters, 1928). Excessively detailed, elaborate, or abstract explanations provide little or no value in communicating the basic idea of how to perform a new skill and often interfere with learning (Hicks, 1975; Renshaw & Postle, 1928). Be mindful that words alone often have little meaning to learners who are acquiring a movement skill for the first time, and usually words have limited value in communicating the general idea of how to move to perform it.

The introduction and explanation should be presented enthusiastically; be brief, simple, accurate, direct, and complement the demonstration.

The explanation should complement the demonstration by giving the learners a general idea of how to perform the skill. It should give them the *big picture* in as few as words as possible. It should inform the learners how to execute the skill by pointing out only one or two of the most relevant informational cues needed for them to understand how to perform it. There is no need to point out too many cues at this stage of learning and *overload* the learners with too much information (Landin, 1994; Hicks, 1975). The remaining cues can be introduced later in acquisition when the learners are capable of processing this additional information. Keep in mind that some cues are more easily communicated with words than demonstrating the skill. For instance, it is easier to tell learners to "put your weight over the balls of your feet," "keep your eyes on the ball," or "grip the bat with less pressure" than it is to demonstrate these informational cues.

## Select the Best Words to Use in the Explanation

Some words more effectively explain how to perform skills than others. Quite often, the words chosen will *directly and literally* communicate what the learners should do. For example, when describing a wrestling stance a coach might say, "Stand with your feet shoulder-width apart, knees slightly bent, head up, and back straight." Sometimes, however, a direct, literal description becomes

The best words to use in an explanation are those that produce the desired result, regardless of whether they are literal or figurative.

too awkward and detailed, giving way to a *figurative explanation,* which can be much more effective (Harrison, 1958; Holding, 1965). For instance, when teaching basketball players how to follow through on a shot, a coach could literally describe the action of the arm, wrist, and fingers in this way: "After you release the ball, be certain that your arm is extended at the elbow, your wrist is bent (flexed), and your fingers are relatively straight (extended) just above and toward the rim of the basket." However, the coach is likely to get better results if he or she used the following figurative description: "After you release the ball, dunk your fingers over the rim and into the basket."

In some instances a combination of literal and figurative explanations is useful. Remember, literal descriptions or explanations work best for some skills, figurative descriptions work best for others, and sometimes a combination of the two is the best choice. When selecting the words or type of explanation to use, the most important consideration is the effect produced, that is, whether the words or type of explanation will result in the learners performing the desired movements.

## Where to Direct the Learners' Focus of Attention

Focusing attention on performing one's movements during their execution can interfere with the performance of well-learned skills (e.g., Bliss, 1892–1893; Boder, 1935; Schneider & Fisk, 1983). Evidence also exists that suggests that self-focused attention can interfere with learning new movement skills (e.g., Masters, 1992; Wulf & Weigelt, 1997). In fact, Wulf and Weigelt found that providing instructions to learners that directed their attention to a feature of their own movement coordination considered essential for successful performance on a slalom ski simulator (see Figure 8.5 on page 246) was even more detrimental than no instruction at all.

This finding especially held when learners were under increased stress to perform successfully. Based on their research and that of Vereijken and colleagues (Vereijken, 1991; Vereijken et al., 1992), Wulf and Weigelt suggested that sometimes learning by discovery might be more effective in acquiring a complex movement skill than giving an explanation or instruction that directs attention to a particular essential movement feature of the skill to be learned.

Sometimes learning by discovery is more effective than instruction that directs attention to important movement features of the skill.

The suggestion of learning by discovery by Wulf and Weigelt is based on evidence from the learning of closed movement skills in which the environment is not changing appreciably. However, their suggestion also may be appropriate for open movement skills that must be performed in response to an environment that is changing (e.g., actual slalom skiing not on a simulator, hitting pitched baseballs/softballs, or returning tennis shots). Learning the regulatory (predictable) features of the environment to which such skills must respond is important to successful performance. For instance, to successfully return shots, a tennis player must repeatedly perform the appropriate return strokes (e.g., forehand, backhand strokes) with the racket head positioned in the *right place* and the *right time* for each of the shots. To perform return shots successfully, the player must be able to learn to predict where the ball will be and when it will be there. Magill (1998) has proposed that learning the environmental regulatory features can, and probably should, be learned implicitly rather than by explanations or instructions that direct attention to regulatory features. In other words, letting performers acquire the regularities by **discovery learning** rather than direct explanation or instruction may be more effective for open movement skills.

Subsequent research (Shea & Wulf, 1999; Wulf, Höss, & Prinz, 1998; Wulf, Lauterback, & Toole, 1999) revealed that learning to perform various movement tasks (e.g., slalom ski simulator, stabilometer, pitch shots in golf) could be facilitated by directing the learners' attention away from their own movements (**internal focus of attention**) and toward the effects these movements have on the environment (**external focus of attention**). In two follow-up experiments, Wulf, Shea, and Park (2001) found further evidence in learning a stabilometer balancing task that supported the benefits of external attentional focus over internal focus. In both experiments, participants who adopted an external focus in learning a stabilometer task displayed better balance performance in retention than those who adopted an internal focus. Therefore, independent of whether participants were assigned to an external focus condition as in previous studies by Shea and Wulf (1999) and Wulf et al. (1998, 1999) or asked to try different attentional foci and make their own decision as in the Wulf et al. (2001) study, an external focus of attention produced superior performance and learning than an internal focus. See highlight, The Learning Advanges of an External Focus of Attention in Golf, on page 232.

The findings from the Wulf et al. (2001) study seem to provide evidence against the idea that individual differences play an important role in the relative effectiveness of an external versus internal focus of attention. Instead, the positive effects of an external focus of attention on learning appear to be more a general phenomenon. Their findings also are consistent with the **constrained action hypothesis** proposed by Wulf, McNevin, and Shea (2002). This hypothesis holds that an internal focus of attention results in a conscious attempt to control movements, which interferes with the automatic motor control processes and negatively affects performance and learning. An external focus of attention enables the motor system to self-organize more naturally (e.g., Kelso, 1995), unconstrained by conscious attempts to control movements. External focus of attention might allow for more natural control processes to take over and self-organize the motor system, liberating conscious attention to be directed to other aspects of the movement task, resulting in a positive effect on performance and learning.

Sometimes focusing attention on the effects of movements rather than on essential features of the movements promotes more effective learning.

## Relate What Is Being Taught to the Learners' Background

How rapidly and well learners acquire a new movement skill and relevant knowledge greatly depends on the extent of their understanding of the skill and knowledge to be learned (e.g., Farr, 1987; Gentner, 1980, 1982; Gentner & Stevens, 1983; Kieras & Boviar, 1984; Mayer, 1975). Of course, acquiring this understanding depends on how effectively the practitioner relates the new skill and knowledge to their previously learned skills and past experience or knowledge. For example, the practitioner may need to explain:

- Why the parts of the new skill must be performed in a particular way
- The relationship of the parts to the whole skill
- How and in what way the new skill is related to what the learners already know

# HIGHLIGHT

## The Learning Advantages of an External Focus of Attention in Golf

In a series of studies conducted in a laboratory setting, Wulf and colleagues (Wulf & Weigelt, 1997; Wulf, Höss, & Prinz, 1998) have provided strong evidence that learners who adopt an external as opposed to internal focus of attention when learning a new motor skill demonstrate significantly better learning. As persuasive as these laboratory findings might be, however, can they be generalized to the learning of more "real-world" sport skills outside of the laboratory (Christina, 1987, 1989)?

To address this very question, Wulf, Lauterbach, and Toole (1999) recruited a group of young adults with no previous golfing experience to learn the skill of pitching in golf. An outdoor setting with a lawn surface was chosen as the site for the experiment. Following basic instruction on how to grip a nine iron club and address the ball, participants were randomly assigned to an internal focus of attention or external focus of attention group. Participants in the internal focus group were instructed to focus on the arm swing during the performance of each pitch shot. Participants in the external focus group were instructed to focus on the movements of the club head during the swing. Pitching the golf ball a distance of 15 meters into a circular target was the goal for each learner.

During a single practice session, each participant performed 80 practice trials in blocks of 10 trials each. Both groups were reminded of their focus at the beginning of each block of trials. The following day, participants returned to the study site and performed 30 additional trials. No instructions about any aspect of the stroke were given. The external focus group performed the skill with greater accuracy during both the practice and retention sessions. On the basis of these findings it appears that the beneficial effects of an external focus of attention can be generalized to the learning of sport skills learned under more real-world conditions.

In a more recent study, Perkins-Ceccato, Passmore, and Lee (2003) also investigated the benefits of an external focus of attention on the performance of a pitching stroke in golf but added the variable of skill level to their study. They compared the performance of highly skilled golfers (mean handicap of 4) to low skilled golfers (mean handicap of 26). Participants were assigned to one of two groups. The internal focus of attention group was instructed to focus on the form of the swing and force generated during the swing; the external focus of attention group was instructed to concentrate on hitting the ball as close to the target pylon as possible. In contrast to the earlier findings of Wulf et al., this group of researchers found that the performance of the low skilled golfers group was more consistent when the focus of attention was internal versus external while an external focus of attention resulted in more consistent performances among the high skilled golfers.

How might we reconcile these apparently contradictory findings? The answer might lie in just how far the focus of attention is directed away from the learner's own movements. In the Wulf et al. study, the unskilled participants in the external focus group were instructed to focus on the movements of the clubhead during the swing, whereas in the study conducted by Perkins-Ceccato et al. the low skilled external focus group was instructed to focus attention well beyond any aspect of the swing to a target location. Perhaps it is a question of how far the learner's attention is directed away from his or her own body movements during the initial stages of learning? In the more recent study, the external focus of attention may have been too remote for the low skilled golfer to derive sufficient benefit when performing the skill. Future research will need to resolve this issue so that practitioners can appropriately select external focus of attention cues for learners at different skill levels.

Teaching any physical or cognitive skills to learners often will produce better results if the explanation relates the new skill and knowledge to ones that they have already learned and have in memory. This approach is likely to enhance the learners' understanding of the movement skill and knowledge to be learned by meaningfully connecting it with their existing knowledge and skills, which provides a strong foundation for promoting effective learning. Actually, this approach takes advantage of the performer's ability to transfer previously acquired skills and knowledge to the learning of the new skill and knowledge. Performers who understand how a previously learned skill or a part of that skill can be transferred or relates to the new skill can usually learn the new skill more quickly than if they lacked such understanding. For example, when students are learning a new tennis serve and are having difficulty moving the racquet through the proper sequence of arm and body movements, comparing these movements to a previously learned skill—such as throwing a baseball overhand—may be helpful.

> Relating the new skill being learned to the learners' background often facilitates learning.

Thus, there appear to be at least two benefits of including one or more mechanical principles or features as part of the explanation to learners who are acquiring a new movement skill. One benefit is that it facilitates the learning of the new skill (e.g., Hendrickson & Schroeder, 1941; Judd, 1908; Mohr & Barrett, 1962; Papscy, 1968; Werner, 1972). Gallahue, Werner, and Luedke (1975) recommended that a variety of examples be provided when teaching a biomechanical principle and that similarities between movement patterns of the new skill and previously learned skills be explicitly pointed out. Another benefit is to facilitate the learning of *other* new skills that make use of the newly explained and acquired principle. Understanding a principle inherent in one skill and applying it to performing that skill should transfer to the learning and performance of other skills that make use of the same principle. Understanding the principle of stability, for instance, as it applies to wrestling and utilizing it during matches should be transferable to learning linebacker skills in football. If a wrestler has learned to lower his center of gravity for increased stability against an opponent, that principle should be available to teaching the linebacker how to increase his stability or balance against an offensive lineman who is trying to block him.

In summary, explanations that help learners relate previously acquired skills and knowledge to new ones can increase their chances of transferring similar skill and knowledge parts of their previous learning to learning of the new skill and knowledge. If these relationships can be communicated effectively, the likelihood that learners will efficiently integrate the previously acquired parts and the newly learned parts into a series of parts that make up the skill, strategy, principle, or play to be learned will increase. One thing seems very clear: To maximize the chances of transfer of learning between previously learned knowledge and skills and the learning of new ones, instructors must teach for it directly and not leave it to chance. (Chapter 12 provides more detailed information about transfer of learning.)

## Demonstrating the Skill to Be Learned

Although there are a variety of ways to present skill-related information to a learner, visual presentation is usually chosen. That is, the skill or movement pattern to be learned is **modeled** or demonstrated a number of times for the observer. In such **observational learning,** learners watch another individual perform the movement before attempting to reproduce the action themselves. Unlike lengthy verbal descriptions, a visual demonstration of the skill quickly provides the learner with a meaningful image of the act. In choosing a visual model to set the stage for learning, the practitioner must first consider a number of important variables that have been shown to influence the effectiveness of this instructional technique.

## Variables That Influence the Effectiveness of Modeling

A number of variables appear to influence how well a modeled skill is initially performed and ultimately retained by the observer (McCullagh & Weiss, 2001). These variables have been identified and incorporated in a model of observational learning developed by McCullagh, Weiss, and Ross (1989) that is presented in Figure 8.2. It is beyond the scope of this chapter to discuss all the variables identified in this model, but we will look at some of them, particularly those that one should consider before introducing a new movement pattern to a group of observers. These include the developmental characteristics of the observer, elements of the demonstration (e.g., augmented information, cognitive task elements, and model characteristics), and the type of rehearsal strategies used. We will begin our discussion by considering the characteristics of the observer that appear to affect how the information conveyed by the model is processed.

*Characteristics of the Observer.*    One has only to watch a group of children try to reproduce a movement pattern that has just been demonstrated by a skilled model to realize that few observers processed the modeled information in the same way. While some first attempts are very accurate, others bear little resemblance to the actual skill modeled. A glance at the model proposed by McCullagh et al. provides some clues to why the performances of the observers vary so greatly. First, it may be that not all of the children observing the model are at the same stage of cognitive and memory development. These differences can be expected to influence both the amount of information that is extracted from the modeled performance and the manner in which it is then organized for later recall (Thomas, 1980). Research has shown that younger children (4–7 years) do not effectively organize information derived from a modeled performance, that they fail to label it in a manner that might facilitate later recall, and that they do not spontaneously rehearse the information presented (Thomas & Gallagher, 1986; Winther & Thomas, 1981). Research has also shown that if children of this age are to be successful in reproducing the modeled skill, it is necessary to instruct them to rehearse cognitively before attempting the skill (Weiss & Klint, 1987).

Just as we can expect differences in cognitive ability to influence how effectively an observer extracts and organizes the information derived from a model, differences in children's levels of physical and motor skill development will also influence how well each child is able to reproduce the skill physically during practice. The changing size and composition of a child's body affect how

An observer's level of cognitive and memory development influences both the amount and the type of information extracted from a modeled performance.

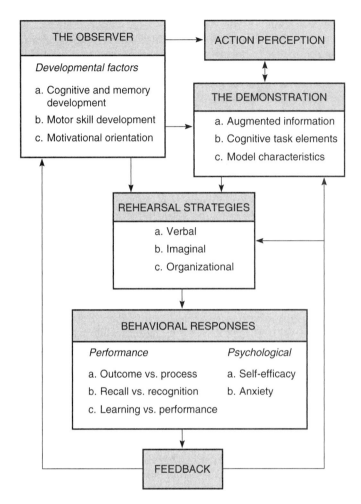

**Figure 8.2**   A number of observer and model characteristics influence the overall effectiveness of demonstrations.

well a skill is performed, as does the level of coordination, strength, and balance the child has achieved at the time the skill is introduced. A review of the motor development literature (Clark & Ewing, 1985; Halverson, Roberton, & Langendorfer, 1982; Seefeldt & Haubenstricker, 1982) also suggests that gender differences exist in the quality of motor skill development. Although the differences in motor development observed between males and females are quite small during the preschool and early elementary school years, they become larger with increasing age. It is therefore important to consider these

An observer's level of physical and motor skill development influences the observer's ability to physically reproduce the modeled action.

differences when modeling new skills in mixed-gender settings. It has also been shown that the level of exposure children have had to organized sports plays a major role in their performance of certain sport-specific skills.

An individual's level of motivation to learn the skill is another factor that must be considered. As Brooks (1986) aptly points out, "Neither a balky child nor a disinterested adult learns easily or improves motor skill" (p. 24). Whereas some individuals need little or no encouragement to learn a new skill or movement pattern because they are already intrinsically motivated, others need repeated words of encouragement or incentives to learn. Thus, a physical therapist often rewards a patient who has worked very hard during a rehabilitation session with the opportunity to choose an activity he or she enjoys at the end of the session, and a physical educator may reward a class of children who have been attentive during a skills practice with a few minutes of game play. Yet another effective way of boosting a learner's motivation to learn a particular skill is to explain how the acquisition of that skill will contribute to his or her overall game-playing versatility or (in the case of a patient) ability to perform certain daily activities.

> Peer models can be used to enhance an observer's confidence in his or her ability to perform the modeled skill.

The use of peer models in classroom (Schunk, 1987; Schunk & Hanson, 1985; Schunk, Hanson, & Cox, 1987) and motor skill settings (McAuley, 1985; Lirgg & Feltz, 1991; Weiss, McCullagh, Smith, & Berlant, 1998) has been shown to enhance the observer's confidence in his or her own ability to perform the modeled skill. The skilled adult model's ability to perform the skill far exceeds that of younger observers, but the peer model who is perceived as similar to the learner in ability can positively influence the observers' perception of their own ability to perform the skill. The end result is usually enhanced motivation to learn the skill. Although its role in the learning of movement skills has often been overlooked in the motor learning literature, motivation is a fundamental prerequisite to both the learning of movement skills and continued participation in activity settings.

### Elements of the Demonstration.

There are several characteristics of the model and of the demonstration itself that one should consider in planning to introduce a new movement pattern via modeling.

### Skill level of the model.

> The use of a model appears to be more effective when an observer is required to learn a new pattern of coordination.

Although research studies have demonstrated superior performance among observers who first watch a skilled model before practicing (Landers & Landers, 1973), Scully and Newell (1985) point out that an equal number of studies have demonstrated no such effect (Martens, Burwitz, & Zuckerman, 1976). Theorists aligned with an information-processing paradigm attribute these equivocal findings to differences in information load among the tasks modeled (Gould, 1980), but Scully and Newell argue that examining the dynamics of the task being modeled provides a more reasonable account of the contrary findings. They suggest that the use of a **correct model** (that is, a skilled model) is more effective when the observer is required to learn a new pattern of coordination rather than to rescale an already familiar movement pattern. If this line of reasoning is accurate, a learner who is being introduced to the Fosbury flop high-jump technique for the first time will benefit more from watching a skilled model than will another performer who is already familiar with this particular style of jumping and is attempting to clear greater bar heights using the technique.

The theoretical assumptions underlying the use of a correct model have been scrutinized by a number of researchers (Lee & White, 1990; McCullagh & Caird, 1990; Pollock & Lee, 1992). In fact, Lee and White have hypothesized that the use of correct models may not be the most effective means of conveying movement skill information during the early stages of skill acquisition. An alternative approach is to have learners watch an unskilled model (that is, a **learning model**) repeatedly practice the skill to be learned. The observer who watches an unskilled model is thought to be more actively involved in the problem-solving activities of the model as the model tries to discover how to perform the skill more effectively. It is further argued that the use of skilled models may undermine the problem-solving process because skilled models offer observers very little error information they can use to develop their own error-detection mechanisms (Pollock & Lee, 1992).

Pollock and Lee had observers watch either a skilled or an initially unskilled model practice a computer tracking game. In addition to watching the model, the observer recorded the model's performance score after each trial. When they compared the performances of both groups of observers to those of the skilled and learning models who demonstrated the skill, the authors found that both groups of observers performed consistently better during practice than any of the learning models who were paired with observers. On the basis of their findings, the authors concluded that observing a model was equally beneficial for the observers no matter what that model's skill level, particularly during the initial performance of a skill.

Extending Adams' (1986) research, McCullagh and Caird (1990) also demonstrated the effectiveness of learning models (see Figure 8.3 on page 238). In addition, they showed that the use of a learning model can positively influence how well the skill is later recalled and generalized to the acquisition of a new movement skill. Specifically, the authors demonstrated that observers who watched a model learn a timing task and received information about the correctness of the model's movement pattern performed as well as a group of subjects who physically practiced the skill and received information about their own performance. This same group of observers also performed much better than a group of observers who watched a skilled model perform the skill before they practiced. It is important to note, however, that simply watching a learning model perform a skill did not provide observers with enough information on which to base their subsequent practice. Participants who watched a learning model but were not privy to the feedback provided to the model about the performance demonstrated little improvement during any of the testing phases. Giving a learner feedback about the model's performance is important, particularly when using learning models.

The importance of receiving feedback about the model's performance when using learning models also was supported by Hebert and Landin (1994). They had inexperienced tennis players observe a correct video demonstration of the forehand tennis stroke that included verbalizations of important movement features. Next players were assigned to one of four groups that received combinations of individual and model feedback. The group that observed a model and received the model's feedback and then received feedback about their own movements performed the best in terms of form and outcome. The group that observed a learning model and received only the model's feedback

*Watching an unskilled model more actively involves the observer in the problem-solving activities of the model than does observing a skilled model.*

*Better retention and transfer of the skill results from providing performance-related feedback to a learning model as the observer watches.*

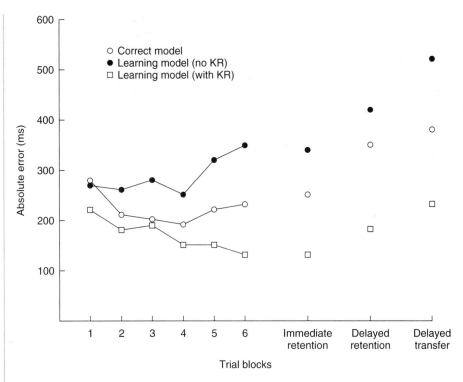

**Figure 8.3**  Influence of model skill level on acquisition, retention, and transfer of a movement timing task.

KR = knowledge of results

performed as well as the group that received feedback solely about its own movements. These findings support the conclusions reached by McCullagh and Caird (1990) that learning models can be an effective tool, especially in situations where students have the opportunity to observe others perform and hear the instructor's feedback about skill corrections.

McCullagh and Meyer (1997) extended the earlier study by McCullagh and Caird by investigating the modeling effects using a free-weight squat in which form as well as outcome could be evaluated. The control group physically practiced and received feedback about its own movements. The correct model group watched correct demonstrations and heard verbal feedback about the model's squat performance. One learning model group observed a model and heard the model's feedback, while another learning model group just observed a model without receiving any model feedback. Form and outcome improved in acquisition, but there were no differences among groups. However, both the correct and learning model groups that received model feedback had better retention of learning from performance than the other two groups. Differences compared to the McCullagh and Caird study could have been due to the type of task and feedback cues. The richer feedback received through knowledge of performance in the McCullagh and Meyer study may have provided additional cues that helped the correct model group.

Based on the research evidence, it is clear that observing a learning (unskilled) model is an effective learning technique, but how can this be explained? At least two explanations have been proposed (Adams, 1986; Lee, Swinnen, & Serrien, 1994; Lee & White, 1990). One explanation holds that if learners view an unskilled model and also receive the model's feedback, they become more cognitively and actively engaged in the problem-solving process than if they viewed a correct model or did not receive the model's feedback about performance. The greater the cognitive and active engagement, the greater the positive influence on learning through observation. The other explanation proposes that people can learn from watching others make mistakes, especially if feedback about performance is provided during the problem-solving process.

***Status, similarity, and age of the model.***   The effects of three additional factors associated with model characteristics have also been investigated. These factors are the perceived status or competence of the model demonstrating the skill (Baron, 1970; McCullagh, 1986), the similarity of the model to the observer (McCullagh, 1987; Gould & Weiss, 1981), and the age of the model relative to that of the observer (Landers & Landers, 1973; Lirgg & Feltz, 1991). In general, although these characteristics of the model appear to influence performance positively by raising the level of attention directed to the model or the motivation exhibited by observers, there is little evidence that any of these model characteristics affect how well a movement pattern or skill is ultimately learned.

> The status, similarity, and age of the model appear to have little effect on how well an observer learns a movement skill.

***Augmented information.***   In certain learning situations, the effectiveness of a visual model can be enhanced by augmenting, or supplementing, the demonstration with verbal cues that convey salient information. Verbal cues that highlight important components of the skill can be very useful additions to a modeled performance (Roach & Burwitz, 1986; Weiss, 1983). Such "show and tell" models are thought to focus observers' attention on the most important features of the skill being modeled. The use of verbal cueing has been shown to be particularly helpful to young children attempting to acquire a new movement pattern or sequence of movement, especially when the verbal cueing is coupled with cognitive rehearsal (McCullagh, Stiehl, & Weiss, 1990; Weiss & Klint, 1987).

> Verbal cueing, coupled with mental rehearsal, is particularly helpful to young children attempting to learn a new skill.

Although the addition of verbal cues has been shown to facilitate reproduction of a modeled action, it is important to consider the form in which these cues are provided, their meaningfulness for the observer, and the frequency with which they are provided. Training the observer to use verbal cues that describe the modeled action prior to its presentation also enhances observational learning (Bandura, Jeffrey, & Bachica, 1974). Gerst (1971) has shown that personally generated cues that are imaged by the observer can be more effective than concrete descriptions of the movement pattern. The issue of meaningfulness also looms large in situations where adults are introducing skills to young children. Often, many of the verbal cues the adult instructor uses to describe an action are too complex for the children to comprehend. Providing opportunities for children to develop their own verbal descriptors of an action may be very useful in the early stages of skill learning.

Reviews by Magill (1993a) and Landin (1994) on the role of verbal cues in movement skill learning acknowledge the importance of verbal cues in conjunction with demonstrations. Magill suggested that modeling and verbal cues may be redundant but also may possess unique characteristics that offer different information that is useful in learning how to perform a movement skill. Further, it has been proposed that the importance of using verbal cues in conjunction with demonstrations to promote observational learning may depend on whether people are trying to acquire new movement skills or modify previously learned ones (Magill & Schoenfelder-Zöhdi, 1996).

Auditory demonstrations may convey more information than visual demonstrations when the skill to be learned involves a high temporal component.

***The type of skill being demonstrated.***    A question that has intrigued one group of researchers interested in modeling issues is whether a visual demonstration constitutes the best method for conveying skill-related information when the skill to be learned is one that has a strong temporal component. In these situations, the use of an auditory demonstration may provide the observer with more salient information about the skill to be learned. To address this question, Doody, Bird, and Ross (1985) examined the performance of subjects on a timing task that was introduced with a visual, an auditory, or a visual and auditory demonstration. A fourth group of subjects simply practiced the skill and received knowledge about their performance after each practice attempt.

The results of an immediate retention test indicated that all the groups that received a demonstration performed better than the physical practice group. Comparing the performance scores of the three demonstration groups, however, revealed that the group that received an auditory demonstration of the timing task performed as well as the group that received a visual and auditory demonstration and both groups performed significantly better than the visual demonstration group. These results suggest that auditory demonstrations can be an effective means of conveying information to observers when timing is important in the task being demonstrated. In another study, Rose and Tyry (1994) manipulated the type of demonstration used to introduce the skill of rapid-fire pistol shooting to a group of experienced single-target shooters. Given that shooters must sequentially fire at each of five targets in a prescribed period of time, this task may be considered to have a strong timing component.

Unfortunately, Rose and Tyry's results were contradictory to those of Doody et al. Participants who received an auditory demonstration exhibited the least effective performance when compared to the groups that received a visual demonstration only or a combined visual and auditory demonstration. Why did the visual demonstration group, who received no auditory information during the demonstrations, perform so well at this task? The answer lies in the fact that timing information was available and could be extracted visually from the demonstration. Each time the model fired the pistol, an opaque puff of air could be observed escaping from the pistol's air ports. Apparently, this recurring visual cue was sufficient to provide the timing information that observers needed to perform the skill successfully. The results of this study suggest that timing information does not always have to come from auditory sources alone. In the case of many skills, timing information can be acquired through other means. This finding has important implications for instructors of people who are deaf, because these instructors cannot exploit auditory sources as a means of teaching the timing components of a skill.

***Rehearsal Strategies.***    The type of rehearsal strategies used by the observer prior to practicing the demonstrated movement pattern are also considered an important determinant of effective modeling. McCullagh et al. (1989) describe different types of rehearsal, two of which will be discussed here. These are verbal and mental, or imaginal, rehearsal strategies. Verbalizing the components of the skill prior to practice has been shown to be particularly helpful to novice performers, but mental rehearsal can also be used to strengthen the observer's perception of the skill to be performed.

*Verbal rehearsal.*  **Verbal rehearsal** has proved to be a particularly effective strategy for increasing the selective attention and recall skills of children with various disabilities who are attempting to learn new skills in classroom settings (Meichenbaum & Goodman, 1971; Tarver, Hallahan, Kauffman, & Ball, 1976). In the area of motor skill learning, Kowalski and Sherrill (1992) also found the use of verbal rehearsal particularly effective for a group of young students with learning disabilities who were asked to perform a seven-part sequence of locomotor movements. The children who were trained to rehearse verbally the information presented by a skilled model reached a criterion level of performance on the task in considerably fewer attempts than those children who simply watched the model perform the task prior to practice.

> Verbal rehearsal is an effective strategy for increasing the selective attention and recall skills of children with various disabilities.

Verbal rehearsal is essentially the same as what was called **verbal pre-training** in the early literature, which also was shown to improve the learning of complex movement sequences (e.g., Adams & Creamer, 1962; Trumbo, Ulrich, & Noble, 1965). Verbal pre-training involved supplying simple word labels that served to prompt learners of the next step in the sequence. Once mastered, these labels identified the steps in the sequence simply and directly and helped learners remember them. Examples of movement sequences include (a) a gymnast learning a new floor exercise routine, (b) a dancer or figure skater learning a new dance routine, and (c) a track athlete learning a triple jump. The key to the successful use of verbal pre-training was to use simple, direct verbal labels that were meaningful to the learners in describing or connecting the movements you wanted them to learn. Collectively, the research findings suggest that training learners, including young children with a learning disability, to use verbal rehearsal or verbal pre-training is an effective strategy for enhancing performance early in learning.

*Mental rehearsal.*  **Imaginal (mental) rehearsal** can also be employed to strengthen the observer's perception of what is required without the need for overt verbalization or, in some cases, physical practice. The effectiveness of this form of rehearsal appears to be influenced by the type of task being rehearsed—that is, whether or not it demands a large amount of cognitive processing. Tasks characterized by a high cognitive component, as opposed to a high motor component, appear to be especially conducive to imaginal rehearsal (Feltz & Landers, 1983). Moreover, individual differences in imaging abilities may influence the degree to which imaginal rehearsal leads to improved performance. Research has demonstrated that the recall of certain movement characteristics (such as distance and location) is affected by an individual's visual imaging abilities (Housner & Hoffman, 1981). Unfortunately, researchers interested in the theoretical underpinnings of observational learning have paid little attention to mental rehearsal, but that appears to be changing. More will be said about this increased interest in the relation between observational learning and mental rehearsal in Chapter 9 in the section titled "Mental Practice" (see page 278).

> Skills that demand large amounts of cognitive processing are well-suited to imaginal rehearsal strategies.

## Evaluating the Effectiveness of a Model

*Form versus Outcome.*    One challenge for the instructor or clinician who must often evaluate the effectiveness of a model is determining whether poor skill reproduction is due to inadequate processing of the salient information or to a lack of motor skill development. Indeed, Scully and Newell (1985) warn that evaluating a model's effectiveness solely on the basis of whether the goal of the movement is achieved can provide misleading information because "observers can pick up information from a demonstration that cannot be immediately realized in producing or mimicking the appropriate action" (p. 183).

Measuring the level of control and co-ordination used to reproduce the skill is a better method of evaluating a model's effectiveness than considering outcome alone.

Scully and Newell suggest that evaluating the level of control and coordination used to reproduce the skill is a better method of assessing the model's effectiveness than simply recording the score achieved by the performer. This may be why some investigators interested in modeling effects have had different results depending on whether they evaluated movement form or outcome (Feltz, 1982; McCullagh, 1987; McCullagh, Stiehl, & Weiss, 1990). Assessing the form of movement as well as its outcome is an important aspect of several modeling studies (Carroll & Bandura, 1990; Meany, 1994; Weiss, Ebbeck, & Rose, 1992).

The type of performance measurement used should also be an important consideration for practitioners who work with a variety of individuals with disabling conditions. A better way to assess the progress of a patient during rehabilitation may be to evaluate form and obtain standard outcome-based measures.

*Performance versus Learning.*    A model's effectiveness may also hinge on whether the observer is asked simply to recognize the correct performance or to recall it from memory without any cues being provided. Similarly, certain characteristics of the modeled performance, such as the model's status and his or her similarity to the observer, appear to temporarily influence only the quality of the immediate *performance,* not the overall *learning* of the skill (McCullagh, 1986, 1987). You will recall from our discussion of these two terms in Chapter 6 that it is inappropriate to use them interchangeably. Learning is a process that cannot be directly observed and must be inferred from changes in performance. If the changes in performance are reliable (durable), then learning is inferred to have taken place. If the changes are unreliable (temporary), they do not qualify as evidence for learning.

In evaluating the influence of verbal cueing and rehearsal on performance and learning, Weiss et al. (1992) recently found that developmental differences exist when the type of model and verbal rehearsal strategies used are evaluated on the basis of immediate performance and later recall. A group of older children (8–10 years) who were provided with a "show and tell" model and verbal rehearsal achieved better performance during early performance trials, whereas those children who watched a visual model only, or such a model combined with rehearsal, performed equally well in later performance and learning trials. Conversely, the use of a visual model combined with verbal rehearsal proved to be the most effective means of teaching younger children (5–7 years) how to perform a sequence of fundamental motor skills. The results of this study are illustrated in Figure 8.4.

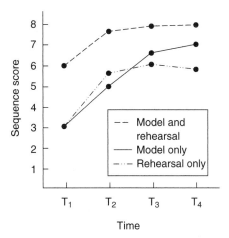

**Figure 8.4**  The use of a visual model combined with verbal rehearsal proved to be the most effective means of teaching younger children (5–7 years) a sequence of fundamental motor skills.

## Guidelines for Using Modeling

The research evidence strongly supports the effectiveness of modeling interventions as a means of facilitating acquisition, retention, and transfer performance for learners of all ages. Learning models, self-observation methods, covert models (imagery), peer models, and coping models are some of the interventions that have been found to be quite effective if used properly. McCullagh and Weiss (2002) have recommended six guidelines for using modeling properly in practical settings.

1. Use methods that maximize the learners' (observers') selective attention and active rehearsal of the demonstrated movements so they are motivated and able to imitate them.
2. The learners' attention and motivation can be addressed by carefully considering the type of model (e.g., learning or correct model, coping or mastery model, and peer or self-model) that is most appropriate for the setting.
3. Ask learners to recall important aspects of the demonstration or to recognize them among several alternatives to ensure they remember them. Also, learners may be asked to use a remembering technique (e.g., self-talk, encoding, labeling) as they view the demonstrated movements.
4. Videotape is the most practical and effective way to demonstrate and model movement skills because learners are able to view the demonstration or selected parts of it repeatedly and conveniently (e.g., teacher's or therapist's office, or learner's home).

5. Providing feedback to the learner during or after demonstrations that imparts information (e.g., focuses attention on a particular aspect of the modeled movement) or serves to motivate the observer (e.g., indicates progress in relation to past performance) is likely to enhance the effectiveness of the modeling technique.

6. Overt and covert (imagery) modeling procedures may be interchanged because they share many of the same cognitive mechanisms. Thus, the same physical and psychological benefits can be achieved regardless of whether learners observe or imagine themselves or similar models on video.

# Theoretical Explanations of the Modeling Effect

How is it that we are able to learn so much simply by watching someone else physically perform a skill? This question has generated considerable controversy in the past and has prompted a number of studies exploring the role of observation in the acquisition of specific behaviors. Two very different theoretical frameworks have guided these research efforts: Bandura's social learning theory (1977, 1986) and a direct perception approach (Newell, Morris, & Scully, 1985; Scully & Newell, 1985; Scully, 1986). Social learning theory attempts to explain how an observer processes the information provided by a model, whereas direct perception theory has been used to identify what type of information is being extracted by an observer. Let's look at the major theoretical assumptions underlying each theory and at their contributions to our present understanding of observational learning.

## Social Learning Theory

Central to social learning theory is the idea that the performance and learning of modeled skills are mediated by cognition.

Although Bandura originally developed a theory that was intended to describe how individuals acquire social skills and behavior through observation, it has since been applied to the motor skills domain (Carroll & Bandura, 1982, 1985, 1990). Central to social learning theory is the idea that both the performance and the acquisition of modeled skills are mediated by cognition. Specifically, four subprocesses are believed to govern skill acquisition. These are attention, retention, motor reproduction, and motivation. The observer extracts the dynamic pattern of the modeled action by selectively attending to certain spatial and temporal features of the skill being modeled. This information is then transformed by the observer into a cognitive representation.

According to social learning theory, the observer uses this cognitive representation to guide his or her first attempts at reproducing the movement skill. It also serves as a perceptual reference against which to judge the correctness of the ongoing performance so that errors can be corrected. Finally, motivational mechanisms facilitate the initial processing of the modeled information by raising both the level of attention directed to the modeled performance and the desire to retain the information presented. For the past several decades, the majority of research findings related to observational learning have been interpreted in terms of this theoretical framework.

## Direct Perception Approach

An alternative approach to the study of observational learning was proposed on the basis of research conducted in the area of visual perception of motion (Cutting & Proffitt, 1982; Johansson, von Hofsten, & Jansson, 1980). The goal of this research was to discover what type of information was being detected by the observers during a modeled action. Using a point-light technique, whereby only an individual's joints were visible to the observer, investigators found that observers were able to identify not only the type of movement pattern represented, such as walking or cycling (Johansson, 1971), but also whether they were viewing a human or a wooden puppet (Johansson, 1976), a male or a female (Barclay, Cutting, & Kozlowski, 1978; Cutting, 1978) or an acquaintance or themselves (Cutting & Kozlowski, 1977) performing the task.

The general conclusion reached on the strength of these varied research findings was that an observer is able to perceive different types of biological motion on the basis of the changing relationships between body parts as a movement is being performed. This **relative motion** of body parts constitutes the "what" being observed during the modeling of an action. These early research findings were later cited by advocates of direct perception (Newell, Morris, & Scully, 1985; Scully & Newell, 1985; Scully, 1986) in support of their claim that modeled actions can be perceived directly from the visual display, without the need for the elaborate cognitive processing described by Bandura. The central tenets of this approach echo those of the ecological approach to perception and action that we outlined in our discussion of the visual system in Chapter 5.

> The relative motion of body parts constitutes the "what" being observed during the modeling of an action.

## Discovery Learning

So far in this chapter, we have focused on the use of dynamic models, whether skilled or initially unskilled, as the primary means of setting the stage for learning. As effective as modeling appears to be during the early stages of learning, some researchers have demonstrated that alternative ways of meaningfully constructing the learning environment can result in equally effective motor skill learning (Pikler, 1968; van Emmerik, den Brinker, Vereijken, & Whiting, 1989; Vereijken & Whiting, 1988). Discovery learning, wherein the learner is required to discover independently the optimal solution to a given movement problem, is one alternative method. Rather than prescribing the appropriate solution for the learner through the use of a dynamic model or a detailed set of verbal instructions, the instructor constructs the learning environment in such a way that the learner is encouraged to employ a variety of different strategies, some more appropriate than others, until he or she finally discovers the best coordination pattern.

> In discovery learning methods, the learner attempts to discover independently the optimal solution to a movement problem.

Despite the limited number of research studies investigating the merits of discovery learning, a group of researchers at the Free University in the Netherlands have provided some empirical evidence in support of this instructional method (van Emmerik, et al. 1989; Vereijken & Whiting, 1988). A ski simulation task was used in each of the studies conducted (see Figure 8.5 on page 246). Each performer made large-amplitude, high-frequency, and

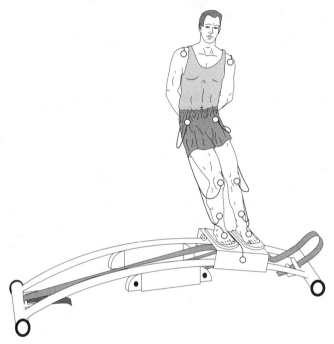

**Figure 8.5**   An illustration of the slalom ski simulation task used to investigate the merits of discovery learning.

fluent skiing movements on a ski apparatus consisting of a platform on wheels that could be moved to the extremities of two bowed, parallel metal rails. When the results were compared, the performance of subjects provided with augmented feedback about critical parameters of the task (e.g., amplitude, frequency, and fluency) was compared to that of a group of discovery learning subjects following four days of training on the task, and no differences were found between the groups. Indeed, the performance of the discovery learning group was superior to that of two of the feedback groups. The finding that discovery learning was more effective than providing instructions on the same ski simulator task that direct the learner's attention to a particular movement aspect of the task to be learned also was supported by Wulf and Weigelt (1997). (Their study was discussed on page 230 in the section "Where to Direct the Learners' Focus of Attention").

In a second study (Whiting, Bijlard, & den Brinker, 1987), the performance of subjects provided with an expert video model either during each training session or between training sessions was compared to that of subjects who were required to learn the ski-like action through discovery. Prior to training, the discovery group was informed only what movement goal was to be achieved. Following a four-day training period, the discovery learning group performed significantly better than either of the two groups provided with a dynamic model.

How is it that a group of learners given very little information about a skill was able to achieve higher levels of performance than groups provided with repeated and correct demonstrations of the skill to be learned? The authors reasoned that the learners who observed the expert model naturally tried to imitate the model's movement form while also attempting to harness the external forces necessary to move the ski platform. Thus their attention was divided between two aspects of performance during training. In contrast, subjects in the discovery learning group had no preconceived idea about the most appropriate movement form to use and could devote all their attention to producing the forces needed to keep the platform moving. As a result, they were more likely to discover the inherent dynamics of the task and exploit them appropriately.

## Applying the Principles of Discovery Learning

From a practical perspective, the use of discovery learning techniques in motor skills settings offers two important advantages. First, it forces the learner to explore the perceptual–motor workspace independently in search of an optimal solution to a movement problem. Second, it shifts the role of the practitioner from that of teacher to that of facilitator, as was once the case when movement education was commonly used in physical education settings. Given that infants learn many phylogenetic skills by means of discovery, it is not unreasonable to think that many ontogenetic skills can be acquired in a similar way. Just how might a practitioner structure a learning environment to promote discovery learning?

> Discovery learning can be promoted by presenting a movement problem and allowing the learner to solve it and by simplifying the learning environment.

***Present a Movement Problem.***   One way for an instructor to stimulate a learner's desire to discover how best to perform a movement is to pose the movement problem verbally and give a brief verbal explanation of the movement goal to be achieved. In introducing the skill of dribbling with a soccer ball, for example, the instructor might simply state that the problem is to move the ball with the foot from one end of the field to the other in such a way that a defender would find it very difficult to steal the ball away. Having outlined the movement problem to be solved, the instructor then leaves the learner to discover the most efficient method of moving the ball with the foot to achieve the goal. No set of verbal instructions and no dynamic model are provided. Following a sufficient amount of practice, the different dribbling techniques can be compared (if several learners are involved) and/or tested by introducing a defender who tries to steal the ball away. A similar approach to the teaching of motor skills is evident in the writings of George Graham and colleagues (Graham, Holt-Hale, & Parker, 1993), whose nontraditional approach to the teaching of physical education emphasizes the use of inquiry (convergent and divergent) and child-designed instructional approaches.

***Simplify the Learning Environment.***   A second way in which an instructor can facilitate discovery learning, particularly when introducing more complex motor skills, is to simplify the learning environment. This can be accomplished by reducing the number of degrees of freedom the learner must control, making it easier for the learner to discover progressively how best to perform the new movement pattern. To illustrate how this might be possible, Vereijken (1991) describes the skill of learning to ride a bicycle. Rather than "teaching" a child how to ride a bicycle, which Vereijken suggests may not be possible anyway, the instructor helps the child keep the bicycle balanced while she or he attempts to discover first how to produce a forward movement and then how to keep the body balanced on the bicycle at the same time. In this way, the level of motor control required in the early stages of learning the skill is significantly reduced while the child discovers the physical laws governing this particular skill's execution.

## Summary

It is common practice to set the stage for motor learning enthusiastically by first briefly, simply, accurately, and directly introducing the skill to be learned and motivating the learners to want to learn it. Next, learners are shown how to perform the movement skill usually by means of a visual demonstration and an accompanying explanation that is brief, simple, accurate, and direct. The explanation should be meaningful to the learners and facilitate their learning to perform the movement skill. Often the explanation should direct the learner's attention to one or two of the movement features that are essential for successfully performing the skill (internal focus of attention). However, sometimes learning is facilitated more by directing the learner's focus of attention to the effects of the movement skill on the environment (external focus of attention) and allowing the essential movement features to be acquired through discovery learning. The explanation should relate the skill to be learned to the performer's previously learned skills that are performed in similar ways in an attempt to facilitate the new learning. Appropriate motivational strategies that encourage learners to want to learn the movement skill and that make use of motivators should be interwoven into the explanation and demonstration, as well as presented before practice begins. Goal setting is one way to effectively motivate people to learn a skill before practice begins. Other variables that play an important role in motivating people to learn are praise, criticism, success, failure, self-esteem, competition, and cooperation.

Before presenting the demonstration the practitioner should consider a number of factors. These include the characteristics of the observer that are most likely to influence what the observer extracts from the modeled performance and how the observer uses that information to guide subsequent practice attempts. The level of cognitive development influences both the amount and the type of information extracted from the modeled performance, and the observer's level of physical and motor skill development influences how well she or he is able to reproduce the skill physically.

Certain characteristics of the model also seem to influence how well the skill is first performed and ultimately recalled. The need for a skilled model does not appear to be as important as previously thought, but the model's ability to convey adequately the strategy underlying the skill to be learned is crucial. Augmenting the information provided by the visual model can be extremely useful, particularly when introducing young children to new skills. Supplementing a visual demonstration with verbal cues that can be readily understood by the learner is particularly helpful in conveying the critical components of the skill. Providing the observer who is watching a learning model with information about the model's performance also appears to increase the effectiveness of this type of model.

Rehearsal strategies are another way to strengthen a learner's perception of a modeled skill. This rehearsal may take the form of verbal "self-talk" or of imaginal (mental) rehearsal. Encouraging young learners to rehearse modeled information verbally before practicing has proved to enhance both immediate performance and later recall of a movement skill.

When evaluating the effectiveness of a model, the practitioner must not take into account only a movement's outcome. Given that the information extracted from a modeled performance does not immediately lead to a successful movement outcome, it is important to find additional ways to measure how much the observer has benefited. Measurements designed to assess the changing levels of control and coordination demonstrated by a learner are therefore necessary when evaluating the overall effectiveness of a model.

Two very different theoretical explanations have been advanced to account for the effectiveness of modeling. The first of these (social learning theory) focuses on how the observer encodes and organizes the visually presented information. The second attempts to identify what the observer extracts from the modeled performance. Proponents of the latter theory contend that the observer directly perceives the relationships among the limbs performing the movement (e.g., relative motions) and uses this perception to guide subsequent physical attempts. Both theoretical accounts will continue to contribute to our understanding of observational learning.

The discovery learning approach is an alternative technique for setting the stage for learning is. Instead of providing the learner with a visual model and thereby shaping the image of the movement to be reproduced, advocates of discovery learning construct the learning environment in such a way that the learner is encouraged to discover independently the optimal solution to a given movement problem. This technique not only shifts the responsibility for learning to the learner but also transforms the role of the instructor from prescription to facilitation.

## IMPORTANT TERMINOLOGY

After completing this chapter, readers should be familiar with the following terms and concepts.

competition
constrained action hypothesis
constructive criticism
cooperation
correct model
criticism
demonstrating [the movement
  skills]
discovery learning
explaining [the movement skills]
external focus of attention
failure
goal setting

imaginal (mental) rehearsal
internal focus of attention
introducing [the movement skills]
learning model
modeled
observational learning
praise
relative motion
self-esteem
success
verbal rehearsal
verbal pre-training

## SUGGESTED FURTHER READING

Landin, D. (1994). The role of verbal cues in skill learning. *Quest, 46,* 299–313.

Magill, R. A. (1998). Knowledge is more than we can talk about: Implicit learning in motor skill acquisition. *Research Quarterly for Exercise and Sport, 69,* 104–110.

McCullagh, P., & Weiss, M. (2001). Modeling: Considerations for motor skill performance and psychological responses. In R. N. Singer, H. A. Hausenblas, & C. M. Janelle (Eds.), *Handbook of sport psychology* (2nd ed., pp. 205–238). New York: Wiley.

McCullagh, P., & Weiss, M. (2002). Observational learning: the forgotten psychological method in sport psychology. In J. L. Van Raalte & B. W. Brewer (Eds.), *Exploring sport and exercise psychology* (pp. 131–149). Washington, DC: American Psychological Association.

## TEST YOUR UNDERSTANDING

1. Briefly explain the role of motivation in movement learning, especially in relation to introducing, explaining, and demonstrating a skill to be learned.

2. Briefly explain the criteria for developing effective learning goals and how setting them can facilitate learning.

3. What is the role of praise, criticism, success, failure, self-esteem, competition, and cooperation in motivating people to learn?

4. Identify the essential ingredients of effective introductions and explanations.

5. Explain why it is important to relate the movement skill being taught to previously learned skills that are similar.

6. Where should the learner's focus of attention be directed when learning a movement skill? Explain why.

7. Briefly describe the observer characteristics that have been shown to influence the effectiveness of modeling.

8. Describe three ways in which an individual's motivation to learn a new skill can be enhanced.

9. Briefly discuss the advantages and disadvantages associated with the use of (a) skilled models and (b) learning models.

10. Briefly describe the various ways in which the information provided by a model can be augmented.

11. How does the type of skill being demonstrated appear to influence a model's effectiveness?

12. Describe two types of rehearsal strategies that can be used to strengthen an observer's perception of the skill to be learned. What factors appear to influence the effectiveness of each of these two types of rehearsal strategy?

13. What variables associated with modeled performances affect the observer's performance? What variables affect the observer's learning?

14. Why is it important to measure both movement form and the outcome of movement when attempting to evaluate the effectiveness of a model?

15. Discuss the two theoretical explanations advanced to account for the modeling effect. In what fundamental way do these two explanations differ?

16. Describe an alternative teaching method that seems to promote effective learning of movement skills. Discuss the various ways in which this technique can be integrated into a learning environment.

# 9

# ORGANIZING THE PRACTICE ENVIRONMENT

*How movement skills are practiced determines not only how well they are learned and retained, but also how well they transfer to real-world situations.*

## CHAPTER OBJECTIVES

After studying this chapter, you should be able to:

- Describe the influence that amount of practice has on the level of performance achieved in original learning, over-learning, and retention.

- Explain how specificity of practice operates in the learning and performance of movement skills.

- Explain how the environment in which a movement skill is learned influences the way the skill should be practiced.

- Identify the factors that determine the type of practice schedule selected.

- Describe the major theoretical explanations that have been used to account for why practice schedules that demand high levels of cognitive effort lead to better retention and/or transfer of motor learning.

- Explain how the distribution of practice within and between practice sessions influences both immediate performance and the eventual learning of different types of movement skills.

- Identify instructional techniques that can be used to increase the effectiveness of a practice session and help the learner reach a criterion level of mastery in a shorter time.

- Describe the various methods of practicing movement skills in parts and the variables that are likely to influence the use of these part-practice techniques.

- Describe mental practice conditions that have been shown to be effective for enhancing performance during original learning and beyond.

Having set the stage for learning by presenting the movement skill to be acquired, practitioners must now make important decisions about what practice conditions are most appropriate and how to effectively organize them to optimize learning. Some of these decisions include the duration of each practice session, the number of practice sessions per week, the types of activities and movement skills to be practiced during each session, the ways in which they are to be practiced in each session, the order in which they are practiced, and the time allotted to practicing each activity and skill. The meaningfulness of any given practice session is further enhanced by the provision of feedback that not only assists learners in identifying and correcting errors in performance, but in motivating them to want to continue to learn movement skills. How often and in what form this feedback should be given will be discussed in Chapter 10.

It is well known that the learning of movement skills cannot take place without practice and that how one practices matters. If the practice conditions are appropriate, they will yield a level of learning that supports the retention of performance even after long periods of disuse, as well as the transfer of that performance to real-world conditions. Of course, this is assuming that the *correct* movement skills are being practiced, the complexity of the movement skill is appropriate for the learner, and she or he is motivated to learn. However, if the practice conditions are inappropriate, they could yield little or no learning or a level of learning that does not strongly support the retention and transfer of performance. Consider, for example, highly motivated athletes who practice the skills of their sport extensively and yet the proficiency of their performance remains unchanged or may even deteriorate. They might be heard saying things like, "I spend a lot of time practicing, but I don't seem to get any better"; "The more I practice the worse I get"; or "I can do it in practice, but I can't do it in the game." Essentially, these athletes are not practicing their skills under appropriate conditions, and as a result their learning and performance suffers. What is practiced determines what is learned, but the conditions under which it is practiced determine how well it is remembered and the extent to which it transfers to real-world situations. Thus, *what* is practiced is as important as the *conditions* under which it is practiced.

This chapter focuses on the conditions of practice, especially how movement skills should be practiced and in what context they should be practiced. A number of key practice variables will be discussed in relation to organizing and structuring effective practice conditions to optimize the learning, retention, and transfer of motor skills. This is followed by a presentation of various instructional techniques that are known to enhance the effectiveness of practice. The chapter concludes with a discussion of mental practice and its role in facilitating motor learning and performance.

# Amount of Practice

Complex movement skills are learned through practice—that is, by performing them repeatedly. They are not acquired quickly. It follows, therefore, that amount of practice is a powerful variable in determining the proficiency level of performance in original learning and beyond (referred to as *over-learning*). When all other important learning variables—motivation, practicing the

When the person is motivated to learn and the conditions of practice are appropriate, performance proficiency will improve as the amount of practice increases, up to the limits of the person's innate ability.

correct movements in the correct ways—are favorable for improving performance, the greater the amount of practice, the more proficient the skill performance up to the limits of the person's innate ability. How does the amount of practice variable affect the level of motor performance achieved in original learning and beyond? What influence does the amount of practice have on the durability or long-term retention of motor learning?

## Level of Original Learning

Assuming that all other important learning variables are in place, then the greater the amount of practice, the higher the **level of original learning** and the better the long-term retention of that learning. Blurring of the learning–performance distinction in the research literature has resulted in the frequent appearance of the phrase *level of original learning* when *level of performance achieved in acquisition* would be the more correct phrase. Because the expression *level of original learning* is just too common in the literature to avoid, it is used here to be compatible with the literature but with the understanding that (a) it actually refers to the level of performance achieved in acquisition and (b) the level of original learning is inferred from the level of performance achieved in acquisition.

There is considerable agreement in the research literature that motor learning and the long-term retention of that motor learning can be improved by increasing the level of original learning or mastery (e.g., Annett, 1979; Farr, 1987; Hagman & Rose, 1983; Hurlock & Montague, 1982; Naylor & Briggs, 1961). Generally, the variable manipulated to increase the level of original learning is the amount of practice. Usually, this manipulation is accomplished by making the criterion of mastery of the motor skill more difficult to achieve so that more practice is needed to achieve it. The additional practice, in turn, enhances long-term retention. For example, suppose a golf coach is training young beginners to putt. She decides that the players should be able to make 25% of the putts attempted from eight feet by the end of three days of training. She could also make the criterion of mastery more difficult to achieve, requiring the players to make 50% of the putts attempted from eight feet or, alternatively, that they make 25% of the putts under more difficult conditions (e.g., simulating competitive conditions). In either case, more practice would be required to achieve the more difficult criterion of mastery, and the additional practice would produce a higher level of original learning and greater long-term retention of that learning.

Thus, one could increase the level of original learning and its long-term retention either by making the criterion of mastery more difficult or by holding the criterion at the same level of difficulty and making the conditions more difficult—both of which increase the amount of practice required. Ways of making the conditions more difficult during acquisition practice include delaying or providing less frequent augmented feedback, using more variable practice within and among motor skills, or increasing the amount of contextual interference during practice by simulating real-world conditions. Appropriate manipulation of such practice variables also should encourage learners to be more cognitively engaged in the learning and performing process (Christina & Bjork, 1991; Lee, Swinnen, & Serrien, 1994). This is likely to produce a higher or more complete level of learning that can enhance the long-term retention and transfer of that learning (Christina & Alpenfels, 2002).

# Level of Over-Learning

Regardless of the level of original learning achieved, one way to become an elite performer and further enhance long-term retention is by providing supplementary practice on movement skills after the criterion of mastery is achieved (Ericsson, 2001). In the previous golf putting example, for instance, the coach could have the players continue to practice putting extensively even though they have achieved the criterion of making 50% of their putts from eight feet. This is referred to as **over-learning,** or *post-mastery learning.* The level of over-learning is usually expressed as the number of practice trials that learners perform after the criterion of mastery has been achieved. It also can be expressed in percentage terms such as 50% over-learning, which means that learners receive half again the number of practice trials that they took to achieve the mastery criterion. The arbitrary nature of the mastery and over-learning criteria can make it difficult to do certain comparisons across studies. A trial that is part of mastery or original learning for one study can be part of post-mastery or over-learning for another study, depending on how one defines and quantifies the level of original learning or mastery to determine when it is complete.

In spite of these complications, it is clear that elite performance and the long-term retention of that performance are better for over-learned or over-practiced tasks (e.g., Ericsson, 2001; Loftus, 1985; Schendel & Hagman, 1982; Slamecka & McElree, 1983). It appears that even the most talented individuals need at least 10 years of practice and involvement before they reach elite levels in activities such as music, chess, sports, science, and the arts (Ericsson, Krampe, & Tesch-Römer, 1993). Informal study of the top nine golfers in the 1900s revealed that eight of them needed approximately 16 years of practice and involvement in golf before they won their first international competition; the other player (Gary Player) took about seven years before he achieved international success (Barkow & Barrett, 1998). Krampe and Ericsson (1996) reported that by the age of 20 years, the best musicians had engaged in more than 10,000 hours of practice, which was 2,500 and 5,000 hours more than two less skillful groups of expert musicians, respectively, and 8,000 hours more than amateur pianists of the same age.

To assume that simply increasing the amount of practice, regardless of its quality, enhances learning and long-term retention and produces elite performance is naive. First, performers must be practicing the correct skills so as not to develop "bad" habits or waste time practicing the wrong skills. For instance, former golfing great Jack Nicklaus (1974) stated that "whenever I do go out with a bag of balls I have a very specific objective in mind and, once I've achieved it, I quit. All my life I've tried to practice shots with great care. I try to have a clear-cut purpose in mind on every swing. I always practice as I intend to play. And I learned long ago that there is a limit to the number of shots you can hit effectively before losing your concentration on your basic objectives" (p. 197).

Thus, a prerequisite for achieving elite performance is a considerable amount of quality practice (deliberate practice) in which the duration of practice is limited by the ability to sustain concentration, a capacity that itself seems to improve with extended practice (Ericsson, 2001). Of course, there are limits to the influence of practice, and a person's innate ability will play an important role in determining the level of performance achieved.

> Elite performance and the long-term retention of that performance are better for over-learned or over-practiced tasks.

Providing too much additional practice on certain aspects of performance can reach a point of diminishing returns.

When to introduce the additional over-learning practice to enhance long-term retention does not appear to be an important factor. The level of performance achieved in over-learning is far more important than the time at which the additional practice is introduced (Schendel & Hagman, 1982). However, providing too much additional over-learning practice can reach a point of diminishing returns (Bell, 1950; McGeoch & Irion, 1952; Melnick, 1971). In other words, increasing the number of over-learning practice trials on an aspect of performance may not produce proportionate increases in long-term retention. In fact, the practice time might be better spent on another aspect of performance or something else. Thus, although 100% additional practice in over-learning may result in better long-term retention than 50%, the slight, if any, gain that results may not be worth the additional time and practice.

## Structuring the Practice Session

One factor to consider in structuring each practice session is the nature of the environment in which the skill is ultimately to be performed. Knowing what environmental demands and/or constraints a learner can expect to encounter during the performance situation makes the task of structuring a meaningful practice environment considerably easier. At one end of the continuum lies a performance environment characterized by stability, whereas the performance environment at the other end is unpredictable and therefore highly variable. In Chapter 1, we discussed stable and variable environments as they influence the demands placed on motor control. We will now consider the role of the performance environment in shaping the structure of practice sessions.

### Specificity of Practice

How similar (or specific) do the practice conditions under which a movement task is learned have to be relative to the real-world conditions under which the movement task has to be performed in order to optimize the transfer of that learning and performance to the real-world conditions (e.g., to games, competitions, occupations, and everyday life activities)? The idea that the practice conditions should match the real-world conditions is one that has been around since Thorndike and Woodworth's (1901) **theory of identical elements.** This theory held that transfer of learning was largely a function of the extent to which two tasks (including the practice and real-world conditions) contained identical elements: the more shared elements, the more similar the two tasks, and the more transfer there would be. Much more will be said about this theory and the transfer of learning in Chapter 12.

The idea of matching practice and real-world conditions was extended to the motor domain by Barnett, Ross, Schmidt, and Todd (1973). They tested the **specificity of practice principle** in a motor skills learning context. Their study emanated from the specificity of training principle in exercise physiology and from Henry's (1958) research and hypothesis that motor abilities underlying successful performance of movement skills are more specific than general. Motor abilities such as balance, strength, endurance, kinesthesis, coordination, and speed are specific to the movement skill being performed. For example, the kind of balance required for successful performance in gymnastics is somewhat different from the type of balance demanded in downhill skiing. Similarly, the kind of speed needed to run a 100-meter sprint is different than the type of speed needed to hit a pitched baseball or a golf ball. Thus, balance and speed are not general abilities that underlie many different movement skills. However, if abilities are specific, then how does one explain individuals who appear to possess general motor ability and are referred to as *all-around athletes*? Henry proposed that these individuals are gifted with so many specific abilities that they appear to have a general motor ability, but the research evidence does not support the notion of individuals with one or more general motor abilities.

The term **motor ability,** often used interchangeably with *movement capability* or *aptitude,* refers to a relatively stable trait that supports or underlies successful performance in a number of movement skills. Abilities are largely genetically determined and developed through growth and maturation and not easily changed through practice. Conversely, movement skills are learned and can be changed through practice. The successful performance of a skill depends on a number of different abilities that are specific to that skill (as shown in Figure 9.1 on page 258) for the complex coordination task (a piloting-type task) in which participants had to manipulate a stick and rudder in response to visual patterns (Fleishman & Hempel, 1954). Further, this figure also reveals that (a) the combination of abilities contributing to performance on the task changed as practice continued; (b) the changes were progressive and systematic and became stabilized later in practice (learning); and (c) a factor (psychomotor performance) specific to performance on the task itself increased with practice and became the major component in the later stages of learning. Using a discrimination reaction time task in a subsequent study, Fleishman and Hempel (1955) also demonstrated a similar shift in the nature of abilities contributing to performance of a discrimination reaction time task as a function of practice and learning.

The finding that different abilities contribute to performance at various stages of practice and learning suggests that those who possess abilities that contribute to successful performance in the early stages will perform at a relatively high level during those initial stages, and those who possess abilities that contribute to performance at the later stages will perform at a high level later in practice (learning). This possibility was studied by Fleishman and Rich (1963), who administered a visual-spatial and a kinesthetic sensitivity test to a large number of participants, and then divided them into low and high groups on each of these abilities. All groups then learned a two-hand coordination task. The results revealed that the high visual-spatial ability group performed better early in practice; but, as practice continued, the low visual-spatial ability group caught up. Conversely, the high and low kinesthetic sensitivity ability groups performed at about the same level early in practice; but, as practice continued, the high group performed better than the low group later in practice. Thus, the successful learning and performance of different movement skills appear to depend on some different underlying abilities that are specific to each of the skills. Further, learning and performance of different skills also appear to depend on some of the same underlying abilities used to different degrees, depending on the stage of practice or learning. (For reviews see Fleishman, 1972, 1978.)

The successful performance of a movement skill depends on a number of different abilities that are specific to that skill.

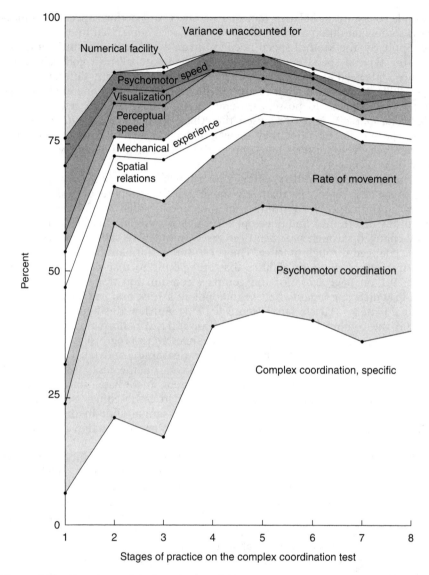

**Figure 9.1**  Changes in ability as a function of acquisition practice (learning) on a complex coordination task (piloting-type task). Percentage of variance accounted for by each factor at various stages of practice.

*Source:* Fleishman, E. A., & Hempel Jr., W. E. (1954). Changes in factor structure of a complex psychomotor task as a function of practice. *Psychometrika, 18,* 239–252.

The practical implication emanating from identical elements theory and the research by Henry and by Fleishman and his colleagues is that one should strive to structure the practice conditions in learning a movement task to simulate (as much as possible) the real-world conditions under which the task must be performed so that there is little or no shift in underlying abilities that would interfere with performance. This is what is referred to as the *specificity of practice principle.* Furthermore, practice conditions must be structured so that all of the elements essential for successful skill performance in the real world—appropriate movements, cognitive processing, strategies, knowledge, and knowledge applications needed to achieve the goal performance—are also practiced and learned. In other words, movement skills must not only be the same in practice (learning) as those that must be performed in real-world situations, but they must be performed in the same ways and under similar conditions in order to achieve the same goal and ensure that the appropriate cognitive processing, strategies, and knowledge applications are being acquired. Thus, an important guiding principle for structuring practice conditions that are most appropriate for optimizing the transfer of learning and performance of movement skills to real-world settings is to *practice those skills in the same ways and under the same conditions that they will have to be performed in real-world settings.*

> The specificity of practice principle holds that practice conditions should match real-world conditions in which the skill will have to be performed in order to avoid a shift in underlying abilities that would interfere with performance.

***Specificity of Sensory Feedback.***      Another specificity of practice issue involves the role of sensory feedback as one learns how to perform a movement skill. Research evidence is largely in agreement that sensory feedback is important throughout learning (e.g., Adams, Goetz, & Marshall, 1972; Elliot, Chua, Pollock, & Lyons, 1995; Elliot & Jaeger, 1988; Proteau, Marteniuk, Girouard, & Dugas, 1987; Proteau, Marteniuk, & Levesque, 1992) and that it does not lose its importance as practice progresses. This research also reveals the **specificity of practice effects for sensory feedback.** It indicates that movement learning is highly specific to the sensory feedback available during acquisition, and more practice encourages the learner to be more dependent on that feedback. The latter evidence extends hypothesis by proposing that as a learner repeatedly performs a movement, a sensory representation of the movements develops that is specific to the sensory feedback, thus providing the greatest accuracy in practice (Soucy & Proteau, 2001; Tremblay & Proteau, 2001).

> Movement learning is highly specific to the sensory feedback available during acquisition, and more practice encourages learners to be more dependent on that feedback.

Learning to use the sensory feedback can be explicit or implicit. That is, regardless of whether one pays attention to a specific sensory feedback source, if it contributes appreciably to the proficiency of movement performance, it will be included in the closed-loop motor control process. The latter explanation is consistent with those of implicit and explicit processes during the learning of movement skill performance (Gentile, 1998). The sensorimotor representation that results is used by the performer to evaluate response-produced feedback and help determine the correctness of the movement performance.

It has been further proposed that error detection and correction procedures develop from any sensory feedback that is useful for improving and controlling movement performance (Coull, Tremblay, & Elliot, 2001). Error detection and correction, which become more efficient with practice, are thought to be controlled by a set of rules that regulate the processing of error estimates. Although efficiency is often thought of in terms of increased movement, speed, or accuracy, in the case of error detection and correction it could include improvements in selecting relevant information from the environment (Abernethy & Russell, 1987a). While Coull and colleagues (2001) favor a closed-loop explanation of movement learning for developing error detection and correction procedures, they do not deny the existence of open-loop

> Error detection and correction procedures develop from any sensory feedback that is useful in improving and controlling movement performance.

control. Clearly, both open- and closed-loop processes are involved in controlling the performance of movement skills (Arbib, Erdi, & Szentagothai, 1998) and skill development (Khan, Franks, & Goodman, 1998).

Although specificity of practice effects for sensory feedback have been found for a number of movement activities such as power lifting (Tremblay & Proteau, 1998), manual aiming (Elliot, Lyons, & Dyson, 1997), and goal-directed locomotion (Proteau, Tremblay, & DeJaeger, 1998), more practice in one sensory condition has not always led to increased interference with the transfer of learning and performance in another sensory condition (Robertson, Tremblay, Anson, & Elliot, 2002). One reason could be that specificity of practice effects result from the development of specific control procedures for using sensory feedback in a given condition. When sensory feedback is changed, these procedures also must be changed to effectively deal with the new sensory feedback situation. Thus, the amount of positive (facilitative) or negative (interference) transfer of learning and performance of a movement skill depends on the extent to which the new procedures for using sensory feedback to improve and control performance of the skill are similar to the procedures practiced and learned during acquisition (Elliot et al., 1995, 1997). The more similar the new and previously learned procedures, the more positive transfer there would be. In some instances the new and previously learned procedures could interfere with each other and produce negative transfer of learning and performance. One practical implication emanating from all of the research finding specificity of practice effects for sensory feedback is that practice conditions should be structured so that procedures for using sensory feedback to improve and control movement performance are the same (or as similar as possible) in learning as in the real-world situation in which one will have to perform.

*Specificity of Context.*   The **specificity of practice effects for the context** in which movement learning and performance occurs also has been studied under the label of **situated learning** (Lave, 1988). This research places emphasis on contextual determinants of learning and performance, especially on social interactions in the task environment, and on the importance of situating the learner in the context of application, as in apprenticeship learning (Lave & Wenger, 1991). Situated learning is similar to the **state-dependent learning** hypothesis, which holds that learning while practicing under conditions that create one physical, mental, and emotional state (e.g., under the influence of physical or mental fatigue or alcohol, being in a particular mood, or under certain environmental conditions) is more effectively demonstrated when the same state is produced in the real world by the same conditions (Davis & Thomson, 1988). If the real-world conditions are different from the practice conditions in acquisition, different states result, and learning is less effectively demonstrated in the real-world setting. Matching the conditions in practice to those in the real world allows the same contextual information to operate and serve as cues to help the individual recall the learned information in the real-world situation.

There is little doubt among cognitive scientists that contextual effects exist in learning, retention, and transfer of knowledge. In verbal learning, for instance, support has been found for the principle of **encoding specificity,** which holds that retrieval of learned information directly depends on

---

*Practice conditions should be structured so that procedures for using sensory feedback to improve and control movement performance are the same in learning as in the real-world setting.*

*Matching conditions in practice to those in the real world allows the same contextual information to operate and serve as cues for retrieval of the learned information in the real-world situation.*

similarities between the retrieval and learning contexts (Tulving & Thomson, 1973). It also has been supported by applied research in which deep-sea divers learned material on land or underwater and were tested in matching and non-matching conditions (Godden & Baddeley, 1975). What makes situated learning different from other approaches is the extent to which learning is claimed to be context specific and the implications for training. Situated learning theorists argue that training (practice) must be situated in the performance context in order to be effective. Thus, it is no surprise that they advance an apprenticeship in the real-world context where training is applied as the best form of learning. One limitation of apprenticeship learning is the potential for variability within that context. Because one cannot always predict the future contexts in which the learner will have to perform, it would seem to be more advantageous to devise a training procedure or program that would optimize performance in various contexts. One way to accomplish this is to develop a training or practice environment that simulates the relevant features of the task. This is often done in sport situations in which coaches use drills that simulate game conditions or scrimmage (practice) games to enhance the transfer of learning and performance from practice to actual game situations.

Although the research evidence for context specificity in motor learning is limited, what is available appears to be consistent with what has been found in cognitive psychology (Wright & Shea, 1991, 1994). Moreover, context specificity research appears to be connected to what has been called the *home-court* or *home-field advantage* in sports. Typically, college and professional teams perform better when playing at home than when playing away on their opponents' court or field (Courneya & Carron, 1992). The question is, why? One possibility is context specificity; that is, certain variables linked to the field or court on which games are played provide an advantage for the home team because the team practices on that field or court. Thus, the practice context for the home team is the same as the game context in terms of the field or court yielding higher context specificity for them than for the visiting team. One variable that might offer an important advantage when games are played on the same field or court is the contextual information provided by the surroundings of the practice area. However, this hypothesis must be viewed with caution because the evidence supporting it is not particularly strong (e.g., Pollard, 1986).

### *Specificity of Cognitive Processing.*   **Specificity of practice effects for cognitive processing** is closely related to the contextual conditions between the practice (learning) and transfer settings, and much more will be said about practice contexts and providing contextual interference during learning later in this chapter (see page 264). However, at this point it is useful to know that the specificity of practice effects for cognitive processing refers to the similarity of the underlying processes between acquisition practice and the real-world setting in which one must perform the movement skill that was learned. The best practice conditions are those that encourage the individual to practice and learn the same underlying processes that will have to be used to successfully perform the movement skill in the real-world setting. Quite often, the best conditions can be achieved by simulating in practice the way in which the movement skill will have to be performed in the real-world setting.

The best practice conditions are those in which the underlying processes learned in practice are the same as those used to successfully perform the skill in the real-world setting.

For example, one way to simulate in practice the way in which golf shots have to be performed during actual play is to actually play a course on the practice range in which successive shots are hit with different clubs rather than the same club. Further, one could hit some of the iron shots from poor lies that are often encountered during play on the golf course. Lastly, one could add some competitive pressure on each of the shots performed by playing a game against an opponent to see who could be more accurate. Such simulation encourages the player to practice and learn the same underlying processes that will be called upon to successfully perform those same golf shots on the golf course. What this simulation example has done is introduce *contextual interference*, or **contextual variety,** as it is sometimes called, into the practice conditions.

Theoretically, practicing under a condition of high contextual interference produces more elaborate and distinctive processing, which enhances retention and transfer of learning and performance (Battig, 1979). Presumably, elaborations during processing produce memory structures for the knowledge or skills learned that are richer and more discernible—and thus, easier to retrieve. The extent to which positive transfer is enhanced is believed to be a function of the degree to which the contextual interference induces processing strategies that are appropriate for learning other tasks (Morris, Bransford, & Franks, 1977; Morris, Stein, & Bransford, 1979). Since contextual variety should lead to more elaborate and distinctive encoding, it is likely to offer stronger resistance to the typical negative performance effects that are found when real-world tasks are changed. In other words, encoding specificity is more likely to be overcome if the original encodings occurred under high contextual variety. Conversely, similar task contexts should induce processing consisting mainly of the development of discriminative and organizational change suited to the specific task demands. In summary, incorporating contextual variety in practice introduces functional interference that makes learning less context dependent and involves learners in processing activity that in turn produces enhanced retrieval from memory and the ability to adapt their performance to different contexts.

## Variability of Practice

One major prediction emerging from schema theory (Chapter 6) is related to the importance of **practice variability.** Schmidt (1975) predicted that practicing a variety of different ways to perform a skill during a practice session would provide the learner with a broader range of movement experiences on which to base the development of a set of rules for action (movement schemas). For example, structuring a practice environment that gives the learner an opportunity to apply different parameters of a movement skill is considered an effective means of facilitating learning. Thus, a learner may practice throwing a ball at targets of different sizes placed at increasingly longer distances from a throwing line or practice hitting objects of different sizes that are pitched at different speeds over the course of a number of practice trials.

The results of several studies provide support for the prediction that practice variability in the acquisition of a movement task facilitates transfer of that learning to the learning of a new (novel) task in the same response class with adults (Catalano & Kleiner, 1984; Margolis & Christina, 1981; McCracken &

Variable practice conditions in learning a movement task facilitate transfer of that learning to the learning of a new task in the same response class.

Stelmach, 1977), and with children (Carson & Wiegand, 1979; Kelso & Norman, 1978; Kerr & Booth, 1977; Moxley, 1979; Shapiro & Schmidt, 1982). However, typically the facilitative effects of practice variability have been more pronounced with children than with adults perhaps because it is easier to find tasks that are truly novel for children than for adults. Margolis and Christina (1981) attempted to resolve this novel-task problem with adults by having them perform a rapid aiming movement with a hand-held stylus to a target distance while wearing prism glasses, which none of them had previously experienced. The glasses enabled them to view the target, which displaced the sight of the target 1.5 inches (5.71 degrees) to the left of its actual location, but not their aiming movement (made with their right hand and arm) or the outcome (how close the stylus came to the target movement distance). The transfer results clearly revealed that the two variable target practice groups performed the transfer task with less error on initial transfer and over all of the transfer trial blocks than the nonvariable target practice groups. This finding clearly supported Schmidt's (1975) schema theory and the prediction that variability of practice in acquisition facilitates transfer to a novel movement task in the same response class, at least with adults.

Promoting variability of practice in a clinical setting is also likely to benefit the patient in terms of **generalizability.** Unlike the carefully structured environment in which the task of walking is practiced during rehabilitation (which includes parallel bars, stable surfaces, and quiet corridors), the real-world context in which the task will ultimately be performed is more variable. Introducing opportunities for patients to practice walking over a variety of different surfaces, in crowded corridors, and while conversing with a second person will better prepare them to return to their former living environments. Also unlike the clinical setting, where a patient is able to perform a task at a self-determined speed, in daily contexts certain external constraints will be imposed on performance of the task (crossing the road in traffic is a good example). Practice that requires patients to manipulate all the various movement patterns of the same task (such as velocity, force, and direction) should also improve their ability to generalize across settings.

Although the findings of a number of research studies provide support for the use of variable practice techniques in the learning of a variety of different movement skills, the practitioner must decide *when* it is appropriate to begin introducing variability into the practice setting. Should practice variability be introduced at the outset of learning or should some initial practice precede its introduction?

Gentile's (1972) two-stage model of motor learning, which was introduced in Chapter 6, provides a partial answer to this question through two guiding principles. The first is that variability of practice should not be introduced until the learner understands the dynamics of the task. Consistent practice of the desired movement pattern may better foster this early understanding of the skill. Second, the type of variability that should be introduced will differ with the type of skill being learned and the environment in which it will ultimately be performed. For example, the pattern of coordination being learned for hitting a ball will eventually be performed within the context of a tennis or racquetball game. Varying that pattern should be an integral component of any practice session once the learner has acquired a global understanding of the skill's dynamics. Recall that Gentile refers to those factors that directly

Practice variability should not be introduced until the learner understands the dynamics of the skill to be learned.

Regulatory conditions are factors that directly influence the way in which a skill is executed.

influence the way a skill is executed as the regulatory conditions. This type of practice variability can be introduced by manipulating variables such as distance, angle, and direction of the stroke during the practice of these skills. By doing this, the instructor can increase the repertoire of possible actions available to the performer in a game situation.

Nonregulatory conditions are external factors that are not directly related to the performance of the skill.

On the other hand, skills that must be performed with a high level of movement consistency in stable environments (e.g., platform diving and gymnastics vaulting) are less well suited to being practiced in a variety of different ways. What *should* be varied during the practice of many of these movement skills is the context in which the skill is practiced, or the nonregulatory conditions. For example, a gymnast must learn to perform a skill or routine in a competition while other performers are simultaneously performing their own routines. The situation is rendered even more potentially distracting by music being played nearby for another gymnast who is performing a floor routine. Opportunities to practice while these nonregulatory conditions are manipulated will better prepare the athlete for the final performance situation. In performance situations similar to this one, then, it is the factors *not* related to movement (e.g., presence of other performers and crowd noise) that should be varied during practice.

## Organizing the Practice Schedule

The previous discussion clearly indicates the importance of organizing a practice environment that engages the learner or patient in practicing variations of a movement task, particularly for those skills that will ultimately be performed in variable performance environments. The next step for the practitioner is to decide exactly *how* this variability should be organized. Fortunately, the issue of how best to schedule practice variability in movement skill settings has been systematically investigated by Magill and colleagues (Hall & Magill, 1995; Lee & Magill, 1983; Lee, Magill, & Weeks, 1985; Magill & Hall, 1990). In the next section, we will review their work and consider its implications for constructing practice sessions.

### Introducing Interference

Contextual interference is functional interference introduced into a practice situation as a result of practicing multiple movement skills.

**Contextual interference (CI)** is functional interference introduced into a practice situation as a result of *several* movement skills being practiced at once. As will be discussed in Chapter 11, introducing high levels of interference into a practice setting is believed to enhance the learner's ability to remember skill-related information. Certainly Battig (1972, 1979) found this to be the case when the concept was applied to the learning of verbal skills. The level of contextual interference present in a movement skill setting has been effectively manipulated by altering the type of practice schedule adopted (e.g., blocked vs. random). In the case of a **blocked practice** schedule, the learner practices multiple variations of a skill, but each variation is practiced for a given period of time before the next variation is introduced. For example, during the course of a volleyball unit, a group of learners may practice setting a volleyball for

10 minutes, then work on bumping techniques for the same period of time, and practice spiking in the final 10 minutes of a 30-minute practice session.

Conversely, practicing according to a **random practice** schedule requires that the performer practice each of the skill variations in random order. Let us consider the same three volleyball skills to illustrate how this type of practice schedule differs from a blocked practice schedule. When the same 30-minute practice session is organized according to a random practice schedule, a learner may practice the setting technique followed by the volleyball spike and the bumping technique on three consecutive practice attempts, and the order in which the skills are practiced constantly changes throughout the practice session. In this latter practice situation, the learner does not practice the same skill for any length of time, as was the case in a blocked practice schedule. This random presentation of skills ensures that the level of CI introduced is considerably higher than that introduced when skills are practiced according to a blocked practice schedule.

Schmidt and Young (1987) questioned whether the variability of practice effects found in previous studies could actually have been due to CI and the influence of blocked and random practice. They proposed that many of the variability of practice effects that were found in studies could be nothing more than random practice effects.

Attempting to resolve this issue, Hall and Magill (1995) designed two studies to determine the practice or skill variation characteristics that differentially influence the variability of practice and CI effects. The results from the first study supported the conclusion made by Wulf and Schmidt (1988) that variability in practice is more influential when the tasks to be learned are parameter modifications of the same generalized motor program. However, the results also were consistent with the hypothesis proposed by Magill and Hall (1990) that contextual factors do influence learning in a variable practice situation when task variations do not belong to the same movement class or generalized motor program.

The findings from their second study indicated that, rather than being at odds with each other, the CI effect and the practice variability hypothesis emanating from schema theory are specific to different situations. The amount of practice variability affected the learning of skill variations when the variations were parameter modifications of the *same* generalized motor program. Conversely, CI variables involving the scheduling of practice affected the learning of skill variations that were controlled by *different* generalized motor programs. Thus, the learning benefits from amount of practice variability are more likely to occur when the movement tasks to be learned are parameter modifications from the same generalized motor program, and the learning benefits of CI are more likely to occur when skill variations are from different classes of movement.

## Influencing Factors

What factors should a practitioner consider when deciding how much CI is appropriate for a given practice situation? In a review of CI research findings, Magill and Hall (1990) identified three important factors that affect the degree to which the practice schedule chosen influences how well a skill is retained

The level of contextual interference is highest when a random practice schedule is used.

Learning benefits from amount of practice variability are more likely to occur when the movement tasks to be acquired are parameter modifications from the same generalized motor program.

Learning benefits of contextual interference are more likely to occur when skill variations are from different classes of movement.

and then later recalled. These include task-related characteristics, learner characteristics, and whether we measure performance or measure learning and/or transfer. We will first consider how the characteristics of the task to be learned influence whether the positive recall effects associated with random practice schedules are observed.

*The beneficial learning effects of random practice schedules are observed more often when multiple skills that require different patterns of coordination are practiced.*

### Task-Related Characteristics.

The beneficial learning effects of practice schedules that promote high levels of contextual interference have been repeatedly observed when multiple tasks that require *different* patterns of coordination are practiced (Lee & Magill, 1983; Poto, French, & Magill, 1987; Shea & Zimny, 1988). Conversely, when only the parameters (such as movement speed and amplitude) of a movement task that involves the *same* pattern of coordination are manipulated, the learning-related benefits of these same practice schedules are less evident (Poto et al., 1987, experiment 2). In laboratory settings, different coordination patterns have been created using multisegment barrier tasks that require subjects to practice knocking barriers down according to different spatial patterns displayed. In one of the few nonlaboratory settings in which the positive recall effects of a random practice schedule have been observed, three different types of badminton serves were practiced (short, long, and drive serves). Each of these different serving techniques involves subtle variations in the pattern of coordination required (Goode & Magill, 1986).

The fact that random practice does not yield learning benefits in situations where only the parameters of a particular set of skills were manipulated during the acquisition phase has been primarily interpreted within the framework of the generalized motor program (GMP) concept first developed and subsequently modified by Schmidt (1975, 1982a,b, 1988a,b). According to Magill and Hall, only those skill variations that are controlled by *different motor programs*, as opposed to the same underlying motor program, will benefit from a random practice schedule. The authors concluded that the same motor program was being used to guide the execution of each skill practiced if "the relative timing, sequence of events, and/or spatial configurations remained constant across the skill variations that were practiced" (p. 254).

### Learner Characteristics.

Several characteristics of the learner also appear to influence whether practicing skill variations in situations of high contextual interference positively influences the retention and subsequent transfer of skill-related information to other movement skill settings. These learner-related characteristics include age, level of experience, intellectual capacity, and learning style.

**Age.**  It is difficult to assess fully the influence of age as it relates to the contextual interference issue, because so little research has been conducted on this topic. Of the few investigations reported in which age was studied, the findings are somewhat mixed. Edwards, Elliott, and Lee (1986) demonstrated superior learning among young children (e.g., 5–8 years) who practiced variations of an anticipation timing task according to a random practice schedule, but some other authors either found no differences in learning to exist as a function of the practice schedule used or found that blocked practice schedules led to superior learning effects (Del Rey, Whitehurst, Wughalter, & Barnwell, 1983; Pigott & Shapiro, 1984).

***Level of experience.***   Del Rey and colleagues (Del Rey, 1989; Del Rey, Wughalter, & Whitehurst, 1982; Del Rey, Whitehurst, & Wood, 1983) have conducted a series of experiments designed to investigate the relationship between previous movement skill experience and practice schedules that incorporate high contextual interference. The authors reasoned that novice performers with little exposure to the types of skills being learned or to the kind of perceptual processing involved would not benefit from random practice schedules as much as a group of more advanced performers. This is not an unreasonable claim in view of our discussion in Chapter 6 of the stages of learning. Recall that learners in the first stage of learning are, among other things, struggling simply to understand the idea of the movement to be learned (Gentile, 1972). As a result, they engage in arduous cognitive processing of the task's demands at one level (Fitts, 1964), while at a second level attempt to "freeze" the many degrees of freedom available to them by constraining multiple joints to act together (Bernstein, 1967). Given that this account was intended to describe what learners attempt to do during the first stage of learning a *single* movement pattern, one can only imagine how much more difficult these various operations would be if multiple skill variations were being practiced concurrently!

> Learners who are limited in their experience with related skills, or with movement settings in general, may not benefit from random practice schedules.

The predictions of Del Rey and colleagues have been partially supported by their own work and that of other authors who also argue that random practice schedules may be inappropriate for learners until they better understand the demands of a particular skill (Goode, 1986; Goode & Wei, 1988). In one particularly interesting study, Goode and Wei introduced a third type of practice condition that combined blocked and random practice schedules. A group of inexperienced females, unfamiliar with sport skills performed in variable environments, began practicing an anticipation timing skill according to a blocked practice schedule before switching to a random schedule of practice. The results of a transfer test indicated that this mixed practice schedule promoted the best performance. From a practical perspective, these findings suggest the need for practitioners to consider a learner's past experience with related movement skills, or with movement settings in general, when deciding how best to organize practice sessions for optimal learning and transfer.

Much of the research investigating the benefits of CI has focused on participants who were inexperienced with the movement task to be learned (that is, they were beginning learners). The question of interest is whether CI can produce similar benefits with experienced performers. In an attempt to answer this question, Hall, Domingues, and Cavazos (1994) studied CI effects using 30 players from a junior college baseball team. Using a pretest, current batting average, and subjective evaluations from the head coach, participants were blocked according to batting skill and then randomly assigned to one of three experimental practice conditions: random, blocked, and control (no extra practice).

The results are shown in Figure 9.2 on page 268. As expected, both random and blocked conditions showed greater improvement in number of solid hits in the practice phase than the control condition, which did not receive any additional batting practice. However, the finding of particular interest was that both transfer order tests revealed better performance in terms of number of solid hits for the random practice condition than for the blocked practice condition. This finding is one line of evidence supporting the benefits of CI with experienced performers. Other studies have found similar benefits with

> Performance benefits of practicing with contextual interference have been found for those inexperienced, as well as experienced, with the movement task.

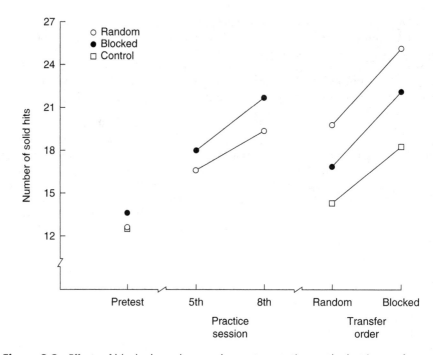

**Figure 9.2**  Effects of blocked, random, and no extra practice on the batting perform-ance of college-level baseball players.

*Source:* Hall, K. G., Domingues, D. A., & Cavazos, R. (1994). The effects of contextual interference on extra batting practice. *Perceptual and Motor Skills, 78,* 835–841.

beginning learners, but Hall and colleagues (1994) provide evidence that these benefits can be extended to experienced participants as well. However, extend-ing contextual interference benefits to experienced performers may not be as simple as it appears at first glance because at least one study tested the idea with golf skills and found only limited support at best (Damarjian, 1997). Clearly, much more research is needed to determine the best ways to manip-ulate practice conditions with experienced performers to optimize the move-ment performance benefits produced by CI.

***Intellectual capacity.***   Although little research has been directed to exploring the effectiveness of random practice for individuals who have impaired intel-lectual capacity, Edwards and colleagues (Edwards, Elliott, & Lee, 1986) com-pared the effectiveness of blocked and random practice schedules for a group of adolescents with Down's syndrome who were learning three variations of an anticipation timing task. Although age-matched control subjects who did not have Down's syndrome and who practiced according to a random practice schedule benefited more than a second group of control subjects who prac-ticed according to a blocked schedule, random and blocked practice schedules produced similar levels of learning among the adolescents with Down's syndrome. Thus the superiority of a random practice environment was not established for these learners.

In order for individuals with reduced intellectual capacity to benefit from practice schedules that introduce high levels of contextual interference, it may be necessary to provide mixed practice schedules similar to those used in earlier studies (Goode & Wei, 1988). Additional research is clearly needed before definitive recommendations can be made with respect to the most effective practice schedules to use when teaching variations of a skill to individuals with reduced intellectual capacity.

*Learning style.*   The degree to which a learner exhibits either a reflective or an impulsive cognitive style, particularly in the performance of skills that require both speed and accuracy, has been explored as it relates to the contextual interference effect (Jelsma & Pieters, 1989; Jelsma & Van Merrienboer, 1989). These authors predicted that a learner exhibiting an impulsive cognitive style who is asked to perform a task as quickly and accurately as possible will tend to ignore the accuracy component in favor of speed. Conversely, the more reflective learner is more likely to place the importance of being accurate above that of being fast. The authors further reasoned that reflective learners would benefit more from practice schedules incorporating high levels of contextual interference than would more impulsive learners. Whereas random practice schedules require high levels of problem solving and therefore greater reflection, blocked schedules require no such reflection. The results of both a retention test and a transfer test provided support for the authors' predictions. The reflective learners benefited more from random practice schedules than learners characterized as impulsive. Although more research is needed in this area, the cognitive style of a learner would appear to be yet another variable that is likely to influence the effectiveness of certain practice schedules.

> Random practice schedules require higher levels of problem solving and greater reflection than blocked schedules.

*Measurement of performance versus learning.*   If the effectiveness of random practice schedules had to be evaluated on the basis of testing the performance of a group of learners at the conclusion of a single practice session, instructors would probably abandon this type of practice immediately. Their decision would be based on seeing a set of performance results similar to those illustrated in Figure 9.3 on page 270. These results clearly demonstrate significantly better acquisition performance for a group of learners who practiced according to a blocked practice schedule (e.g., low contextual interference) than for a second group of learners who practiced according to a random practice schedule (e.g., high contextual interference).

However, when the same two groups of learners are compared again at a later time, perhaps at the start of the next practice session, their respective performances are quite different. In contrast to the earlier performance results, the results of a retention/transfer tests (illustrated on the righthand side of the same graph) indicate that the performance of the random practice group on the same movement skill is now superior to that demonstrated by the blocked practice group. How can we account for this rather dramatic reversal in performance? The answer appears to lie in whether it is performance or learning that is being measured. You will recall from our discussion in Chapter 7 that retention/transfer tests, administered some time after completion of acquisition practice, are assumed to measure the durability of learning. Performers

> Practicing according to a blocked schedule has been shown to produce superior performance but inferior learning and/or transfer.

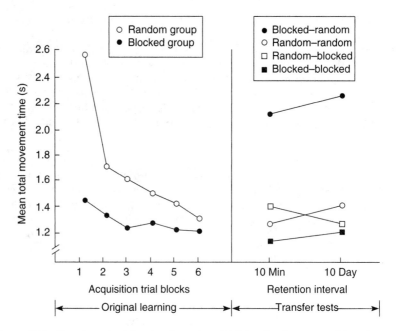

**Figure 9.3**　Practice schedules that introduce high levels of contextual interference appear to affect performance adversely but lead to superior retention of the skill.

*Source:* Shea, J. B., & Morgan, R. L. (1979). Contextual interference effects on the acquisition, retention, and transfer of a motor skill. *Journal of Experimental Psychology: Human Learning and Memory, 5,* 179–187.

practicing under the more difficult random practice conditions do not exhibit the same quality of performance, even though they are developing a better understanding of the skill itself. But when they are asked to perform the skill again after a period of rest, the greater benefits of the more difficult practice schedule become evident.

The same is not true for the blocked practice group, who in some retention situations actually perform more poorly than they did right after the first practice session. The superior performance of the random practice group is also evident when the results of transfer tests are considered. In these tests, the learner is required to perform a new variation of the skill not previously practiced.

Two theoretical explanations for this CI effect have been described in the literature and will be the topic of the next section in this chapter.

## Theoretical Accounts of the Contextual Interference Effect

Practice schedules that introduce high levels of contextual interference (CI) into the practice setting have been repeatedly shown to enhance the learning of a skill among adults, even though the benefits are not readily apparent during the practice session itself. Two very different explanations have been developed to identify the type of cognitive processing that produces the contextual interference effect. The first of these, the **elaboration view,** draws on many of the concepts described in the levels-of-processing framework that was originally developed by Craik and Lockhart (1972) and that we will discuss in Chapter 11. The early ideas of Battig (1972, 1979) related to intertask transfer in verbal learning situations are also encompassed within this theoretical viewpoint. The second explanation, which has been called the **action-plan reconstruction view,** is strongly influenced by motor program theory. We will begin by outlining the major assumptions of the elaboration view.

## Elaboration View

According to the elaboration view, individuals who practice according to a random practice schedule engage in a variety of cognitive processing activities that have the net effect of making the task-related information more distinctive. These multiple processing strategies ensure that the memory representation is also more elaborate, because the information is more "deeply" processed in memory. The learner who practices in conditions of high CI is thought to store all of the variations of the task simultaneously in working memory. This makes the processing more difficult for the learner, but it also provides the opportunity to compare and contrast the different versions during practice. The resulting memory representation for each variation is therefore more distinctive and more likely to be recalled at a later time. In contrast, the learner who practices according to a blocked practice schedule has no opportunity to engage in such complex processing because only one variation of the skill is stored in working memory.

The intuitive logic encompassed in this viewpoint has had great appeal for researchers seeking a theoretical explanation for the contextual interference effect. As a result, a number of research findings have been interpreted according to this view (Shea & Morgan, 1979; Shea & Zimny, 1983, 1988).

> The multiple processing strategies engaged in during random practice ensure that the memory representation is elaborately processed in memory.

## Action-Plan Reconstruction View

An alternative explanation for the CI effect has been advanced by Lee and Magill (1983, 1985). These authors argue that learners involved in random practice are required to regenerate the plan of action each time that particular variation is presented. It is thought to be necessary to regenerate, or reconstruct, the plan because the previous plan is temporarily forgotten between practice attempts. For example, plan A is formulated for task variation A but is needed for only one practice trial. Plan B must then be formulated for task variation B, which is being practiced on the very next trial. Plan C must then be formulated for practicing the third variation of the task. As a result of forgetting plan A in the interim, the learner is forced to regenerate the plan when task A is practiced again. A similar type of regeneration process was proposed by Cuddy and Jacoby (1982), who compared the recall abilities of two groups of children who practiced solving mathematical problems according to a random or a blocked practice format. They also found that children who practiced in conditions of high CI demonstrated superior recall at a later time.

> Because of forgetting, the plan of action must be continually reconstructed each time the skill variation is presented.

## Spacing/Distribution of Practice

Another issue that arises for the practitioner is how to space or distribute practice for optimal learning. The practitioner not only must decide how many practice sessions to schedule each week, but also must determine how practice will be temporally distributed in any given practice session. This second type of scheduling has attracted considerable interest among experimental psychologists and motor learning researchers. The effects of two very different types of practice schedules have been investigated over the years. In **distributed practice,** the amount of time that the learner is resting between practice attempts during any given practice session is equal to or greater than the amount of time that the learner is engaged in the practice of the movement skill. In **massed practice,** the amount of time that the learner is engaged in practicing a movement skill during any given practice session is considerably greater than the amount of time devoted to rest.

Although a number of research studies have been conducted to determine which practice schedule leads to better performance and learning, little consensus has been reached among researchers. Whereas some authors conclude that the massing of practice negatively affects both performance and learning (Oxendine, 1984; Schmidt, 1988b), others argue that the negative effects of massed practice schedules are confined to performance (Adams, 1987; Magill, 1993b; Singer, 1980).

Why do motor learning researchers appear to be so divided on this issue? In a review article devoted to the topic, Lee and Genovese (1988) suggest that the lack of consensus is largely due to the different retention measures that researchers have chosen to assess learning. However, Christina and colleagues (Christina, 1997; Christina & Shea, 1988, 1993) argue that the problem is not with use of different retention measures, but with the misinterpretation of what they actually represent. This issue will be discussed in more detail in Chapter 11.

Distributed practice benefits both the performance and learning of movement skills, but the effect on performance appears to be greater than the effect on learning.

As a result of the review they conducted, Lee and Genovese (1988) concluded that "distributed practice is beneficial to both the performance and learning of motor skills, although the effect on performance is greater than the effect on learning" (p. 282). In their final discussion, the authors raise one point of potential interest to the practitioner that no doubt partly accounts for the conclusion. It involves the type of task that has been commonly used to investigate the spacing-of-practice effects observed. Lee and Genovese point out that in almost all the research studies devoted to this issue, the type of task used has been exclusively continuous—that is, one in which the performer responds to stimulus information presented continuously, such as pursuit tracking. Given that these tasks are, by their very nature, more likely to result in increasing fatigue if continuously practiced without rest, it is perhaps not surprising that the superior beneficial effects of distributed practice compared with massed practice are more evident in immediate performance than after a rest interval.

As Figure 9.4 shows, once the effects of fatigue associated with practicing a continuous task according to the more demanding massed practice schedule have dissipated, the two different practice groups exhibit very little difference in quality of performance. The fact that two studies (Carron, 1969; Lee & Genovese, 1988) using a discrete skill produced quite different performance and

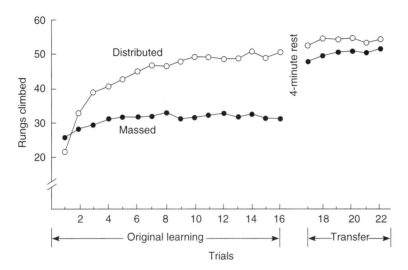

**Figure 9.4**   The effect of a massed versus a distributed practice schedule on the performance in original learning and transfer of a Bachman ladder climbing task.

learning effects from those observed when a continuous task was employed suggests that the effects of a massed or a distributed practice schedule on performance and learning vary as a function of the type of skill to be learned.

According to Lee and Genovese (1988, 1989), the distribution of practice effects for motor tasks is more likely to be found for continuous tasks than for discrete tasks, but some evidence is beginning to emerge which also supports it for discrete tasks (e.g., Dail & Christina, 2004; Shea, Lai, Black, & Park, 2000). The effects to which Lee and Genovese refer involve the manipulation of relatively short rest intervals (e.g., seconds or minutes) between repetitions in a single practice session rather than the spacing of practice over relatively long intervals (e.g., across days). Shea et al. studied the effects of distributing practice sessions across days compared to within days on the learning of continuous and discrete motor tasks. Their findings revealed that distributing practice sessions over days resulted in the enhancement of performance during the remaining practice sessions and enhanced the durability of learning as assessed by a delayed retention test. Thus, the positive effects of distributing practice sessions over longer intervals appears to be a reproducible event that benefits the performance and learning of both continuous and discrete motor tasks. It is interesting to note that this finding is consistent with memory consolidation theory, which was discussed in Chapter 6. Shea et al. also point out that the CI practice effect in which blocked practice usually results in poorer learning compared to random practice may interact with distribution effects such that the negative effects of blocked practice may be lessened when longer intervals separate practice in motor tasks or task variations. Of course, further research is needed to determine the validity of this idea.

The positive effects of distributing practice sessions over longer intervals appear to benefit the performance and learning of both continuous and discrete motor tasks.

# Techniques for Enhancing the Effectiveness of Practice

Although a large amount of practice is necessary for successful learning, practice by itself is not sufficient for many individuals trying to learn or relearn a particular pattern of movement. Fortunately, a number of instructional techniques can be used to increase the effectiveness of any practice session and help the learner reach a criterion level of mastery in a shorter period of time. These techniques may take many forms: verbal instruction, videotape replays of performance, physical guidance, and/or instrumentation designed to amplify a performer's own level of sensory feedback. The next section of this chapter is devoted to a discussion of the utility of each of these techniques in a variety of learning environments.

## Guidance Techniques

Numerous practice techniques are available that are designed to help learners acquire a certain movement pattern with a minimum of error. These **guidance techniques** range from intermittent verbal cues provided to a learner to assist the learner in recalling the steps of a new dance routine to mechanical performance aids such as a harness designed to prevent a gymnast from injuring herself as she practices a difficult somersault. In the absence of these often expensive mechanical devices, an instructor or therapist may physically guide the limbs of a learner through an entire movement pattern or a portion of it. When teaching a child how to perform a forehand tennis stroke, for example, the instructor may stand behind the performer and guide the hitting limb through the desired movement trajectory. During the warm-up before a gymnastics meet, a coach may act as a spotter in the corner of the floor exercise mat and briefly make physical contact with the gymnast's back during the first rotation of a double somersault. This brief moment of physical contact may help the gymnast impart just a little more vertical lift during the rotation or it may simply provide psychological support during certain maneuvers that the gymnast has previously found difficult to complete successfully.

In clinical settings, **physical guidance** is regularly used to assist a patient in a variety of ways. In Bobath's (1965, 1978) neurodevelopmental treatment approach, particular handling techniques are used to guide the patient toward a nearly normal movement pattern in the early stages of rehabilitation. Physical guidance techniques can also be useful for patients who lack confidence in their ability to perform certain activities or suffer from impaired vision and/or hearing. In these situations, a therapist's supportive touch can reduce the patient's anxiety or provide an important means of communication. In general, the use of physical guidance techniques in clinical settings is predicated on the assumption that compensatory or abnormal movement patterns must be eliminated as soon as possible during the relearning of movement patterns. Therefore, therapists often use physical guidance during the cognitive phase of learning (see Chapter 6).

Although the use of physical guidance clearly has many positive effects on the early performance of a new and often complex movement pattern, most motor learning researchers (Annett, 1959) believe that such techniques do little to promote movement skill learning and often result in undesirable dependence on the individual providing the guidance. Schmidt (1991a,b) and Schmidt and Wrisberg (2000) attribute the ineffectiveness of physical guidance as a learning tool to the fact that it does not enable the learner to experience errors during practice. As a result, the learner fails to develop the necessary error detection and correction skills that will be needed for success in later performance situations where guidance is no longer available. In a discussion of treatment strategies designed to improve a patient's motor control, O'Sullivan (1988) further concludes that the "key to success in manually guided movements is knowing when to remove support and to let the patient move independently" (p. 270). In order for learning to occur, individuals must engage in active movement so as to benefit from the rich sources of intrinsic sensory feedback available to them (such as somatosensation and audition). Passively driven movements tend to eliminate and/or distort the quality of these intrinsic sensations.

Physical guidance techniques, though useful for learners who lack confidence, do little to promote movement skill in learning.

If physical guidance does little to promote learning, then why is it used at all? Used intermittently, physical guidance can successfully convey the general idea of a movement pattern not previously experienced. Although the use of modeling techniques can often provide the same information, individuals with visual impairments are much less likely to benefit from a modeled performance. Other learners may simply be unable to derive enough clues from a visual model or set of verbal instructions on which to base their first few practice attempts. Recall that one of the important variables influencing model effectiveness is the degree to which the underlying strategy of the to-be-learned movement pattern is evident to the learner. In these situations, physical guidance can serve such a function.

A second value of physical guidance that has already been mentioned is psychological in nature. Manual guidance, if progressively withdrawn, can be extremely effective in helping a learner overcome any initial fears related to an activity. Feltz (1982) demonstrated the effectiveness of physical guidance in helping a child overcome his fear of diving into a pool head first. No doubt many of us can remember a time when this same activity caused us much nervousness. In fact, physical guidance techniques are still commonly used during the early stages of learning this complex skill. Finally, physical guidance in some form is recommended during the early stages of learning skills that may lead to injury if performed incorrectly. Some gymnastics maneuvers and diving techniques could not be safely taught if mechanical aids were not at first available as a means of constraining the movement pattern and thereby simplifying the learning environment.

## Whole-Task versus Part-Task Practice Strategies

A question that has often proved difficult for the researcher and practitioner to answer is whether it is better for the learner to practice the entire movement pattern from the outset or to practice it in parts until each one has been thoroughly learned. Although part-task practice simplifies the practice environment for the learner, there is some concern that this type of practice will prevent the learner from acquiring a fluent pattern of coordination. To further complicate the issue, a number of research studies have produced equivocal results. The different findings have once again been largely attributed to the type of task used to investigate the issue (Naylor & Briggs, 1961; Wightman & Lintern, 1985).

*Nature of the Skill.*    What is it about certain movement skills that makes part-task training effective or ineffective? Naylor and Briggs (1961) suggest that the inherent complexity (e.g., the number of components involved) and organization (e.g., the extent to which the components are interrelated) of a given movement skill largely determines whether **part-task practice** is appropriate. For example, a dance or a gymnastics floor routine comprises many individual movement skills that are simply combined to form a new movement sequence. These are considered high in complexity but low in organization. Accordingly, the authors consider these movement skills well suited to part-task practice.

Conversely, movement skills that are much less complex but are highly organized in terms of their component parts are better suited to **whole-task practice** methods. Two examples of such skills are hitting a baseball and loco-motion. Both skills comprise components that are temporally linked, in particular (e.g., the backward-swing and forward-swing components in hitting). As simple as it would seem to recommend part-task or whole-task practice on the basis of this simple formula, a closer look at the relationship between these two characteristics of a skill complicates the decision. For example, what type of practice is best in the case of skills that are both high in complexity and high in organization? Serving a tennis ball and serving a volleyball by using an overhead motion might be good examples of such skills.

*Capabilities of the Learner.*    In deciding whether to implement part-task or whole-task practice methods, a practitioner must also consider the capabilities of the learner. It is likely that a novice performer who has little or no experience of the skill being introduced—or of motor skill settings in general—will not benefit from practicing the entire skill. In these practice situations, the higher demands placed on the learner from a processing and control standpoint may actually hinder the learning of the skill. Partitioning a skill into meaningful parts that are practiced first alone and then in combination may be a more suitable practice method to employ in the case of inexperienced performers.

Of course, the extent to which a new movement skill must be partitioned during the early stages of learning can be significantly reduced if the learner has already mastered any of the prerequisite skills that invariably precede more complex skills. For example, a learner who has not yet mastered the skills of dribbling and shooting in basketball will find it extremely difficult to perform the more complex lay-up skill, which requires both of these skills to be reasonably well developed. In many situations, the breadth of the learner's repertoire of known fundamental motor skills (e.g., throwing, catching, running, and hopping) will also determine whether whole-task practices are possible. Finally, the intellectual and physical capacity of the performer will influence the type of practice method chosen. Patients with cognitive deficits and individuals with certain types of physical disabilities may find it extremely difficult to practice skills as a whole during early practice sessions.

---

The inherent complex organization of a skill determines whether part-task practice is appropriate.

---

The extent to which a skill is partitioned can be significantly reduced if the learner has already mastered any prerequisite skills or abilities.

## Part-Task Practice Methods

*Segmentation.*   Wightman and Lintern (1985) have identified three methods of part-task practice that may be appropriate for use in certain movement skill learning situations. They are segmentation, simplification, and fractionization. **Segmentation** involves partitioning the skill according to certain spatial and/or temporal criteria. Once partitioned, the components are practiced separately until a certain level of success has been achieved. These learned components are then combined to form the whole skill. A variation of this method involves practicing the first part of a skill, then the second, and then the combination of the two before proceeding to the third component. This approach is often used in the teaching of dance and gymnastics floor routines. In a clinical setting, this type of part-task practice can be useful when teaching bed-to-chair transfer skills. This method has been called progressive-part practice elsewhere in the literature (Magill, 1989; Schmidt, 1988b).

Segmentation involves partitioning a movement skill according to certain spatial and/or temporal criteria.

*Simplification.*   A second method of part-task practice is called **simplification.** In this method, various aspects of the skill and or environment are simplified. This might involve the removal of accessory parts that are normally used when the whole skill is performed or the use of equipment that reduces the level of control required to perform the skill. For example, a ski instructor often has the novice performer practice without ski poles, thereby simplifying the level of coordination needed to perform the skill. The use of scarves instead of balls when first teaching juggling to beginners also serves to simplify the practice environment and give the learner more time to catch the slower-moving scarves. When first teaching a CVA (cerebrovascular accident) patient to walk again, the therapist often provides the patient with a walking frame or wide-based cane. The use of such assistive devices reduces the level of dynamic balance and lower-extremity strength required to walk.

The complexity of various aspects of the skill and/or environment are reduced in the part-task practice method known as simplification.

*Fractionization.*   The third method of part-task practice involves **fractionization** of the skill, whereby two or more components of the skill that are normally performed simultaneously are practiced in isolation. An example is to practice the diagonal-stride leg action independently of the arm action when first learning cross-country skiing techniques. Unfortunately, this method of part-task practice has proved to be the least successful means of fostering learning of the whole skill. This is not surprising, given that two components performed simultaneously in an entire skill would be highly interdependent and therefore largely invariant from a timing perspective.

Fractionization of a skill involves practicing in isolation those skill components that are normally performed together.

## Attentional Cueing and Whole Practice

Perhaps a compromise approach is one that allows performers to practice the skill in its entirety while their attention is directed to one or two important aspects of the skill. For example, an instructor might direct the learner's attention to particular aspects of the skill, such as the transfer of weight from the rear to the front foot as the ball is contacted during performance of the forehand tennis stroke. Similarly, a therapist may ask the patient to focus on moving the trunk forward over the base of support before attempting to stand from a chair or bed. Although the performers' attention is focused on one or (at most) two parts of the skill while they practice, the whole skill is continually being performed.

Both the spatial and the temporal patterns of a skill are maintained when it is performed as a whole while attention is directed to one or two parts of the skill.

One possible advantage of this **attentional cueing** technique over other part-task practice methods is that both the spatial and the temporal patterns of coordination are maintained when the skill is performed as a whole. One has only to observe a number of recreational players who were taught the tennis serve using part-task practice methods such as fractionization to see how much the temporal fluency of the serving motion has been compromised.

Whatever method of part-task practice is used, it is important that learners understand how the part or parts they are currently practicing are related to the whole skill. Newell and colleagues (Newell, Carlton, Fisher, & Rutter, 1989) found this to be an important component of part-task practice in a study that compared two groups of novice performers attempting to learn a rather sophisticated video game. Both groups practiced the skill in parts, but one group was also privy to the overall strategy needed to be successful when performing the whole skill. Needless to say, those who had this additional information learned the task considerably better than those who were not aware of how the various parts of the skill being practiced related to the performance of the whole game. In teaching the group of learners about the game's strategy, the authors had fostered the learners' understanding of the skill to be learned. You will learn from our discussion of memory in Chapter 11 that using such a teaching technique also fosters the long-term retention and transfer of the skill-related knowledge that is acquired.

## Mental Practice

In addition to physical practice, mental practice is also available when learning how to perform movement skills. **Mental practice** has been defined as "the symbolic rehearsal of a physical activity in the absence of any gross muscular movement" (Richardson, 1967, p. 95). Examples include mentally rehearsing how to perform (a) a motor skill—golf swing, tennis serve, or how to walk or use one's arm and hand again following a stroke—or (b) a movement routine—gymnastics floor exercise routine; steps required to change a tire, shut down a nuclear power plant, or log on and off a computer to access the Internet. **Motor imagery** is a term that is often erroneously used interchangeably with mental practice, but they are not the same. Motor imagery is a more specific form of mental practice. Jeannerod (1994) defined it as the mental representation of us performing a movement skill without any actual movement. Motor imagery is a conscious experience in which we use all of our senses to create or recreate the execution of a movement skill in our mind (Vealey & Greenleaf, 1998).

More often than not, people use motor imagery that relies on visualization (seeing the movement skill being performed in one's mind). However, it has been pointed out that sensory experiences mediated through senses other than the visual sense (e.g., auditory, kinesthetic) also can operate in motor imagery (Anderson, 1981). Perhaps the term *motor imagery* is more appropriate to use when imagery scripts explicitly set forth the practice session as an imaginary movement sequence and specify the content of the image. Without such specification, the more generic term *mental practice* is more appropriate to use.

Evidence from early research was inconclusive with regard to whether mental practice enhanced motor performance (Richardson, 1967). It was not until the 1980s when meta-analyses (quantitative reviews) were used that mental practice was found to enhance motor performance (Feltz & Landers, 1983; Hinshaw, 1991). The benefits of mental practice on motor performance have been found in (a) laboratory studies using novel motor tasks, (b) studies using sport skill performance among high school and college athletes (Feltz & Landers, 1983) and among elite Olympic athletes (Kim, 1989), and (c) rehabilitation settings involving relearning (Linden, Uhley, Smith, & Bush, 1989).

*Mental practice and motor imagery, used as a supplement to physical practice, have been found to enhance movement performance.*

## Mental Practice Conditions

Just as for physical practice, the effectiveness of mental practice for enhancing motor performance largely depends on the conditions used. Some of the conditions that have been studied include (a) how long to mentally practice, (b) how much mental practice to use, (c) external versus internal imagery, (d) form versus outcome focus of attention, and (e) when to mentally practice. Let's look more closely at how each of these conditional variables can influence the effectiveness of mental practice.

***Duration of Mental Practice.***   How long one should mentally practice is closely connected to the extent to which the motor skill that has to be performed contains cognitive components (Driskell, Copper, & Moran, 1994; Feltz & Landers, 1983; Hird, Landers, Thomas, & Horan, 1991). For example, playing golf or tennis or the position of quarterback in football appear to be higher in cognitive components (e.g., plays, strategies) than running in track or swimming or playing the position of a defensive lineman in football. Meta-analyses have revealed that performance of motor skills high in cognitive components can benefit with as little as 3 to 5 minutes or 5 to 6 rehearsals of mental practice. However, performance of motor skills low in cognitive components may require at least 15 minutes or 30 rehearsals of mental practice. Driskell et al. (1994) also found that the performance of participants who were inexperienced in motor skills (novices) benefited more on motor tasks that were high in cognitive components. They also found that the performance of participants experienced in motor skills benefited about the same from mental practice regardless of the extent to which cognitive components were involved in the skills. Lastly, the optimal amount of time one should mentally practice a motor skill before attempting to perform it appears to be about the same as the amount of time it takes to perform the skill (Etnier & Landers, 1996).

*Less mental practice time is needed to enhance performance of movement skills that are higher in cognitive components.*

***Amount of Mental versus Physical Practice.***   The research literature indicates that for a given amount of practice time or repetitions, decreasing the amount of physical practice relative to the amount of mental practice decreases motor and sport performance (Feltz, Landers, & Becker, 1988; Hird et al., 1991). For example, Hird and colleagues compared six different conditions of mental and physical practice and found three major results (see Figure 9.5 on page 280). First, posttest performance was better on both tasks for mental practice than no practice (control group). Second, as the proportion of physical practice increased relative to mental practice for both tasks,

*Mental practice and motor imagery should be used as a supplement to physical practice.*

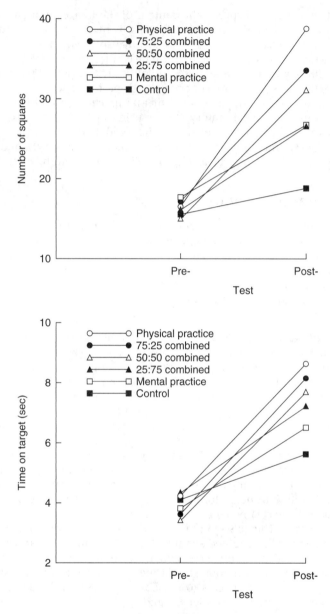

**Figure 9.5**  Effects of various combinations of physical and mental practice on cognitive and motor task performance. The top graph shows the pretest and posttest results for the pegboard task, and the bottom graph shows the results for the pursuit rotor tracking task.

*Source:* Hird, J. S., Landers, D. M., Thomas, J. R., & Horan, J. J. (1991). Physical practice is superior to mental practice in enhancing cognitive and motor task performance. *Journal of Sport & Exercise Psychology, 13,* 281–293.

performance on the posttest increased. Third, physical practice was found to result in better posttest performance on both tasks than a combination of mental and physical practice or mental practice alone. These findings suggest that as long as participants are able to physically practice, mental practice should not be substituted for physical practice. If participants are injured, fatigued, or for some other reason unable to engage in physical practice, then time for mental practice should be allocated during physical practice sessions. Thus, based on the available research evidence, it is recommended that the time allocated for mental practice should be supplemental to and not take away from the time allotted for physical practice.

***Type of Imagery.*** Imagery can be external or internal (Mahoney & Avener, 1977). When you imagine yourself performing a motor skill from the perspective of an external observer, you are using **external imagery.** In terms of visual imagery, it would be like watching yourself perform a motor skill on videotape. You would be able to see the form of your motor skill execution. When you imagine yourself performing a motor skill from your own perspective (the performer's perspective), you are using **internal imagery.** In terms of visual imagery, it would be like watching yourself perform with a camera on your head. You would see only what you can see when you perform, but you would not be able to see the form of your motor skill execution.

Research evidence (e.g., Hinshaw, 1991) reveals that both types of imagery can enhance motor performance if used properly, but greater effects have been found for internal imagery. Some scholars have misinterpreted this finding and recommended that performers only use an internal form of imagery when both types appear to be important for improving performance. In fact, whether a performer uses external or internal imagery may be less important than using the type that produces the most clear, controllable images. Elite archers reported that they routinely use both types, but use internal more than external imagery (Landers, Wang, Daniels, & Boutcher, 1984). It seems that performers should be encouraged to use both types of imagery not only because they both can enhance performance, but also because changing from one imagery perspective to the other could be helpful in developing skill in imagery control.

> The limited research available suggests that both external and internal forms of imagery should be encouraged.

***Focus of Attention.*** Should performers focus their attention on their form when executing a motor skill or on the outcome of the skill performance when mentally practicing to enhance performance? For instance, in golf should performers focus more on the form of their swing (stance, posture, swing plane, etc.) or more on where they want the ball to go (outcome) when mentally practicing? One study investigated this problem using a golf swing (Lutz, Landers, & Linder, 2002) in which the researchers examined what performers should think about or imagine while mentally practicing a golf putt. **Form focus of attention** was on the biomechanical elements required for successful putting performance (e.g., stance, ball position, keeping body and head still during putt, and how the arms should move in executing the putt). **Outcome focus of attention** was on the path of the ball as it rolled into the hole. The findings revealed that participants who focused their attention on the outcome while imaging performed better than those who focused on their putting form. Based on this finding, focusing on the outcome is better than focusing on

> The appropriate use of *form* and *outcome focus of attention* is still a matter of some uncertainty.

form—at least for self-paced motor tasks that demand a great deal of accuracy for success. However, these researchers do not report whether the putting form improved more for the participants who had form focus than for those who had outcome focus. It could be that improvement in form occurs best when focusing on form and improvement in outcome occurs when focusing on outcome. Clearly, further research is needed to determine if this or some other recommendation is best.

*Mental Practice Schedule.*    Should you mentally practice before or after a session of physical practice? Should you physically practice a motor skill and then imagine it before performing it, or should you imagine the skill first and then physically practice it before you perform it? Research seeking the answer to this question was conducted by Etnier and Landers (1996). They used college-age participants with previous basketball experience and formed three groups: (a) mental practice before physical practice, (b) physical practice before mental practice, (c) and a control group. The motor skill participants had to mentally practice and perform was a 3-minute basketball shooting task (outside an arc that was 15 feet from the basket). On trial 1, participants simply physically performed the task. Prior to physically performing the task on trials 2 and 3, they practiced either mentally or physically. The groups of participants who experienced mental practice performed better than the control group, and mental practice before physical practice performed better than physical practice before mental practice. The implication from this research is that it appears to be better for participants to engage in mental practice before engaging in physical practice. However, much more research is needed before the validity of this or other recommendations can be ascertained.

The limited research available suggests that it is better to engage in mental practice before, rather than after, engaging in physical practice.

## Variables Limiting Our Understanding of Mental Practice Effects

There are at least three variables that need to be studied further to better understand how mental practice operates to enhance motor performance. These variables are (a) the amount of mental practice, (b) mental practice procedures, age, and skill level, and (c) modeling and mental practice. Let's examine the issues surrounding each of these variables next.

*Amount of Mental Practice.*    It has been known for some time that, other things being equal, motor learning and its long-term retention can be improved by increasing the level of original learning (level of proficiency of motor performance) in acquisition (for a review see Christina & Bjork, 1991). Most often, the variable manipulated to increase the level of original learning is the amount of physical practice. Whether increasing the amount of mental practice improves motor performance and its long-term retention in the same way that increasing physical practice does is still a matter of some uncertainty. Several neuropsychological researchers have proposed that mental practice generates functionally equivalent cognitive and physiological processes as those found during motor task performance (Cooper, 1995; Jeannerod, 1994; Johnson, 1982). If this proposal is correct, then increasing the level of original learning by increasing the amount of mental practice in acquisition should improve performance just as it does for physical practice. However, studies

Whether increasing the amount of mental practice improves learning and retention is still unclear.

investigating this problem have not found this to be the case (Etnier & Landers, 1996; Lutz et al., 2002; Weinberg, Hankes, & Jackson, 1991). Consequently, any recommendations regarding the optimal duration or amount of mental practice are based more on opinion than on scientific facts, at least at the time of this writing.

*Mental Practice Procedures, Age, and Skill Level.*    Another matter of some uncertainty involves the application of mental practice procedures to people of different ages and skill levels. Much of the research on mental practice has been conducted using younger people who are relatively inexperienced performers (low skill level). Thus, it is unclear whether the mental practice procedures found to enhance motor performance with younger, inexperienced performers actually hold for older and/or more experienced performers (high skill level). Moreover, it is unclear how much introducing new ways to mentally practice or imagine motor performance will interfere with the old ways that experienced performers have relied on for many years. Thus, recommendations involving the use of new mental practice or imagery procedures with experienced performers should be offered with great care because they may interfere with old mental practice routines and actually impair physical performance. Clearly, more research is needed on this problem to better understand the mental practice procedures that are most appropriate for people of different ages and different skill levels.

*Modeling and Mental Practice.*    Some studies investigating the effects of mental practice or imagery on motor performance have involved modeling (observational learning) in the procedures. In these studies, it is difficult to determine the extent to which the effects on motor performance are due to mental practice, modeling, or some combination of both. Both mental practice and modeling have been shown to enhance motor performance in acquisition (motor learning) and in post-acquisition (Driskell et al., 1994; Feltz & Landers, 1983; McCullagh & Weiss, 2001).

Generally, research attempting to untangle the mental practice and modeling effects has found that imagery alone is not very effective for enhancing performance during the motor learning of a new skill. This finding suggests that when performers have no prior experience with the motor skill they are attempting to learn, it is difficult for them to use imagery to create an image of how to execute the skill that will promote learning. However, improvements in motor performance for both form and outcome during learning can be achieved with imagery when it is combined with modeling. Modeling does provide an external stimulus to facilitate imagery via a live demonstration or videotape of the motor skill performance to be learned. So, it should be no surprise to find out that modeling combined with imagery or modeling used alone may be the most effective way to enhance performance during motor learning or for motor skills in which form is important.

The available findings emanating from research that combined imagery with modeling suggest that the size of the imagery effects on motor performance during learning may have been due more to modeling than to imagery. However, further research is needed to determine the validity of this explanation and to separate the effects of imagery per se from the effects of modeling (Martin, Moritz, & Hall, 1999).

---

*The application of mental practice procedures to people of different ages and skill levels is yet to be determined.*

*Research attempting to separate the effects of mental practice from modeling has found greater benefits for modeling than for imagery.*

## Physiological Basis of Mental Practice

Are there physiological changes that occur with mental practice or imagery? If there are, what are they? Are they similar to or do they reflect the physiological changes that take place when the motor skill is performed physically? If the answer to the last question is yes, it would suggest that mental practice or imagery of the execution of a movement skill and actual physical execution of that skill are "functionally equivalent." Evidence for functional equivalence would begin to enhance our understanding of how mental practice and imagery operate to enhance movement performance and provide another line of evidence justifying its use (see highlight, The Role of Mental Practice in the Relearning of Movement Skills). Let's look at a sample of the research investigating the physiological changes associated with mental practice and the **functional equivalence of imagined and physically executed movements.**

Changes in heart and respiratory rates during imagery were similar to those found during actual execution of the movement.

Are the heart and respiratory rates during imagery of the execution of a movement similar to those that are activated during the actual physical execution of the movement? The answer to this question appears to be yes (Decety, Jeannerod, Germain, & Pastene, 1991; Jeannerod, 1994). Increased heart rate and pulmonary ventilation proportional to the imagined walking rate has been found, but at a rate less than actual walking. Also heart and respiration rates have been found to increase with increased levels of imagined exercise (Decety, Jeannerod, Durozard, & Baverel, 1993).

Imagery of the execution of a movement activates many of the same physiological responses and subcortical and cortical areas of the brain as does the actual physical execution of the movement.

Research investigating cortical and subcortical areas during imagined and executed movements has found that many of the same physiological responses and areas are activated during imagery of the execution of a movement as during the actual execution of the movement, but always to a lesser degree than found during actual movement (e.g., Decety, Perani, Jeannerod, Bettinardi, Tadary, Woods, Mazziotta, & Fazio, 1994; Roland, Larsen, Lassen, & Skinhöf, 1980; Pfurtscheller & Neuper, 1997; Roth et al., 1996). This finding may be interpreted as one line of evidence justifying the use of mental practice or imagery of movement skills during motor learning. Also, because research has shown that higher level motor areas of the brain, such as the primary motor cortex and supplementary motor area, are activated during imagery of the execution of a movement, it has been proposed that motor imagery and the actual execution of the movement activate the same motor programs (Bonnet, Decety, Jeannerod, & Requin, 1997). However, during motor imagery the passage of motor signals probably is controlled somewhere at the subcortical level.

EMG activity during imagery appears to "prime" the muscles rather than mirror what happens during movement execution.

Electrical activity associated with functioning skeletal muscle (electromyography, or EMG) has also been studied in relation to mental practice and motor imagery (Jeannerod, 1994). The skeletal muscles responsible for producing a specific movement are activated during imagery of the execution of the movement, and the rate is proportional to the imagined effort (Wehner, Vogt, & Stadler, 1984). Monosynaptic tendinous reflexes in the leg involved during motor imagery were increased more during imagery than during rest (Bonnet et al., 1997). Many studies have found EMG activity slightly above baseline levels during imagery for simple movements (e.g., Bakker, Boschker, & Chung, 1996; Slade, Landers, & Martin, 2000). Thus, motor imagery does produce some activation of the skeletal muscle(s) involved in the execution of the movement being imagined. However, there does not appear to be any evidence

# HIGHLIGHT

### The Role of Mental Practice in the Relearning of Movement Skills

The positive benefits of mental practice in the performance and learning of sport skills has been well documented. Clinical researchers also have begun to explore the efficacy of mental practice in the relearning of movement skills (Page, 2000; Page, Levine, Sisto, & Johnston, 2001; Stevens & Stoykov, 2003).

Page and colleagues (2001) compared the efficacy and feasibility of a treatment program that combined therapy and imagery to a traditional therapeutic program in a group of 13 patients who had experienced a stroke sometime within the previous year. In addition to receiving traditional therapy for 3 hours per week over 6 weeks, 8 of the 13 patients also received an additional 10-minute guided imagery session following each therapy session. They were also instructed to practice imagery at home an additional two times per week. The remaining 5 patients participated in educational sessions in lieu of the imagery sessions.

What the authors of the study found following the 6-week intervention was that the patients receiving the combined program improved their scores on two commonly used tests of motor function by as much as 12 to 16 points, while the group receiving traditional therapy showed very little if any improvement on the same tests. The authors concluded that adding mental imagery to a patient's treatment program is both clinically feasible and cost effective. The hypothesis being advanced by some researchers to explain the improvements observed in the motor performance of their patients is that the motor

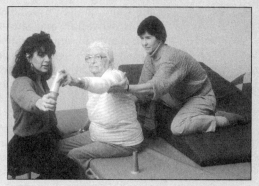

Patients receiving a combination of traditional therapy and mental practice performed better on tests of motor function when compared to patients who received traditional therapy only.

system is being primed at a central command level that eventually leads to movements being executed more quickly and with greater control (Stevens & Stoykov, 2003). The proposed physiological processes that are believed to result from mental practice were also discussed in the mental practice section of this chapter. Although larger randomized, controlled trials are needed to replicate and extend the findings reported in this and other published case reports, the use of mental practice techniques in clinical settings will likely serve as an innovative and effective adjunct to traditional therapeutic techniques for selected patient populations.

*Source:* Carr & Shepherd (1998).

showing that EMG activity is associated with the phasing action between agonist and antagonist muscles involved in the actual execution of the movement during imagery (Hale, 1981, 1982; Slade et al., 2000). Without such evidence, the EMG findings seem to suggest that the benefit derived from motor imagery at the skeletal muscle level is to "prime" the muscles (get them ready) rather than to mirror (to a lesser extent) what happens during the actual execution of a movement as other physiological measures have done.

To summarize, one consistent finding in much of the research investigating the functional equivalence of imagined and physically executed movements is that imagery of the execution of a movement activates many of the same physiological responses and cortical areas of the brain as does the preparation and actual physical execution of the movement. However, the degree of this activation and the observed physiological responses associated with mental practice and imagery of a movement are considerably less than those associated with actual physical execution of movement. Further, the pattern of physiological activity for cortical measures found with imagined movements has not been found to exactly mirror the pattern found for physically executed movements, but it is much closer than for skeletal muscle measures of EMG. The question remains as to what extent the imagined and actual movements are functionally equivalent. The physiological changes associated with mental practice and imagery that *have* been found are promising in that they indicate the presence of related physiological changes during mental practice and imagery. However, more research is needed to determine the extent to which these physiological changes associated with mental practice and imagery are directly related to improvements in actual movement performance.

## Summary

The influence of the amount, specificity, and type of practice on the learning or relearning of any given movement skill has been the subject of a considerable amount of research in the area of movement skill learning. The primary goal of this research has been to identify various theoretical principles that can be used to facilitate the learning of movement skills by improving the quality of each practice session. The collective results of these research endeavors can be used to guide practitioners in structuring meaningful and efficient practices.

For example, the practitioner knows that it is important to structure practice conditions to match (as much as possible) the real-world setting in which movement skills will have to be performed so that the motor abilities, procedures for using sensory feedback, environmental context, and cognitive processing are the same (or similar) in both settings. The practitioner also knows that it is important not only to introduce practice variability, whatever the type of skill to be learned, but also to consider organizing that variability according to the principles of contextual interference. Although practicing a skill under conditions of high contextual interference (random practice) does not always promote good initial performance of that skill, it often leads to superior movement skill learning and transfer. In determining what level of contextual interference is most appropriate for any group of learners, however, the practitioner should first consider the past experiences of the learner with respect to open movement skills in particular and movement skills in general. The intellectual capabilities of the learners and their predominant learning style (reflective or impulsive) must also be considered. The type of movement skill to be learned has also been shown to influence the extent to which high levels of contextual interference promote learning.

The elaboration view and the action-plan reconstruction view have been advanced to explain why high levels of contextual interference often promote superior learning. The two accounts differ with respect to exactly *how* the interference produced by the practice situation influences the nature of the processing operations performed by the learner. But the proponents of both views agree that making the practice more difficult requires the learner to adopt a more active and independent role in the processing of skill-related information.

Finally, the spacing, or distribution, of practice between and within sessions must be considered when structuring an efficient practice environment. Whether a practitioner should use massed or distributed practice schedules depends on a number of factors. These include the characteristics of the skill, the individual characteristics of the learner, and the external constraints that are imposed in a practical setting.

Attempts by practitioners to help learners or patients achieve a level of skill mastery in a shorter period of time have also prompted the use of a number of different practice techniques. Two of the more commonly used are guidance techniques and part-task practice strategies. Manual guidance techniques are effective in minimizing the amount of error produced by learners and the tendency for patients to enlist abnormal or compensatory movements early in rehabilitation. When overused, however, they are likely to hinder the learner's development of error detection and correction skills that will be needed when the guidance is removed. The importance of engaging in active movements in order to benefit from the rich sources of intrinsic feedback they offer is another reason for quickly reducing the amount of guidance provided to a patient or young learner.

Part-task strategies are also used to boost the speed with which a particular skill is mastered by reducing its overall complexity. Various part-task methods can be implemented, depending on the characteristics of the skill to be learned and the capabilities of the learner. Three part-task practice methods are fractionization, segmentation, and simplification. An alternative practice strategy—attentional cueing—provides for practice of the whole skill while the learner's attention is directed to specific aspects of the skill. The primary advantage of this technique may be preservation of the spatial and temporal coordination of the skill during practice.

Mental practice and motor imagery, used to supplement physical practice, have been found to enhance movement performance. Mental practice is the cognitive rehearsal of a movement performance without any actual movement. Motor imagery is a more specific form of mental practice and usually relies on visualizing the movement sequence being performed. It involves the use of imagery scripts, which explicitly set forth the practice session as an imaginary movement sequence and specify the content of the image. Similar to physical practice, the effectiveness of mental practice in enhancing motor performance depends on the conditions such as (a) duration of mental practice, (b) the amount of mental practice used relative to physical practice, (c) external versus internal imagery, and (d) when to mentally practice. The available research suggests that less mental practice time is needed to enhance performance of movement skills that are higher in cognitive components. It also suggests that the optimum amount of time to mentally practice a movement skill before attempting to perform it is about the same as the amount of time it takes to actually perform the skill. Further, the time allocated for mental practice should be supplemental to and not take away from physical practice time. The limited research available on whether focus of attention should be external or internal when using imagery suggests that both types of imagery should be encouraged not only because both can enhance performance, but also because changing from one imagery perspective to the other could be helpful in developing skill in imagery control. And lastly, it appears that it is better to engage in mental practice before rather than after engaging in physical practice. However, much more research is needed before the validity of these recommendations can be ascertained. Further, more research is needed to determine the extent to which the physiological changes associated with mental practice and imagery are directly related to improvements in actual movement performance.

## IMPORTANT TERMINOLOGY

After completing this chapter, readers should be familiar with the following terms and concepts.

action-plan reconstruction view
attentional cueing
blocked practice
contextual interference (CI)
contextual variety
distributed practice
elaboration view
encoding specificity
external imagery
form focus of attention
fractionization
functional equivalence of imagined
    and physically executed
    movements
generizability
guidance techniques
internal imagery
level of original learning
massed practice
mental practice
motor ability

motor imagery
outcome focus of attention
over-learning
physical guidance
part-task practice
practice variability
random practice
segmentation
simplification
situated learning
specificity of practice effects for the
    context
specificity of practice effects for
    cognitive processing
specificity of practice effects for
    sensory feedback
specificity of practice principle
state-dependent learning
theory of identical elements
whole-task practice

## SUGGESTED FURTHER READING

Christina, R. W., & Alpenfels, E. (2002). Why does traditional training fail to optimize playing performance? In E. Thain (Ed.), *Science and golf IV: Proceedings of the World Scientific Congress of Golf* (pp. 231–245). London: Routledge.

Ericsson, K. (2001). The path to expert golf performance: Insights from the masters on how to improve by deliberate practice. In P. Thomas (Ed.), *Optimising performance in golf* (pp. 1–58). Brisbane, Australia: Australian Academic Press.

## Test Your Understanding

1. Explain how level of original learning, over-learning, retention, and elite performance are each a function of the amount of practice.

2. Provide an example of how a practitioner could structure practice so that it was consistent with the specificity of practice principle. Use a particular sport skill or activity of daily living in your example, and be certain to design practice conditions that are appropriate for the specificity of motor abilities and procedures for using sensory feedback, as well as context and processing specificity.

3. Briefly explain why the introduction of large amounts of practice variability is believed to enhance the learning of movement skills.

4. According to Gentile's two-stage model of motor learning, at what stage in the learning of a movement skill is the introduction of practice variability considered most appropriate? Explain your answer.

5. Identify ways in which variability of practice can be introduced in the learning of different types of skills (i.e., closed skills vs. open skills) in a physical education or clinical setting. In what way does the type of variability introduced differ in different learning situations?

6. Briefly describe how the principle of contextual interference is related to the concept of practice variability.

7. Describe how a practitioner might structure a practice session that introduces a high level of contextual interference. Choose a particular sport skill or activity of daily living to illustrate your answer to this question.

8. Identify the various factors that a practitioner must consider when deciding how much contextual interference is appropriate for a given practice situation.

9. How does the type of measurement used to evaluate the benefits of contextual interference influence the conclusions that are reached?

10. Compare and contrast the assumptions underlying the two theoretical accounts advanced to explain the contextual interference effect.

11. Briefly describe the controversy that exists with respect to the spacing, or distribution, of practice within a particular practice session.

12. Briefly describe the advantages and disadvantages associated with the use of guidance techniques in physical education and clinical settings.

13. Outline certain guidelines that you, as a practitioner, would follow when considering the use of guidance techniques in any movement skill learning environment.

14. When are part-task practice strategies most likely to be used in the teaching of movement skills? Describe three common part-task practice methods that are used to help learners reach a level of skill mastery in a shorter period of time. Provide examples of skills that are most suited to each type of part-task practice method.

15. Describe an alternative practice method that appears to combine the advantages of part-task practice with those associated with the whole-task practice of movement skills.

16. Based on the available research evidence, describe the mental practice conditions that you would recommend to help learners acquire new movement skills in original learning and after original learning.

17. Identify the major variables that limit our understanding of mental practice effects, and explain why they impose limits.

18. What is the physiological basis of mental practice, and why is it important to search for such a connection?

## PRACTICAL ACTIVITIES

To help you better understand the concept of contextual interference, we have designed the following experiment:

- Divide into three small groups of 4–5. Group 1 will practice the skill according to a blocked practice schedule, group 2 will practice the skill according to a serial practice schedule, and group 3 will practice the skill according to a random practice schedule.
- Place 3 targets on the floor at 5, 10, and 15 feet from a starting line.
- The task is to throw an object (e.g., bean bag, ball), using an underarm throwing action, into each target according to the practice schedule assigned.
- The task is to complete 30 trials divided into 3 blocks of 10 trials.

Write down how each member in your group should perform the 30 trials based on the practice group to which he or she has been assigned. Also consider how you might design a retention or transfer test to see which practice group may have learned the task better. Do you think the three different tasks (using different target distances) you were asked to perform belonged to the same class of actions or a different class of actions? If you think the skills you just performed belonged to the same class of actions, design a follow-up experiment that now includes three tasks that you think belong to a different class of actions. Share your ideas with each other, and then actually conduct the proposed experiment.

# 10

# AUGMENTED FEEDBACK AND MOTOR LEARNING

*Feedback is information arising as a consequence of performance, which is essential for motor learning not only because it provides a basis for evaluating the correctness of performance, but also because it can serve as incentive to influence one's motivation to learn.*

## CHAPTER OBJECTIVES

After studying this chapter, you should be able to:

- Explain and provide examples of how intrinsic (internal) and augmented feedback can function as information, reinforcement, punishment, and motivation to promote motor learning.

- Describe the various types of augmented information feedback used to facilitate motor learning.

- Explain and give examples of the various forms of augmented information feedback that focus on kinematic aspects of a performance and with those forms that emphasize the unobservable kinetic parameters of movement.

- Describe the type of augmented sensory feedback that is used to promote better motor

control and learning by providing the learner with information about internal physiological events.

- Describe the various factors that must be considered when deciding how precise the augmented information feedback that is provided to a learner should be.

- Explain how the frequency with which information feedback is provided to the learner influences motor learning and performance.

- Explain how the timing of information feedback following a practice attempt influences motor learning.

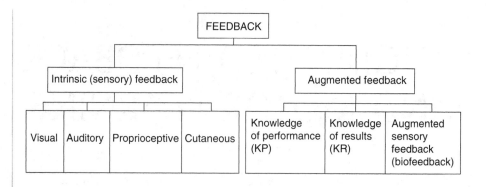

**Figure 10.1**   Feedback is available from two primary sources: Intrinsic (sensory) feedback arises as a natural consequence of the movement itself via the learner's sensory receptors, whereas augmented feedback originates from an external source.

Now that we have considered the many issues involved in organizing the practice environment, let us turn to a discussion of how the practitioner can further shape the quality of each practice session by providing information to the learner about the nature of his or her practice performance. We read in Chapter 4 that learners possess a sophisticated repertoire of **intrinsic (sensory) feedback** mechanisms (such as vision, audition, and somatosensation) that acquaint them with many aspects of a movement. We will now consider a second source of movement-related information that can be provided to the individual. This second and external source of feedback, called *augmented feedback,* can be used to supplement the feedback already available from intrinsic sensory sources. (Figure 10.1 illustrates the relationship between these two categories of feedback.)

**Augmented feedback** consists of information provided to the learner from an external source. Three characteristics of this feedback are notable. First, it may be provided in a verbal or nonverbal form. Second, augmented feedback may be provided during (**concurrent feedback**), immediately following (**terminal feedback**), or some time after a movement has been completed (**delayed feedback**). Third, the augmented feedback may describe the outcome of the movement and/or the movement pattern itself.

Augmented feedback that is provided after the completion of a movement and describes the *outcome* is called **knowledge of results (KR),** whereas information specific to the *quality* of the movement pattern produced is known as **knowledge of performance (KP).** These two components of augmented feedback have inspired a number of research endeavors during the past several decades. This chapter discusses the general findings of these numerous studies and their practical relevance.

Providing meaningful augmented feedback to a learner during practice is one of the most important responsibilities of an instructor or clinician. Not only can augmented feedback help the learner identify and correct

Augmented feedback is information provided to a learner from an external source that describes the outcome and/or quality of a performance.

performance errors, but it can also serve as an important incentive to motivate the learner during practice and to reinforce the performance being learned. Four important aspects of feedback will be discussed in the remaining sections of this chapter: (a) the functions of feedback in motor learning, (b) the form of feedback provided to the learner, (c) the precision of the feedback, and (d) the frequency with which it is presented during practice.

# Functions of Feedback in Motor Learning

During the process of learning a motor skill, feedback, whether intrinsic or augmented, can operate to serve four functions: (a) information or knowledge, (b) reinforcement, (c) punishment, and (d) motivation. Depending on how the learner perceives the feedback, it can serve one or more of these functions at a time. Let's examine more closely how feedback can work to serve each of these functions.

*Feedback can serve four important functions: information or knowledge, reinforcement, punishment and motivation.*

## Feedback as Information to Correct Performance Errors

Feedback that provides information or knowledge (**information feedback**) can carry a message about the effectiveness of a skill performance, the errors that were made, and how to correct them. More specifically, information feedback has the potential to carry a message to learners about:

*Information feedback provides knowledge about the execution and outcome of movement skills.*

- The outcome of their skill performance (KR)
- The movement-produced sensations that accompany their skill performance (proprioceptive feedback)
- Which parts of the skill they performed correctly and incorrectly (KP)
- The explanation of the cause(s) of their error(s)
- Changes in technique that must be made to correct the error(s)
- The reasons why these particular changes are recommended

When a learner executes an action plan and produces a movement, commands (nerve impulses via the central nervous system) tell the muscular system which muscles are to contract and how they are to contract to successfully generate the goal movement. Simultaneously, a copy of the neural commands (action plan, or efference copy) that were sent to the muscular system is stored in the brain for action evaluation. As the muscles contract and the movement is produced, sensory receptors in the muscles (muscle spindles), tendons (Golgi tendon organs), and joints (joint receptors) are stimulated and provide kinesthetic feedback through the learner's sensory system for movement evaluation. The learner's brain uses a copy of the commands along with the kinesthetic feedback to evaluate whether the movement was performed as he or she intended to perform it. Regardless of the proficiency of the outcome of the movement or the correctness with which it is executed, if it was performed as intended, the learner experiences a feeling that it was correct; and if the movement was not performed as planned, the learner experiences a feeling that it was incorrect. The more advanced the learner is in performing the response, the greater the accuracy of the movement evaluation. The movement evaluation of learners who are in the beginning stages of learning a new motor skill is less accurate because they have not yet developed a memory for how the skill should feel when performed correctly.

In addition to intrinsic feedback from kinesthetic receptors, learners also receive intrinsic feedback about the movement from other sensory receptors, such as their cutaneous receptors (touch pressure, heat, cold, and pain), eyes (visual) and ears (auditory), and augmented feedback from external sources such as teachers, coaches, clinicians, teammates, spectators, and opponents. For example, if an experienced basketball player misses a well-learned basketball shot in practice, the movement will feel wrong, and the player will see the ball miss the basket, even hear it hit the rim of the basket, and might also receive augmented feedback from the coach and teammates. All of these sources of feedback enter through the appropriate sensory receptors and tracts of the player's sensory system and travel to the brain, where the information is sensed, perceived, and used to evaluate the correctness of the movement that was just performed. If an error is detected, the next time the movement is made the player attempts to change the action plan and correct the previous commands that were sent to the muscular system to produce the missed shot. If no error is detected, the player will attempt to use the same action plan and send the same commands that were sent to generate the previous movement.

## Feedback as Positive Reinforcement to Strengthen Correct Performance

Feedback also can function as **positive reinforcement** to strengthen a movement skill. Such feedback has pleasant properties that a learner will pursue if at all possible. However, for it to serve as positive reinforcement, it must follow the movement, preferably immediately, and increase the likelihood that it will occur in the future under the same or similar conditions.

An example of internal feedback that may serve as positive reinforcement is the satisfaction of seeing the soccer ball you kicked or a golf ball you hit go exactly where you planned for it to go and sensing (via kinesthetic feedback) that your body moved precisely as you planned to perform the kick or golf swing. Internal feedback consisting of this type of information can be quite rewarding; and, to experience it again, you will try to execute the kick in the same way in the future under similar conditions.

Examples of augmented feedback that may act as positive reinforcement for a learner are verbal compliments or praise from a teacher, coach, or clinician like "Good try," Great move," or "Your form was perfect—keep up the good work," and nonverbal types of communication, such as a smile or nod of approval or a pat on the back. Receiving this kind of augmented feedback soon after a learner performs a skill can be very rewarding. To obtain it again, the learner will try to perform the skill in the same way in the future under similar conditions. Some practitioners believe that if they use augmented feedback as a reward for a movement, it always will function as positive

For feedback to serve as positive reinforcement, it must follow shortly after the movement and increase the likelihood that the movement will be repeated in the future under the same or similar conditions.

reinforcement. However, this is true only if the movement skill is strengthened (that is, if the chance that the skill will be repeated in the future is increased), and that depends on whether the learner, not the practitioner, perceives the augmented feedback as reward. What is perceived as positive reinforcement by one person may be interpreted quite differently by another. For example, changing a baseball player's field position may be perceived by the coach as evidence of the player's all-around athletic ability, but the player may be upset with the move because he or she interprets it as a failure to play the first position well.

## Feedback as Negative Reinforcement to Strengthen Correct Performance

**Negative reinforcement** feedback possesses unpleasant properties that a learner will avoid if at all possible. For this type of feedback, its removal or avoidance must strengthen the movement you want the learner to acquire. An example of internal feedback that may serve as negative reinforcement is a player's dissatisfaction at seeing the basketball miss the basket and at sensing kinesthetically that his or her body did not move as intended in performing the shot. Because such feedback is unpleasant, the learner will attempt to avoid it on future shots by changing his or her shooting technique. If the change results in internal feedback that serves as positive reinforcement (the satisfaction of seeing the basketball go into the basket) and the removal of internal feedback that acts as negative reinforcement (the dissatisfaction of seeing the basketball miss the basket), the new technique is likely to become strengthened with practice and eventually learned.

> For feedback to serve as negative reinforcement, its removal or avoidance must strengthen the movement you want the learner to acquire.

Augmented feedback also may act as negative reinforcement. For instance, the coach of a boys' baseball team was trying to improve a right-handed player's batting technique. The coach had been trying to get the player to learn to become more consistent in taking a shorter rather than longer step (stride) with his leading leg as he swung at each pitch. The coach had talked to the player about shortening his step, showed films, and called attention to the error every time it was made. Nothing seemed to work. The coach decided to try using negative reinforcement to correct the error. The coach placed a wooden barrier on the ground about 12 inches in front of where the player's left leg was striding. The wooden barrier, which was too high to step over when batting, was placed at the maximum distance that the player should stride with his leg when performing the skill correctly. At first on each swing the player's left foot contacted the barrier because his stride was too long. The player perceived the barrier to be annoying or unpleasant because it was in the way of his left foot when he took his step to swing the bat. Eventually, the player learned to avoid the unpleasantness of hitting the barrier by decreasing the length of his stride. Avoiding the negative feedback of the barrier associated with the long stride (incorrect movement) reinforced the learning of the shortened stride (correct movement) and increased the probability that he would keep it short when batting in the future.

## Feedback as Punishment to Suppress Errors

For feedback to operate as punishment it must follow the incorrect movement and decrease the likelihood of that movement being made in the future under the same or similar conditions.

Like feedback that functions as negative reinforcement, feedback that acts as **punishment** also possesses unpleasant properties that a learner will avoid if possible. In fact, the same unpleasant and aversive feedback can be used to produce either negative reinforcement or punishment, depending on whether it strengthens or weakens a movement. For feedback to operate as punishment, it must follow (preferably immediately) the undesirable movement that we want the learner to decrease the likelihood of making in the future under similar conditions. Essentially, the punishing feedback is avoided by learning not to perform the undesirable response in the future.

An example of internal feedback that serves as punishment is the unpleasant experience of feeling a severe pain in your elbow each time you throw a certain pitch, such as a "slider" in baseball, or each time you hit a "slice" serve in tennis. This kind of internal feedback is very painful and unpleasant, so you will try to avoid it in the future by not throwing that particular pitch or serve.

Following is an example of augmented feedback that operates as a punishment. A basketball coach decides to use feedback as punishment to stop a player from making the repeated error of taking an unnecessary dribble (bounce) of the ball immediately before taking a shot. The coach could punish the error in a couple of ways. One way is to express (nonverbally and verbally) his or her disproval of the unnecessary dribble immediately after the player performs it. Another possibility is for the coach to threaten to withdraw positive reinforcement immediately after the player makes the error. For instance, the coach could threaten to give the player less playing time in games until he or she learns to eliminate the unnecessary dribble.

Regardless of which way feedback is used as punishment, however, it is important to note that the coach punished the undesirable response (the unnecessary dribble) and not the player. The problem with punishing the player or being perceived as punishing the player is that it could lead to feelings of rejection and, as a result, could produce emotions of resentment, aggression, hostility, or avoidance. On the other hand, if only the undesirable movement is punished and effort is praised (if deserved), the player is likely to take the punishment in stride.

## Feedback as Motivation for Motor Learning

Feedback can have a very strong influence on a person's motivation to learn motor skills.

Various aspects of motivation and learning were introduced in Chapters 6 and 8. In this chapter we will focus on feedback, which can have a very strong influence on a person's **motivation** to learn motor skills. Suppose a person's goal is to learn to perform a motor skill exactly as it was explained and demonstrated by the instructor or clinician. Assume that the learner, Lynn, is motivated to achieve this goal because the instructor/clinician convinced her that it is one prerequisite for fulfilling her need to feel competent, successful, and worthy as a human being and to have fun. After each attempt to perform the skill, Lynn receives internal and augmented feedback that informs her about how far her present performance is from the goal performance and how to correct the errors. Knowing these factors enables her to modify her actions to reduce her performance errors until eventually, through practice and learning, her performance matches the goal performance. In this context, feedback is providing information/knowledge to Lynn that influences her **directive function of motivation.**

Feedback also can have an effect on the learner's **arousal function of motivation,** that is, how much energy the learner will expend on future attempts to learn a new motor skill. For example, if information feedback (internal or external) indicates that the difference between Lynn's performance and the goal performance is decreasing with practice, she is likely to perceive that she is improving and that progress is being made. Feedback conveying this kind of information can be very rewarding to the learner and act as an incentive to continue to use the available energy to try to improve until the goal performance is reached. Conversely, if the feedback reveals that the difference between the learner's performance and the goal performance is unchanged or increasing, the learner will probably think that little or no improvement or progress is being made with practice. Feedback carrying this message can be quite frustrating. It may serve as an incentive either to reduce the amount of energy used in future attempts to learn the goal performance or not to use any energy at all to learn it in the future. That is, Lynn may not try very hard to learn the skill or may completely give up trying.

It is important that the practitioner consider when feedback should be used to give the learner error-correction information about the performance and when it should be used to motivate the learner. Although it is now clear that learners require less augmented feedback than was previously thought, that should not preclude the use of less specific feedback intended to motivate learners or patients to keep up their good efforts. When deserved and sincerely conveyed, simple phrases such as "You are really working hard to improve your performance" and Nice try!" can do much to improve or maintain a learner's interest in the movement skill being taught. The use of bandwidth KR schedules (see page 306) would also seem to provide an opportunity to motivate performers. Remember that instructors who use this schedule provide learners with error-correction feedback only when their performance does not fall within a predetermined range of acceptable performance. Therefore, on those practice attempts for which an instructor does not provide any feedback, he or she is conveying the idea that the performance was within the acceptable range. This type of KR schedule, then, not only serves as a valuable method of conveying error-related information, but also offers a way of motivating the learner.

# Form of the Feedback

A practice session affords many ways to provide learners with information about their performance. The forms most commonly used are verbal instructions, videotape playbacks of performance, and augmented feedback. Verbal feedback provided by a teacher or clinician still tends to be the form most commonly used in sport and clinical settings. A variety of alternative feedback techniques have also been shown to facilitate the learning and/or relearning of movement skills. The discussion that follows focuses on a variety of alternative forms of augmented feedback that can be conveniently divided into those methods that emphasize the kinematic aspects of a performance and those that focus on the unobservable kinetic parameters. As we will see, kinematic feedback can be provided by using videotape replays of actual performance or graphic displays of limb displacement, velocity, and/or acceleration. Kinetic aspects of a performance can be revealed by using similar types of graphic visual displays or auditory signals associated with EMG activity, torque output, and/or ground reaction forces. One or both of these forms of augmented feedback may be presented to the performer for any given performance. And either form may be provided while the performance is occurring or following its completion.

## Kinematic and Kinetic Visual Displays

Traditional forms of KR can specify only what *not* to do on a subsequent trial whereas kinetic and/or kinematic feedback can specify what *to do*.

Newell and colleagues (Newell & McGinnis, 1985; Newell, Quinn, Sparrow, & Walter, 1983) have demonstrated the effectiveness of using both **kinetic** and **kinematic feedback** in the learning of a variety of movement skills that involve rapid limb movements or the generation of criterion levels of force. Newell and Walter (1981) argue that the use of traditional forms of KR (such as movement time and peak force) can specify only what *not to do* on a subsequent trial following an incorrect attempt, whereas the use of kinetic and/or kinematic representations of movement can provide useful information about what *to do* on the next trial (p. 246).

Unfortunately, the value of these types of displays is often limited to describing only one, or at most two, parameters of performance. This may be viewed as a drawback when the movement skill to be acquired is considerably more complex because of the number of degrees of freedom involved. In these situations it may be necessary to represent the dynamics of the movement by using a display that combines multiple segments. Alternatively, one or more parameters of performance might be identified that, if specifically practiced, will benefit the overall performance of the task. Of course, identifying these critical parameters requires a thorough understanding of exactly what parameters are being manipulated to produce a particular coordination pattern. Given that a primary focus of the dynamic systems approach is to identify the equations of motion that govern both the stability and the instability of a particular pattern of coordination, it will become easier to identify the critical parameters that can be represented either kinematically and/or kinetically.

Global information about a movement's outcome may be more effective when the skill to be learned involves a high number of degrees of freedom.

Although kinematic representations of a movement's dynamics have been shown to benefit learners performing single-degree-of-freedom movements, Swinnen and his co-investigators (Swinnen, Walter, Lee, & Serrien, 1993) provided empirical support for the use of feedback based on movement outcome (KR) rather than detailed kinematic information in more complex skill situations. In a series of three experiments, the authors demonstrated that subjects provided with general information on outcome were better able to learn a bimanual coordination task that required them to perform different limb movements than were subjects provided with detailed kinematic feedback (Figure 10.2).

The authors reasoned that because the movement goal was made clearly apparent to the performers, "they were largely capable of comparing what was done with what should be done, using the limited amount of extra KR feedback" (p. 1341). These findings of Swinnen et al. are also in agreement with

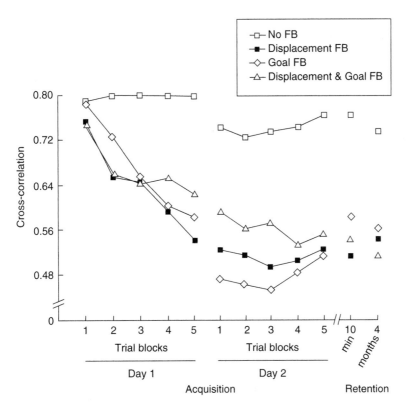

**Figure 10.2**  The relative effects of feedback based on movement outcome versus performance-based kinematic feedback in the learning of a bimanual coordination task. FB = feedback

those described earlier by Young and Schmidt (1990), who suggested that global information about a movement's outcome may be more effective when the skill to be learned involves a greater number of degrees of freedom.

## Videotape Feedback

The effectiveness of videotape replays focusing on the kinematic aspects of performance appears to be influenced by a number of factors. These include the skill level of the learner, the period of time over which the videotape feedback is used, and whether it is supplemented with additional verbal feedback. In reviewing a number of studies in which videotape feedback was used, Rothstein and Arnold (1976) found that skilled performers tended to benefit more from the use of unguided videotape feedback than did novice performers. It has been argued that the large amount of information available from videotape feedback has a tendency to overwhelm the novice performer who has not yet learned how to attend selectively to the important aspects of the performance (Newell & Walter, 1981). Rothstein and Arnold did find, however, that in those studies in which the videotape feedback provided to novice learners was supplemented with specific skill-related verbal cues, considerably more benefit was derived from the videotape feedback.

Kernodle and Carlton (1992) further explored the role of attention-focusing cues in optimizing videotape feedback by providing one of two different types of cues to a group of performers attempting to learn the overhand throw. One group received cues intended to focus attention on important aspects of the throwing action ("Focus on the initial position of the body" and "Focus on the hips during the throwing phase"); a second group was presented with error-correction transitional cues that were intended not only to help the learner identify what component of the skill to change, but also to tell the learner how to change the movement in order to accomplish the intended coordination pattern. Performers in this group were likely to receive cues such as "Align your body so the right shoulder faces the target area" and "Rotate the hips from left to right during the throwing phase." The type of cue provided to each learner was based on the type of error made on the previous attempt.

As Figure 10.3 shows, the learners who received the error-correction transitional cues ("Transition") or attention-focusing cues ("Cue") before watching the videotape demonstrated significantly greater improvement in the distance they were able to throw the ball after four weeks of practice when compared to two other groups of learners who received KR or KP alone. More important, the transitional-cues group received the highest movement form rating across all practice sessions when compared to all other feedback groups. The transitional cues were clearly helping these learners modify their movement patterns to achieve the desired action. On the basis of their findings, Kernodle and Carlton concluded that providing KR or KP alone may not be the most potent form of feedback when the skill to be learned is one that involves multiple degrees of freedom.

Allowing a sufficient period of time for learners to view the videotape feedback has also been shown to be important. Learners need time to familiarize themselves with this form of augmented feedback and learn to extract the most useful information. Using videotape feedback over an extended period of time also ensures that the skill to be learned is adequately practiced. On the basis of their review, Rothstein and Arnold recommended that videotape feedback should be presented for at least five weeks in order to be effective. Studies in which videotape feedback was used for a shorter period of time did not result in improved performance.

One final issue related to the use of videotape feedback is that of skill level. On the basis of a number of unpublished doctoral studies, Rothstein and Arnold suggest that novice performers gain less from the use of videotape feedback than players at a more advanced level of performance. Unfortunately, although a number of recent studies have attempted to determine whether this is indeed the case, the results of these studies are inconclusive. Although Rikli and Smith (1980) concluded, on the basis of their findings with novice performers, that videotape feedback may be more effective for intermediate performers attempting to learn the tennis serve, van Wieringen and colleagues

Novice performers derive greater benefits from videotape when it is supplemented with attention-focusing and error-correction verbal cues.

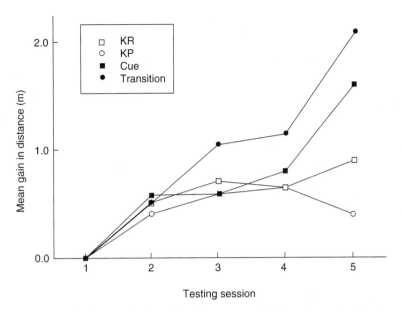

**Figure 10.3** The mean gain in throwing distance was significantly greater for the group that received error-correction transitional verbal cues in addition to the videotape feedback.

(Emmon, Wesseling, Bootsma, Whiting, & van Wieringen, 1985; van Wieringen, Bootsma, Hoogesteger, & Whiting, 1989) found no benefits of videotape feedback training with a group of intermediate tennis players. The researchers found that neither serving form nor serving accuracy improved to any greater extent for players who received the videotape feedback training than for players who received more traditional tennis training. The authors of both studies generally conclude that videotape feedback training may not be as effective as practitioners would like to think. On the basis of these two studies, at least, there is little evidence to suggest that its use is superior to existing teaching methods.

## Augmented Sensory Information: Biofeedback

Unlike the more general category of augmented feedback, **augmented sensory feedback** is specifically designed to amplify and display different types of internal physiological events, both normal and abnormal, in an effort to help an individual learn how to control these events. **Biofeedback** is the clinical term often used to describe this form of feedback. In rehabilitation settings, biofeedback is commonly used to inform patients about their own joint

Augmented sensory feedback is designed to amplify different types of internal physiological events.

displacement, level of muscle activity, force generation, and/or movement of the center of mass. This internally generated information is subsequently presented to the patient in a visual or auditory form and can be used to modify the performance in progress or a subsequent attempt.

Biofeedback devices provide patients with important feedback that is often more relevant and accurate than that provided by the clinician.

Biofeedback techniques are commonly used during the rehabilitation process as a means of facilitating neuromuscular reeducation. They are considered a generally effective supplementary tool for patients with different types of muscle paresis, chronic pain, foot drop following a stroke, cerebral palsy, and Parkinson's disease (Inglis, Campbell, & Donald, 1976; Wolf, 1983). By far the most popular techniques are EMG recordings, goniometry, and various kinetic feedback devices. These different types of devices can provide the patient with feedback that is often more relevant and accurate than that provided by the clinician. The information provided is often more immediate for the performer and can be used to correct errors in performance in a more timely fashion.

Shumway-Cook and colleagues (Shumway-Cook, Anson, & Haller, 1988) found that the use of visual biofeedback—providing information about the kinetic aspects of postural sway—was particularly effective in the postural retraining of stroke patients. The authors compared two groups of hemiplegic patients who were being taught how to develop a more symmetrical stance. One group received conventional therapy emphasizing tactile and verbal cues, whereas the second group received kinetic biofeedback in the form of foot center of pressure. The results of this study indicated that patients provided with the visual kinetic biofeedback were much more successful in developing a more symmetrical stance. Specifically, the patients in the kinetic biofeedback training group began to increase the loading of their involved limb in order to maintain standing balance more than those patients who received conventional treatment. The authors attributed their findings to the fact that it is extremely difficult for the therapist to infer loading patterns accurately just from observing patient postures or reductions in overall body sway.

### Guiding Principles for the Use of Biofeedback.

As effective as certain types of biofeedback appear to be in the rehabilitation process, it is important that certain principles associated with its use be followed. First, the patient must understand the relationship between the signal presented and the task to be performed. For example, the young child with cerebral palsy who is participating in gait training must know whether the presence of an auditory signal indicates acceptable or unacceptable heel contact performance. Kinetic feedback devices attached to the heel of the child's involved limb may be programmed to emit an auditory signal when the child contacts the floor with the heel during gait (positive feedback) or may emit a continuous signal until the time that the child does contact the floor, at which time the signal stops (negative feedback).

Once the patient understands the relationship between task and signal, practice at controlling the signal should follow while the clinician provides positive verbal reinforcement. Given that this period of the training can often be very tiring and frustrating for the patient, it is also important to limit the use of the biofeedback device to manageable time periods. Finally, once introduced, the device should be used until the task has been learned and the device is no longer needed. At this point in the reeducation process, the patient should have begun to equate the biofeedback signal with the appropriate movement sensation.

# Precision of Augmented Feedback

Another factor that must be considered when deciding what type of augmented feedback to provide to the learner is the level of precision associated with the feedback. One can logically expect that as the level of precision associated with the augmented feedback increases, so too does the amount of processing required of the learner. It should logically follow, therefore, that as the level of precision associated with the feedback increases, so too should the time provided for the learner to process the information. A number of research investigations devoted to the investigation of the issue of feedback precision (Reeve & Magill, 1981; Rogers, 1974; Smoll, 1972) have also demonstrated that increasing the level of precision associated with the feedback enhances learning only up to a certain point, beyond which performance is negatively affected.

The skill level of the learner has also been shown to be an important consideration in how precise the information feedback should be. Magill and Wood (1986) nicely illustrated this relationship by manipulating the **precision of the augmented feedback** provided to a group of subjects attempting to learn a six-segment movement pattern. The goal of the task was to perform each of the six segments in a particular criterion movement time. One group of subjects received information about the direction of the error (too fast or too slow); a second group also received information about the amount of error produced (number of seconds too fast or too slow).

Figure 10.4 on page 304 demonstrates two interesting findings that emerged from this investigation. First, both groups performed with similar amounts of error during the early practice trials, irrespective of the type of augmented feedback provided. Second, during the later practice trials, the group receiving the more precise information feedback began to perform significantly better than the group receiving the less precise form of feedback. The performance of the high-precision feedback group was also significantly better during a no-KR retention test, which indicated that providing feedback that was more precise positively influenced the learning of the task.

On the basis of their findings, the authors concluded that providing more precise levels of feedback early in the learning of a movement skill did not lead to better performance of the task. They suggested that more precise feedback should be withheld until the learner has had enough practice on a task to benefit from detailed information. During the early stages of learning it may be more appropriate to provide general information about the learner's performance until the skill level of the learner and her or his knowledge of the skill's dynamics improves.

*As the level of KR precision increases, so too should the time provided for the learner to process the more precise information.*

*More precise feedback should be withheld until the learner has completed a sufficient amount of practice.*

# Frequency of Augmented Feedback

How often should an instructor or clinician provide augmented feedback? If we were to consider only the experimental findings of studies conducted more than thirty years ago, the answer would be "the more the better." This was the conclusion that emerged from a series of studies conducted by Bilodeau and colleagues (Bilodeau & Bilodeau, 1958a,b; Bilodeau, Bilodeau, & Schumsky, 1959) in which the amount of KR provided to a group of learners was

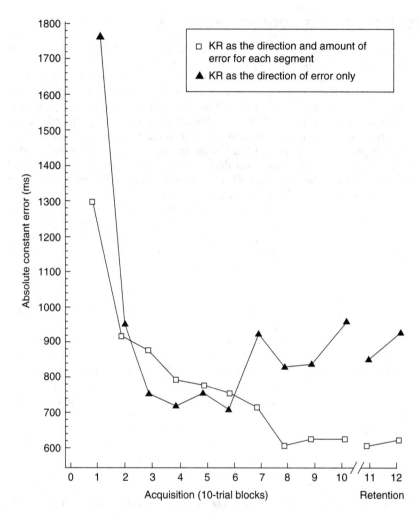

**Figure 10.4**  The more precise KR (direction and amount of error) resulted in better performance in later acquisition and retention trials than did the less precise KR (direction of error).

*Source:* Magill, R. A., & Wood, C. A. (1986). Knowledge of results precision as a learning variable in motor skill acquisition. *Research Quarterly for Exercise and Sport, 57,* 170–173.

manipulated. In one study (Bilodeau & Bilodeau, 1958a), participants attempting to learn a simple lever-pulling task were provided with KR after every third or fourth trial or after every trial. At the conclusion of the practice phase, a comparison of the performances of both KR groups on the task revealed significant differences: The group that received KR after every trial exhibited the least amount of performance error.

The story is somewhat different, however, when the results of later studies are considered (Ho & Shea, 1978; Johnson, Wicks, & Ben-Sira, 1981). Two aspects of the earlier studies were altered during these later studies, and these changes largely account for the reversal of findings observed. First, no-KR retention tests were included in the later studies, which made it possible to differentiate performance from learning effects. Second, the **absolute frequency of KR** (the total number of trials after which KR was provided) was no longer held constant but rather was allowed to vary with the **relative frequency of KR** (the percentage of trials after which KR was provided). This second change eliminated the problems that arose in Bilodeau and Bilodeau's earlier study because the groups received different amounts of practice. Despite the fact that all groups received the absolute amount of KR, the group receiving KR after every trial practiced the task only 10 times, whereas the group receiving KR after every fourth trial received 40 practice trials.

Although the results obtained by Ho and Shea were similar when the immediate-performance findings were reviewed, the exact opposite was true when the no-KR retention test results were compared across the different KR frequency groups. The group receiving KR after every trial now performed the task with significantly higher performance error than the other two groups who had received KR less frequently during the acquisition phase. Thus it appears that the benefits associated with providing large amounts of KR are limited to immediate performance. Once the KR is no longer available, the quality of the performance deteriorates quickly. Two theoretical explanations for these disparate findings will be discussed later in this chapter.

The traditional view, that "the more KR the better," is no longer tenable.

## Fading-Frequency Schedules of Knowledge of Results

In an attempt to design a KR schedule that might optimize the beneficial effects of low-KR-frequency practice conditions, Winstein and Schmidt (1990) conducted a study in which the schedule of KR and no-KR trials was manipulated. Rather than providing KR after a set number of trials during the acquisition phase, they experimented with a **fading-frequency schedule of KR** that employed a higher frequency of KR during the early acquisition trials but then a reduced relative KR frequency during later trials. For example, the 50%-relative-frequency-KR group received a relatively high frequency of KR (such as 100%) during the early practice trials, but then the frequency was systematically reduced (to 25%, for example) during the later trials. Although the authors found that the 50%-relative-frequency-KR group performed the complex spatial-temporal movement task only marginally better on an immediate no-KR retention test, the findings were somewhat different when a second no-KR retention test was administered one day later. In the case of this second retention test, the performance of the 50%-relative-frequency-KR group was significantly better than that of the high-relative-KR-frequency group. The results of this study are presented in Figure 10.5 on page 306.

## Bandwidth Knowledge of Results

Sherwood (1988) developed an alternative instructional strategy for providing KR during the early stages of learning that is also designed to produce practice characterized by reduced KR relative frequency. This alternative method

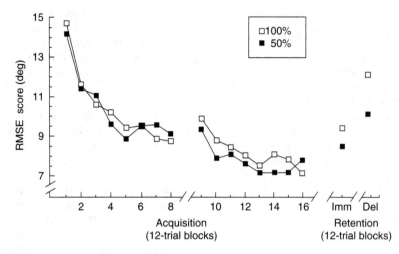

**Figure 10.5**  The effects of different KR-frequency schedules on the acquisition and retention of a tracking task.

RMS = root mean square, Imm = immediate, Del = delayed

During bandwidth KR practice conditions, a learner who does not receive KR after a practice attempt is being indirectly told that the performance was satisfactory.

Bandwidth KR practice conditions promote greater movement consistency.

of providing feedback is known as **bandwidth KR.** During practice conditions in which bandwidth KR is used, augmented feedback is provided only if errors in performance are outside a given error range. In this practice situation, the learner is informed that the absence of KR after a given trial indicates that his or her performance on the previous trial was acceptable. Not only does the augmented feedback provided during bandwidth practice conditions serve an informational function, but also its absence motivates and/or reinforces the performer. According to Sherwood (1988), learners who do not receive KR after a given practice attempt are being indirectly told that their performance is satisfactory and should be repeated.

The results of a number of research studies (Lee & Carnahan, 1990; Reeve, Dornier, & Weeks, 1990; Sherwood, 1988) devoted to investigating the possible benefits of this practice strategy have demonstrated that, compared to high-KR-frequency schedules, bandwidth KR promotes significantly better long-term retention of a skill. Moreover, the superior retention performance demonstrated by subjects who received bandwidth KR has been attributed to more than just a KR-frequency effect. Lee and Carnahan (1990) have also demonstrated that subjects receiving bandwidth KR achieved higher levels of performance consistency during acquisition when compared to subjects who practiced in conditions of reduced KR frequency. Within-subject variability was also significantly lower among subjects in the bandwidth KR group as measured by a later retention test. It appears that a second major advantage of bandwidth KR practice conditions over those designed simply to reduce the relative frequency of KR is that the former promote greater consistency of movement.

In a review article devoted to a discussion of the application of various motor learning principles to physical therapy, Schmidt (1991) points out yet another beneficial feature of bandwidth KR that should make it easy to implement in practical settings. He suggests that bandwidth KR actually provides a fading schedule in that early practice attempts are more likely to produce performance errors that exceed the established error range. Larger errors will therefore result in a higher frequency of KR being provided. As practice continues, however, and performances become more consistent, the sizes of the performance errors are reduced to the extent that they now fall within the band of acceptable performance. The frequency with which augmented feedback is provided to the learner therefore decreases, producing a low relative frequency of KR. Thus the primary responsibility of the practitioner using this type of feedback condition is choosing a bandwidth that is large enough to ensure that only the positive guiding effects of KR are evident. Reducing the bandwidth as practice progresses may serve a similar function.

## Reversed Bandwidth Knowledge of Results

A group of researchers has begun to explore a variation of bandwidth KR in which augmented feedback is provided when a learner is performing within a given range of error as opposed to outside of that range (Cauraugh, Chen, & Radlo, 1993). These researchers were particularly interested in comparing the effectiveness of traditional bandwidth KR with that of **reversed bandwidth KR** in the learning of a simple timing task. Unlike the traditional bandwidth method, which produces a low-KR-frequency schedule (such as 35% relative frequency) because augmented feedback is provided only when the performer exceeds a range of error, the reversed bandwidth KR condition would create a considerably higher KR frequency condition (such as 65% relative frequency). Although a review of the changes in absolute performance that occurred during acquisition indicated that the two bandwidth groups adopted different performance strategies for improving their performance accuracy, both groups performed equally well on a no-KR retention test. Cauraugh et al. concluded that whether augmented feedback was provided after an accurate response (reversed bandwidth KR) or after an inaccurate response (traditional bandwidth KR) was immaterial: Both groups of learners demonstrated similar levels of learning.

## Summary Knowledge of Results

A third method of reducing the frequency of augmented feedback was first investigated by Lavery (1962) and involved the withholding of feedback from a learner for a number of practice attempts. When finally presented to the learner, the information described the outcome achieved on each of the trials in which no feedback was provided. In some movement situations, the learner performed as many as twenty trials on a given movement task before any feedback was provided. This augmented feedback schedule came to be known as a **summary KR** schedule. This type of schedule differs from schedules based on the relative frequency of KR, in which a learner practices a skill for

The amount of information provided to a learner after a given trial is what primarily differentiates summary KR from reduced-frequency-KR schedules.

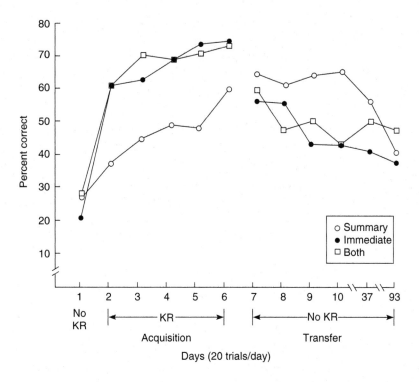

**Figure 10.6** The effects of different KR schedules on performance during acquisition and on no-KR transfer trials. The performance of a group receiving KR after every 20 trials (summary) was compared to that of a group receiving KR after every trial (immediate) and to that of a third group receiving both KR schedules (both).

a certain number of attempts before receiving feedback related to the last practice trial only. The amount of information provided to the learner after a number of no-feedback practice trials have been completed is what differentiates these two feedback schedules.

Lavery and several other investigators (Schmidt, Young, Swinnen & Shapiro, 1989; Schmidt, Lange, & Young, 1990) have since found that the effectiveness of providing augmented feedback according to a summary schedule is most evident when performances on a no-KR transfer test are compared (see Figure 10.6). As Lavery's results demonstrate, the performance of the summary KR group was significantly better on no-KR transfer tests conducted on days 7 through 10 when compared to a second group who received feedback after every trial or to a third group who received a combination of both schedules (KR after every trial in addition to summary KR after twenty trials). If one were to consider only performance during the course of six days of practice, however, the same conclusion would not be reached. During the acquisition phase, the performance of the summary KR group was significantly worse than that of either higher-frequency-KR group.

Schmidt and colleagues (Schmidt et al., 1989) extended the early work of Lavery by searching for the optimal number of trials to summarize. They varied the length of the summary KR period from five to 15 trials, and then compared the relative effectiveness of each summary KR interval to that of an immediate-feedback schedule. The most effective learning was observed in the group that practiced according to the longest summary KR schedule (15 trials), and the least effective learning was associated with the immediate-feedback group. Providing a 15-trial summary schedule was not as effective as shorter summary periods (such as five trials), however, when a more complex task was to be learned in a subsequent study (Schmidt, Lange, & Young, 1990). In fact, in these more complex learning situations, an inverted-U relationship was evident between the length of the summary KR period during acquisition and performance during a no-KR retention phase. The optimal summary KR length is therefore influenced by the characteristics of the skill to be learned.

In addition to exploring how task difficulty might influence the optimal summary KR length, researchers also have begun to study how the characteristics of the learner interact with different summary KR schedules. Carnahan, Vandervoort, and Swanson (1996) were interested in determining whether older learners (mean age of 75 years) use summary KR to learn a new motor skill in the same manner as do younger adults. This is an important question to ask, given the age-associated changes in cognitive processing (Salthouse, 1991) and motor control (Spirduso & McCrae, 1990) that have been described in the literature.

Interestingly, the authors found that the older adult learners used summary KR provided after five practice trials in a manner that was very similar to the younger adult group. Moreover, they demonstrated that both the older and younger summary KR groups performed the task with significantly greater accuracy when compared to a younger and older adult group who received KR after every trial during acquisition. At a practice level, it would appear that summary KR schedules may also be effective when teaching older adults certain types of motor skills. Of course, as the authors point out, much more research needs to be conducted with older adult groups to determine whether the complexity of the task to be learned and the length of the summary KR period interact with age. In the study described, the task to be learned was a self-paced key pressing task, and the length of the summary KR interval was quite short. It remains to be determined, among other things, whether the current findings hold true when tasks that are externally paced and/or more complex in terms of their motor control requirements must be learned and/or the length of the summary KR schedule increases (see highlight, Applying Motor Learning Principles to Clinical Settings, on page 310).

> Older adults use summary KR in a manner similar to that of young adults.

## Average Knowledge of Results

Although the collective findings of these laboratory-based studies provide support for the use of summary KR schedules, the usefulness of this type of feedback schedule in more practical settings is questionable. How likely is it, for example, that a practitioner will watch a performer practice a movement skill

# HIGHLIGHT

### Applying Motor Learning Principles to Clinical Settings

A technique that clinicians commonly use when teaching partial-weight-bearing skills to patients is to provide concurrent augmented feedback (through auditory feedback devices worn in the shoe, for example, or bathroom scale monitoring of limb loading) during the acquisition phase. Unfortunately, providing concurrent augmented feedback has proved to be an unsatisfactory method of teaching such skills. This is perhaps not a surprising outcome in light of what we now know about the effectiveness of different KR presentation schedules in the learning of various motor skills.

Although providing KR to a learner during and/or after every practice trial appears to enhance *performance* of a skill, it does little to facilitate *retention* of that skill. In fact, a number of researchers have concluded that providing KR on every practice trial fosters over-dependence on the externally presented feedback at the expense of the learner's attending to her or his internal sources of feedback.

Applying motor learning principles, particularly those related to the provision of augmented feedback, Winstein and colleagues (Winstein, Christensen, & Fitch, 1993) conducted a clinical study in which they attempted to teach a group of 40 healthy adults how to put no more than 30% of their total body weight on one leg while learning to walk with crutches. During the 80-trial acquisition phase, the researchers manipulated the amount of KR provided according to four different summary KR schedules (KR after 1, 5, 10, or 20 trials). KR was presented in the form of a bar graph similar to the one shown on the facing page, which indicated the degree to which the subject overshot or undershot the 30%-weight-bearing goal. Two days after completion of the acquisition phase, each adult completed a no-KR retention test. Recall that this test is commonly used by researchers to measure the degree to which a particular skill has been learned.

In contrast to previous laboratory studies, the results of this more applied study indicated that the weight-bearing performance of *all* the KR groups improved significantly during the acquisition phase, irrespective of the summary KR schedule followed. Both the absolute amount of error (AE) recorded and the variability of that error (VE) decreased significantly during acquisition. The KR-1 group did, however, demonstrate significantly lower amounts of error when compared to the group that received KR after 20 practice trials during acquisition. How did the results for the retention trials compare to those of previous studies investigating the effectiveness of different

---

When average KR schedules are used, only one piece of information is provided to learners following multiple no-KR practice attempts.

for a number of trials and then provide information about his or her performance on each of the attempts just completed? It is much more common for a practitioner to watch portions of several trials, and then provide one or two pieces of information that describe the essence of the learner's overall performance.

A variation of summary KR is currently being investigated by a group of researchers who share a similar practical concern. Rather than information about each no-KR trial being provided at the conclusion of a summary KR period, in an **average KR** schedule only one piece of information representing an averaged performance score is provided to the learner after several no-KR practice attempts. The effectiveness of average KR schedules has been demonstrated by Young and Schmidt (1992), who compared the retention test performance of an average KR group with that of a group who received KR

HIGHLIGHT, CONTINUED

summary KR schedules? Once again, the retention results were at odds with previous studies in that no significant differences for AE or VE were observed among the four summary KR groups during the retention phase. Although the group receiving KR after every five practice trials now performed with the highest level of performance accuracy, the difference was not significant.

Although the learning of the partial-weight-bearing task used in this study did not appear to be influenced by the frequency with which the feedback was provided, the findings do suggest that the task can be learned as efficiently with less feedback than is commonly provided in clinical settings. Receiving feedback as little as once every twenty practice attempts resulted in the same level of learning as that observed for a group receiving KR after every practice trial. This finding alone certainly proves that more is not always better.

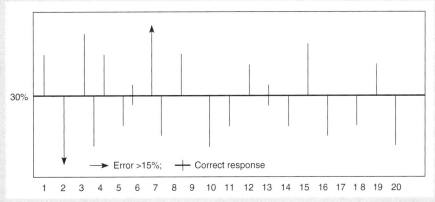

Example of a KR summary graph. KR was presented in the form of a bar graph that indicated the degree to which the subject overshot or undershot the 30%-weight-bearing goal. KR was provided according to four different summary KR schedules.

in the form of a kinematic visual display after every trial. Wood and colleagues (Wood, Gallagher, Martino, & Ross, 1992) also found average KR schedules for a group of experienced golfers attempting to improve the dynamics of their golf swing to be more beneficial when compared to a second group of golfers who received no feedback at all during practice.

Weeks and Sherwood (1994) directly compared the effectiveness of average KR to summary KR schedules in the acquisition of a static force production task. Kinetic feedback describing the level of force generated was provided either after every trial, following a block of five no-KR practice trials according to a summary KR schedule, or at the completion of the same number of no-KR trials according to an average KR schedule. In general, the findings for both an immediate-retention and a delayed-retention test indicated greater response consistency among the two groups receiving either a summary or an average KR schedule when compared to the group receiving KR after every trial.

In contrast, the level of response bias demonstrated among the groups was significantly different only for the test of short-term retention. In comparing the relative effectiveness of the two lower-frequency-feedback conditions alone, the authors concluded that a summary KR feedback schedule and an average KR feedback schedule were equally effective in promoting greater response consistency and less response bias among the group of subjects tested. Given the unlikelihood that a teacher or clinician can devote enough attention to a single learner during practice to implement a summary KR schedule, it is comforting to know that a practice already in widespread use among practitioners appears to be equally effective.

## Self-Regulated (Controlled) Augmented Feedback Schedules

In self-regulated (controlled) augmented feedback schedules, learners decide when, during a set of practice trials, they will receive feedback.

Over the course of the past decade, the learning benefits of a new type of augmented feedback schedule have been investigated (Janelle, Kim, & Singer, 1995); Janelle, Barba, Frehlich, Tennant, & Cauraugh, 1997). Unlike the practitioner- or experimenter-determined augmented feedback schedules described in this chapter, it is the learner who decides when, during a set of practice trials, he or she will receive the augmented feedback. The development of this type of feedback schedule is predicated on the notion that, by giving learners the opportunity to have some control over the learning process, they will be more actively engaged in learning the skill and retain it better as a result (Hardy & Nelson, 1988; Zimmerman, 1989).

Janelle et al. (1995) were the first to examine the efficacy of this type of **self-regulated augmented feedback schedule** when applied to movement skill settings and found not only that it benefited learning, but that providing feedback in the form of KP and KR as opposed to KR alone was most beneficial. In a follow-up study, Janelle et al. (1997) investigated the learning benefits of this type of schedule on the performance of a throwing skill. These researchers found that when given the opportunity to control their augmented feedback schedule, people require relatively less feedback to learn skill performance and retain it at a level equivalent to or better than those who are given more feedback but are unable to control their schedule. This clearly supports the idea that giving people more control over their own skill learning process by allowing them to control their own augmented feedback schedule encourages them to be more actively engaged in learning the skill, which results in enhanced learning and retention.

People who have more control over their learning will process the skill-related information more deeply and also be more motivated to learn the skill.

What is quite interesting and perhaps somewhat of a surprising finding of this study is that participants in the self-regulated group requested augmented feedback, on average, on just 11.15% of the total number of acquisition trials. This is a much lower frequency of feedback than used in previous studies that explored relative and absolute frequency of KR schedules. Why is it that self-controlled augmented feedback schedules that resulted in so little feedback being requested produced such positive effects on skill learning and retention? The authors proposed that people who have more control over their learning will process the skill-related information more deeply and also be more motivated to learn the skill. They further argue that a self-regulating learning style allows the learner to develop more effective learning strategies as a result of being able to request augmented feedback when they feel it is needed rather than when the instructor or coach chooses or is available to provide it.

# Theoretical Explanations of the Frequency Effect

## Guidance Hypothesis

Several theoretical explanations have been advanced to account for the KR frequency and scheduling effects just described. Let's look at two of the more contemporary views developed to explain exactly why the learner benefits from practice conditions wherein less augmented feedback is provided. The first hypothesis developed to account for the superiority of practice conditions that feature a low frequency of KR is the **guidance hypothesis** (Salmoni, Schmidt, & Walter, 1984). According to this hypothesis, the presentation of KR may have both beneficial and detrimental effects on learning. That is, although practice conditions that include high frequency of KR guide the learner toward the correct performance very quickly, such practice conditions may also lead to overdependence on this form of augmented feedback. The provision of too much augmented feedback is thought to prevent the processing of other information related to the inherent dynamics of the task. Remember that the overuse of manual guidance techniques (discussed in Chapter 9) also produces negative consequences. Certainly, the type of cognitive processing used will be different in these two diverse practice conditions. Whereas low-KR-frequency practice conditions seem to foster increased problem solving and independent exploration of a task's dynamics, high-KR-frequency practice conditions apparently do little to promote such activities on the part of the learner.

> Low-KR-frequency practice conditions foster more problem solving and independent exploration of the skill's dynamics than do high-KR-frequency conditions.

## Consistency Hypothesis

The **consistency hypothesis** is a second theoretical explanation advanced to account for the learning benefits associated with fading-frequency and bandwidth KR practice conditions. According to this hypothesis, providing learners with high relative frequency of KR leads them to adjust their performance continually on the basis of each new piece of information provided to them. This constant short-term correction of performance is believed to prevent the learner from developing a stable plan of action and is reflected in a high level of performance variability. You will recall that participants in the Lee and Carnahan (1990) study who practiced according to a bandwidth KR schedule not only performed the timing task as accurately during a retention test as subjects who received KR after every trial, but also demonstrated less within-subject variability in their performance. The benefits of bandwidth KR were therefore twofold: increased performance accuracy and greater consistency.

> Providing learners with large amounts of KR causes them to make continuous short-term corrections that hinder the development of a stable action plan.

# The Timing of Knowledge of Results

Yet another issue that has been investigated by a number of researchers interested in the area of knowledge of results is when to provide KR following a given practice trial. To investigate this issue, researchers have systematically manipulated the time that elapses between the completion of a practice trial and the presentation of performance-related feedback. This interval of time has been referred to as the **KR delay interval.** It has been hypothesized that the longer the KR delay interval, then as a result of increased forgetting, the more detrimental that delay will be to the learning of a task. Alternatively, it has been suggested that very short KR delay intervals may be equally detrimental to learning by not allowing sufficient time for the learner to engage in important cognitive operations necessary for developing error-detection and -correction abilities (Salmoni, Schmidt, & Walter, 1984). Providing a KR delay interval that optimizes the amount of time available for the learner to engage in important processing activities, while preventing the tendency to forget what has just been practiced, is clearly an important issue for the practitioner.

**Increasing the KR delay interval does not negatively affect learning.**

Fortunately, the results of a number of research studies generally indicate that increasing the KR delay interval does not negatively influence learning (Bilodeau & Bilodeau, 1958b). Conversely, Swinnen and colleagues (Swinnen, Schmidt, Nicholson, & Shapiro, 1990) have demonstrated that very short KR delay intervals can have a detrimental effect on learning. When the retention test performance of a group of participants who received KR immediately following each practice trial was compared to that of a group who received KR following an 8-second unfilled interval, the delayed-KR group performed significantly better, particularly when the retention test was conducted two days after the acquisition phase.

**Providing KR immediately after a practice attempt prevents the learner from engaging in the important process of error detection and correction.**

What is of perhaps greater interest to the practitioner is the fact that a third group who was asked to estimate their error verbally during a similar 8-second delay interval performed significantly better than the first two groups during the same retention test (see Figure 10.7). This finding suggests that providing KR immediately following a practice attempt prevents the learner from engaging in important error detection and correction during practice. The negative effects of this practice become apparent, however, only when the learner is asked to perform the skill again in the absence of that feedback. In contrast, delaying the presentation of KR during practice also encourages learners to evaluate the accuracy of their previous practice attempt during the delay, and it results in considerably better performance when augmented feedback is no longer provided. This particular result supports a similar finding reported in a much earlier study by Hogan and Yanowitz (1978). These researchers were particularly interested in knowing whether subjective estimates of error facilitated the learning of a motor skill. They also demonstrated superior retention performance for a group of subjects who were required to estimate the amount of error following each practice trial.

**Subjective evaluation of movement form facilitates the learning and retention of a skill.**

Not only has it been found that the estimation of a movement's outcome during the KR delay interval facilitates the learning of a motor skill, but so too does the subjective evaluation of form during that same period. Liu and Wrisberg (1997) have demonstrated that learners who are asked to rate their movement form either before or after they receive KR following a practice attempt are not only able to estimate their movement outcome more accurately, but

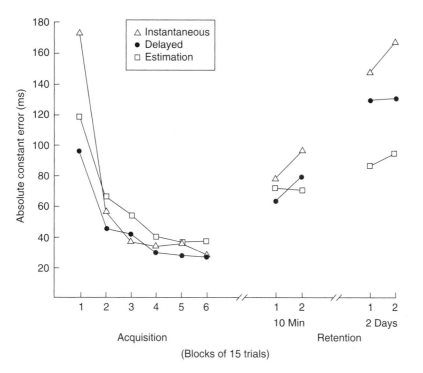

**Figure 10.7** Delaying the presentation of KR during practice, while encouraging learners to estimate their error during the delay, resulted in the best performance on the no-KR retention trials.

*Source:* Swinnen, S. P., Schmidt, R. A., Nicholson, D. E., & Shapiro, D. C. (1990). Information feedback for skill acquisition: Instantaneous knowledge of results degrades learning. *Journal of Experimental Psychology: Learning, Memory, and Cognition, 16,* 706–716.

also are able to perform with significantly greater accuracy once the KR is removed (during the retention phase).

These findings carry important implications for teachers, coaches, or clinicians, particularly as they relate to when augmented feedback should be provided to learners or patients. On the basis of their findings, Liu and Wrisberg believe that instructors/clinicians need not be concerned if they are not able to provide augmented feedback on a regular basis during a practice or treatment session as long as they encourage the learner to try to subjectively evaluate movement form after each practice attempt. Whether the subjective evaluation occurs before or after augmented feedback is provided also does not seem to be a cause for concern.

Motor learning as a function of the **post-KR interval** also has been investigated. This interval is the time between augmented feedback being given and the onset of the next trial or response. No evidence was found indicating either an optimum duration or an upper limit for this interval. However, the available evidence indicates that learning is negatively affected if this interval is too short and that the minimum duration of this interval may depend on the type of skill being learned. (Gallagher & Thomas, 1980; Rogers, 1974; Weinberg, Guy, & Tupper, 1964). The implication for practice is that the post-KR delay interval needs to be long enough for learners to process the augmented feedback received from the previous response and plan how to execute the next response.

The influence of *activity* during the post-KR interval is similar to that of the KR delay interval. Some types of motor (making an arm movement through three barriers in a time slower than the criterion time) and cognitive (number guessing) activities had no effect on learning an arm movement through three barriers in a criterion time (Lee & Magill, 1983). Certain types of cognitive activity (mathematics problem solving task and subjective estimate of another person's movement time error) were found to interfere with motor learning (Benedetti & McCullagh, 1987; Swinnen, 1990, experiment 3). Apparently, these types of cognitive activity were so demanding that they interfered with the learners' ability to cognitively interpret the feedback received from the previous response and plan how to execute the next response during the post KR interval. Only one study was found that indicated that certain types of motor activities (mirror tracing and arm movement tasks) facilitated the learning of a two-component arm movement task (Magill, 1988). These types of motor activities may have facilitated learning because the cognitive and motor processing required for their successful performance of the motor activities was similar to the processing required for successful performance of the two-arm movement task. Thus, the processing learned to successfully perform the motor activities could have transferred to the processing needed to perform the two-arm movement task. However, further research is needed before the validity of this explanation is ascertained.

> The post-KR delay interval needs to be long enough to process the feedback received from the previous response and plan how to execute the next response.

## Summary

Feedback provided to learners from an external source (such as an instructor or video) is intended to augment, or add to, the information that is naturally available to the learners from their own internal sensory sources. Augmented feedback may be provided in many different forms (verbally, via graphical displays, and so on), and it may be offered during performance (concurrent feedback), immediately following a movement (terminal feedback), or some time after a movement has been completed (delayed feedback).

Information provided about the outcome of an action is called knowledge of results (KR), whereas knowledge of performance (KP) is information provided about the quality of the movement pattern produced. Whether it is desirable to provide one or both types of augmented feedback is largely determined by the characteristics of the learner (skill level, past experiences, and the like) and the nature of the task being learned (such as whether the movement involved entails one or several degrees of freedom).

The secret to using augmented feedback effectively is to understand how it functions as information/knowledge, reinforcement, motivation, and punishment. Information feedback conveys a message to the learner about the effectiveness of the performance, which usually includes the parts of the performance that were correct, the errors that were made, and how to correct them. Feedback that acts as positive reinforcement must be perceived by the learner as pleasant and follow (preferably immediately) the performance you want to strengthen. For feedback to serve as negative reinforcement it must be perceived by the learner as unpleasant, which can be avoided by making the correct performance instead of the incorrect one. Feedback can motivate people to learn movement skills if it provides information about their errors and how to correct them (directive function of motivation) and about the extent to which their performance is improving (arousal function of motivation). For feedback to function as punishment it must be perceived as unpleasant by the learner and follow the performance you want to suppress.

Information feedback describing the kinematic and/or kinetic aspects of a movement can give the performer useful information about what to do on the next practice attempt, whereas more traditional forms of KR (such as movement time and absolute error) provide only information about what *not* to do on a subsequent attempt. This latter type of feedback appears to be less effective as the number of degrees of freedom associated with a particular skill increases.

The use of augmented sensory information, or biofeedback, has proven to be a valuable technique in clinical settings because it conveys information to a patient about otherwise unobservable events (level of muscle activity, force generation, movement of the center of mass). This type of feedback gives patients immediate information about their performance, and that information is often more relevant and accurate than information provided by the clinician.

Recent research into the optimal amount of feedback to give a learner suggests that "more is not better." Although the initial performance of a skill is facilitated when augmented feedback is provided after every practice attempt, its subsequent removal leads to diminished performance and poor retention. According to the guidance hypothesis, although high-KR-frequency practice conditions guide the learner toward the correct performance very quickly, such practice conditions also promote overdependence on this externally presented information. In contrast, low-KR-frequency practice conditions foster increased problem solving and independent exploration of the skill's inherent dynamics and results in better retention of the skill in the long term.

Feedback schedules that provide learners with more feedback during the early stages of learning, and with less as they progress in the learning of the skill, are particularly useful. Fading-frequency and bandwidth schedules of feedback are examples of such schedules. According to the consistency hypothesis, these types of schedules promote the development of a stable plan of action, which, in turn, leads to increased accuracy and consistency of performance. Bandwidth KR schedules also provide learners with two different types of feedback: (1) feedback that motivates and/or reinforces the performer by virtue of its not being presented and (2) feedback that serves an important error-correction function when a particular performance falls outside a predetermined error range.

Summary KR and average KR schedules have also been shown to enhance the learning of movement skills. Unlike other low-KR-frequency schedules, a learner practices a skill for a certain number of attempts before receiving feedback related to the last practice trial (summary KR) or information that provides an averaged performance score of all no-KR practice attempts (average KR). Research has demonstrated that each of these schedules promotes greater performance consistency and less response bias. Although considerably more research that explores the efficacy of the different types of augmented feedback schedules with populations other than young adults is needed, it does appear that older adults use summary feedback in a manner similar to younger adults.

Self-regulated or controlled augmented feedback schedules also have been demonstrated to be beneficial for learning. Unlike other augmented feedback schedules, the learner controls how much feedback is provided during a practice session. It is believed that these types of feedback schedules foster deeper levels of processing, greater confidence in the ability to perform the task, and a higher level of motivation to perform well.

Finally, the KR delay interval needs to be long enough to allow learners to engage in the process of error detection and correction. The post-KR delay interval needs to be long enough for learners to process the feedback received from the previous response. Encouraging learners to subjectively estimate performance error and/or form during the KR delay interval is particularly beneficial for learning. This instructional strategy provides learners with the opportunity to engage in important cognitive activities associated with error detection and correction. Encouraging learners to be actively engaged in the learning process also places the responsibility for learning more under their control.

## IMPORTANT TERMINOLOGY

After completing this chapter, readers should be familiar with the following terms and concepts.

absolute frequency of KR
arousal function of motivation
augmented feedback
augmented sensory feedback
average KR
bandwidth KR
biofeedback
concurrent feedback
consistency hypothesis
delayed feedback
directive function of motivation
fading-frequency schedule of KR
guidance hypothesis
information feedback
intrinsic (sensory) feedback
kinematic feedback
kinetic feedback

knowledge of performance (KP)
knowledge of results (KR)
KR delay interval
motivation
negative reinforcement
positive reinforcement
post-KR interval
precision of the augmented
    feedback
punishment
relative frequency of KR
reversed bandwidth KR
self-regulated augmented feedback
    schedule
summary KR
terminal feedback

## SUGGESTED FURTHER READING

Moreland, J. D., Thomson, M. A., & Fuoco, A. R. (1998). Electromyographic biofeedback to improve lower extremity function after stroke: A meta-analysis. *Archives of Physical Medicine and Rehabilitation, 79,* 134–140.

Swinnen, S. P. (1998). Age-related deficits in motor learning and differences in feedback processing during the production of a bimanual response coordination pattern. *Cognitive Neuropsychology, 15,* 439–466.

Winstein, C. J. 1991. Knowledge of results and motor learning—Implications for physical therapy. *Physical Therapy, 71,* 2, 140–149.

Wrisberg, C. A., Dale, G. A., Liu, Z., & Reed, A. (1995). The effects of augmented information on motor learning: A multidimensional assessment. *Research Quarterly for Exercise and Sport, 66,* 9–16.

## TEST YOUR UNDERSTANDING

1. Identify each of the different types of augmented feedback and provide one example of each type.

2. Explain and give examples of how augmented feedback can function as information, positive reinforcement, negative reinforcement, motivation, and punishment.

3. Briefly explain why kinetic and kinematic visual displays are a more valuable form of augmented feedback than traditional forms of augmented feedback. In what types of learning situations are these displays likely to be less effective?

4. Outline three guidelines a practitioner should follow when using videotape as a form of augmented feedback.

5. Briefly describe the advantages associated with the use of kinetic biofeedback devices. Provide one research example that demonstrates the advantage of these devices.

6. Cite four principles that one should follow when using biofeedback devices in clinical settings.

7. What factors should be considered by a practitioner when deciding how precise the augmented feedback that is provided to a learner should be?

8. Briefly explain how the research findings that emerged from studies conducted in the 1950s differed from those presented in later studies investigating the issue of how often to provide KR to learners. What may account for these differences?

9. How does a fading-frequency schedule differ from a bandwidth KR schedule? Outline the major benefits associated with the use of each of these KR schedules in the acquisition of movement skills.

10. Briefly describe how augmented feedback is provided according to a summary KR schedule. How does the use of this feedback schedule affect the quality of performance and learning of movement skills?

11. Briefly explain why self-regulated augmented feedback schedules are believed to be beneficial for learning.

12. Compare and contrast two theoretical explanations advanced to account for the KR frequency and scheduling effects.

13. Briefly explain why the subjective estimation of performance error and/or movement form is beneficial for learning.

14. Briefly describe how augmented feedback can be used to motivate the learner.

15. Identify five general guidelines a practitioner should follow when providing augmented feedback to a patient in a clinical setting or to students in a physical education class.

# 11

# MEMORY AND FORGETTING

*Memory is the storage and retrieval of what is learned, forgetting is its loss,*
*and retention is observable evidence of its durability over time.*

## CHAPTER OBJECTIVES

After studying this chapter, you should be able to:

- Explain the contemporary concepts of human memory that have guided research during the past three decades.

- Identify the areas within the central nervous system that appear to play important roles in memory-related functions, and explain how they operate.

- Explain and give examples of the different types of memory and how they contribute to the learning of movement skills.

- Distinguish among the terms memory, forgetting, retention, and learning.

- Explain and give examples of how memory, forgetting, and the retention of motor skills are scientifically studied.

- Explain how to control for variables that can confound temporary performance effects with the effects due to memory and forgetting.

- Explain the theories of forgetting, and provide examples of how they work.

- Explain and be able to describe the factors that influence the long-term retention of movement skills.

- Explain and give examples of the techniques and strategies a practitioner and/or clinician can employ to enhance the learning and retention of movement skills.

How is it that we are able to remember hundreds of seemingly unrelated events, countless procedures for assembling equipment or operating a computer, and the abstract rules associated with playing a particular game or solving a complex mathematical equation? The answer to this question appears to lie in a construct known as *memory*. Gordon (1989) states that "the term *memory* is most often defined as an internal record or representation of some prior event or experience" (p. 9). Thus it is intimately related to learning, which we discussed at length in Chapter 6.

In this chapter you will learn about memory and its role in the learning and forgetting of movement-based skills. In Chapter 6 we described *motor learning* as a process by which the capability for producing movement performance (an internal state that cannot be directly observed) and the actual movement performance (which can be directly observed) are reliably changed through instruction, practice, and/or experience. The storage and retrieval of this learned capability for producing the reliable change in movement performance is the process of **memory.** Thus, motor learning is the acquisition of the capability for generating the reliable change in movement performance, while memory saves it over time and retrieves it when needed.

In contrast, **forgetting** is a process that refers to the loss of the ability to effectively store and retrieve the learned information needed for producing a reliable change in movement performance. The persistence with which learned changes in movement performance can be demonstrated over time without practice (**retention interval,** or **RI**) is referred to as **retention.** Remember that motor learning, memory, and forgetting are internal processes that operate within the learner and, therefore, cannot be directly observed and measured. What *can* be directly observed and measured is the learner's motor performance in acquisition and on tests of retention. Thus, we use the motor performance directly observed and measured in acquisition and retention as evidence from which to make inferences about the memory and forgetting of learned movement skills. For instance, acquisition performance that is retained on a retention test following an RI is inferred to be learned. Conversely, acquisition performance that is not retained over an RI on a retention test is inferred to be forgotten. Whether this retention loss and inference about forgetting actually represents a memory loss of the learned capability for producing the acquisition performance or whether the learned capability is at full strength in memory and simply can't be retrieved is a matter of some uncertainty and continued debate.

Is memory a structure that can be traced to a particular area of the brain or somewhere else in the nervous system? Or is memory best conceptualized as a cognitive process that enables us to act upon a continual flow of externally and internally generated information in a meaningful way? This is just one of the many questions addressed in this chapter. No doubt many more questions will emerge as the discussion unfolds, and some will remain unanswered at its conclusion. Let us begin our discussion by describing two contemporary yet contrasting views of the construct called memory.

## Contemporary Concepts of Memory

Numerous attempts by researchers to describe the intricacies of human memory have yielded a variety of theories and models over the years. One has only to read the literature to encounter descriptions of memory that range from reverberating circuits in the brain (Hebb, 1949) to computer analogies wherein memory is likened to a central processing unit consisting of a set of structures through which all information must pass. Two contemporary concepts of memory that have contributed to a renewed research interest in human memory over the past three decades are discussed in this section. The first of these two concepts

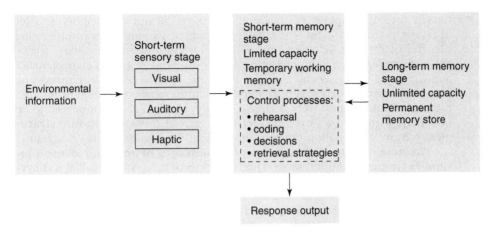

**Figure 11.1**   The Atkinson and Shiffrin multistore stages of memory consolidation model.

*Source:* Atkinson, R. C., & Shiffrin, R. M. (1971). The control of short-term memory. *Scientific American, 225,* 82–90.)

represents a more structural view of memory. The second proposes an alternative view that emphasizes a more functional approach to the study of memory.

## Atkinson and Shiffrin's Multistore Model

One of the most highly developed multistore models of memory was proposed and empirically tested by Atkinson and Shiffrin (1968, 1971). Their model was based on the **consolidation theory** of memory that was originally proposed by Müller and Pilzecher (1900). In the earlier theory, it was suggested that information is initially stored in some pattern of dynamic electrical activity that gradually leads to structural changes in the brain. The idea that learning and memory could involve changes in the neuronal circuits was incorporated in a conceptual framework that was developed by Hebb (1949) and described in his book, *Organization of Behavior*. Essentially, he hypothesized that the memory for something learned is due to activity in a *cell assembly,* in which nerve cells are connected together in special circuits and that, when a nerve cell is active, its synaptic connections become more effective. This effectiveness may be reflected in a temporary increase in the synapse's excitability, as in short-term memory, or it may involve some long-lasting structural change in the synapse, as in long-term memory.

According to the multistore model, human memory consists of clearly defined structures in which various types of processing occur.

The ideas that plastic changes at synapses are the underlying mechanisms of learning and memory and that brain functions are mediated by cell assemblies and neuronal circuits have become widely accepted. Although the specific details of consolidation theory have varied somewhat among scholars, there were enough common elements for Atkinson and Shiffrin (1968, 1971) to propose their multistore model of memory (see Figure 11.1). Drawing heavily on the computer analogy, they conceived of human memory as a set of clearly defined structures (hardware) in which various types of processing occurred (software). Atkinson and Shiffrin distinguished among these hypothesized memory stores on the basis of their different retention characteristics and the types of processing activities that took place in each. The processing activities included such things as memory coding, rehearsal, organization, and retrieval of information from memory. Each process was also considered to be under the control of a processor that used each of these **mnemonic strategies** to move information through the system in a highly regulated fashion.

According to the **multistore model of stages of memory consolidation,** environmental information enters the first of three stages, called a **short-term sensory stage (STSS).** This relatively large-capacity store is responsible for registering the physical features of an environmental display provided by any and all of our sensory systems (e.g., visual, auditory, haptic). These features registered might include the shape of an object, the feel of a surface, and sound coming from a nearby location. In order to preserve the information entering the STSS, however, an individual must attend to it or it will decay and be lost in a period of 30 seconds or less.

Once the selected information is transferred to the next stage of this multistore model, we become consciously aware of its presence. In this second memory stage, which the authors refer to as **short-term memory (STM),** much of the active processing necessary to transfer the selected information into the third stage for more permanent storage takes place. Unlike the STSS, the STM is much more limited in its capacity but capable of more sophisticated processing. One control process in particular serves an extremely important function in this stage of memory. This process, called **rehearsal,** is important for the maintenance and/or elaboration of information reaching the STM and for its subsequent transfer to the third memory stage.

Much of the active processing necessary to transfer information to LTM occurs in STM.

This final stage, known as **long-term memory (LTM),** is viewed as a relatively permanent store with an essentially unlimited capacity for storing information. It is here that the individual is thought to store knowledge of the world in various forms. These various forms include important facts (declarative knowledge), operations (procedural knowledge), and/or concepts (semantic knowledge). Although it is represented only once in the model constructed by Atkinson and Shiffrin, the STM is actively involved in the flow of information before it actually reaches LTM. For example, information entering the STSS cannot be labeled or categorized until it is compared with information already stored in the LTM. Similarly, the strategies that govern the movement of information through the system must first be represented in the LTM in the form of rules or principles.

The multistore model developed by Atkinson and Shiffrin has guided research in the area of human memory during the past three decades. It has been used to describe how adult memory operates and has also proved to be an effective framework for interpreting age-related changes in various aspects of memory capability (Chi, 1976, 1977; Ornstein, Naus, & Liberty, 1975).

# Levels-of-Processing Framework

Despite the evidence compiled in support of Atkinson and Shiffrin's multistore model of memory, a growing number of researchers began to question the usefulness of this approach. Two particularly avid critics of structural accounts of memory were Craik and Lockhart (1972; see also Craik 1977; Cermak & Craik, 1979), who viewed the phenomenon of memory very differently. Unlike other cognitive psychologists of that time, they believed that research attention should be directed solely toward better understanding of the processes used to acquire, store, and then recall memories. They further argued that clear demarcations between the various structures of memory were not so distinctive as previously thought and that the projected capacity of each store could be significantly influenced by other variables. These might include the type of information processing necessary or the time available to process the incoming information. Craik and Lockhart were to develop an alternative memory framework—the **levels-of-processing framework**—that focused on how information was processed at different levels within a unitary memory structure.

The levels-of-processing framework focuses on the processing of information at different levels within a unitary memory structure.

Craik and Lockhart proposed that memory of an event (e.g., movement skill) depends on the *depth* to which the event is processed. The greater the depth of processing, the more elaborate and durable the memory of the event. They believed that two primary factors determined how much information was eventually stored in memory. These were (a) the number of memories an individual was capable of processing at any one time and (b) the depth to which the incoming information was processed. The authors realized that not all the information presented to an individual at any given time could be processed and that, therefore, the learner needed to choose which information would be processed. Craik and Lockhart hypothesized that although the most recently presented information was more likely to be processed, given its importance in changing the nature of the problem being explored or the action being performed, the performer could also choose to continue processing previously presented information. Information processed by the learner constituted *primary memory;* the remaining, unprocessed information occupied *secondary memory.* An individual could then choose to process the information at a shallow level or at progressively deeper levels that provided a greater opportunity for elaborating the information or rendering it more distinct in some way.

They envisioned shallow levels of processing as being concerned with analysis of the sensory or physical features of the incoming information related to the event. Deeper levels of processing involved matching the incoming event information with a stored abstraction from past learning. Based on this concept of a hierarchy of processing levels, memory of an event depends on the depth of processing, as well as other variables such as the amount of attention devoted to the event, its compatibility with the analyzing structures, and the processing time available. Memory was linked to levels of processing and was viewed as a continuum extending from simple sensory analysis to abstract associative functions; therefore, memory depended on the depth to which sensory events were analyzed, rather than the amount of processing. Later, Craik (1977) and Craik and Tulving (1975) modified the original framework by proposing that it was the degree to which the sensory event was elaborated rather than the depth to which it was processed that determined whether it became a persistent memory trace.

Addressing the relevance of the level-of-processing approach to memory for movement skills, Lockhart (1980) indicated that the ability to remember a movement skill is influenced by the degree to which the performer can make use of his or her existing skills to structure and perceive meaning in the skill. Memory depends upon the degree to which the performer's skills and the structure of the movement skill itself allow processing of increasing depth. If the levels-of-processing approach has relevance for the memory of motor skills, it is to point out that movement skills have meaning in the sense that they have internal structure, purpose, and function. The extent to which the performer's perception provides an analysis of this meaning and the capacity to reconstruct it will determine the memory of a movement skill.

Like Atkinson and Shiffrin's model, Craik and Lockhart's alternative framework for studying memory has had its critics (Baddeley, 1978; Morris, Bransford, & Franks, 1977). The major criticisms include there being no way to measure the depth to which information was processed, a problem Craik and Tulving (1975) were unable to solve, and the framework's preoccupation with how information is encoded in memory as opposed to how it is retrieved. Finally, one of the strongest criticisms of this framework came from Glanzer and Koppenaal (1977b), who argued that it was not actually a rival of consolidation theory or the multistore model proposed by Atkinson and Shiffrin. They considered both theories as representing a single approach to the study of memory with the term *stages* heavily used in consolidation theory and the Atkinson-Shiffrin multistore model, and the label *levels* heavily used in the levels-of-processing framework.

## Neurobiology of Memory

A question one might aptly raise at this point is whether there is any neurological evidence in support of Atkinson and Shiffrin's structural claims or any areas within the nervous system capable of serving the type of processing functions described by Craik and Lockhart. Certainly, the interest in human memory has not been confined to a psychological level of analysis. It has fascinated an equal number of neuroscientists, who have attempted to identify regions within the nervous system that might subserve memory. A review of their research efforts and limited findings is the topic of this section.

The search for neuroanatomical sites corresponding to memory dates back to ancient times and the study of phrenology, a pseudoscience whose adherents traced the contours of the skull in an attempt to reveal an individual's character and mental faculties. Today, the experimental paradigms and measurement techniques used to study memory are not only more sophisticated, but also more extensive in scope. They range from the ablation and lesion techniques used to study memory in animals (Lashley, 1950; Mishkin, 1982) to the use of contemporary brain mapping and scanning techniques, such as positron emission tomography (PET), functional magnetic resonance imaging (fMRI), and transcranial magnetic stimulation (TMS) that were discussed in Chapter 2. These imaging techniques have made it possible to identify areas within the brain that are active during the performance of different types of memory tasks (Ungerleider, 1995). Systematic clinical observations of patients with neurological damage that has caused different types of amnesia have also helped researchers identify areas in the human nervous system that may be involved in several important memory functions.

One early pioneer in memory research was Karl Lashley (1929, 1950), who spent a number of years trying to identify specific brain structures that might be responsible for coding and storing mnemonic information. Using an animal model to study memory, Lashley systematically ablated or introduced lesions to increasingly large areas of an animal's cortex. The results of his work indicated that how well the animal was able to remember a given task was determined primarily by the total amount of cortex destroyed rather than by the specific region affected. Lashley's conclusions were to become the cornerstone of a memory principle called **equipotentiality:** the idea that no one area of the cortex is more likely than any other to be involved in the storage of memories.

Early research revealed that no one area of the cerebral cortex is more involved than any other in the storage of memories.

Although this same distributed view of memory still exists today, researchers have begun to identify distinct anatomic structures and areas within the CNS that support different types of memory. These different memory systems have been broadly divided into two categories: **declarative (explicit) memory** and **nondeclarative (implicit) memory** systems (Squire & Knowlton, 1994; Squire & Zola, 1996). Before identifying the different neural structures associated with each of these different memory systems, let us first discuss how these systems differ from each other. First, declarative memory involves the memory for events, facts, and concepts. These memories might involve activities that you can remember doing on a particular day last week, the rules of a sport or game you play, or what happened on a certain date in history. These memories are consciously remembered. In contrast, nondeclarative memories are acquired at a subconscious level and are associated with such things as learned skills or procedures that can be easily performed but not as easily described verbally. Habits that we acquire are also examples of nondeclarative memories.

Neural structures identified with the storage of declarative memories include the medial temporal lobe and structures within the diencephalon that include the hippocampus and the parahippocampal, perirhinal, and entorhinal cortices. In contrast, the neural structures involved in the storage of nondeclarative memories include the striatum, the cerebellum, and the prefrontal, somatosensory, motor (M1), and occipital cortices. The occipitotemporal cortex, amygdala, and spinal cord have also been identified in the storage of nondeclarative memories as well as different types of learning (associative and nonassociative).

Specific neural structures have been identified as being involved in the storage of different types of memory and learning.

How is it that these different types of memories are stored in the brain? The general consensus among researchers is that highly selective changes in the strength of synaptic connections between neurons are at least partly involved in the development of memories. Although it is beyond the scope of this book to describe the exact mechanisms involved in the storage of memories, a number of animal studies suggest that changes in the existing neural circuitry are associated with short-term forms of memory while the storage of long-term memories is associated with a sequence of processes that culminate in the growth of new synaptic connections. (See Baxter & Baxter, 1999, for a more detailed review of the neural mechanisms associated with learning and memory.)

# Types of Memory

## Short-Term and Long-Term Memory

The temporary storage of information in short-term memory enables us to compare and contrast stored items.

Short-term memory, or working memory (Baddeley, 1981) as it is often called because of its active role in the processing of information, is assumed to contain all the information we are currently thinking about or are conscious of at any particular point in time. How much information is this component of memory capable of storing at any given time? Miller (1956) proposes that we are capable of temporarily storing as few as five separate units of information to as many as nine individual units. Given this limited capacity of working memory, it is fortunate that phone numbers rarely exceed seven digits in length and that social security numbers are limited to nine! The temporary storage of information in working memory also enables us to compare and contrast the items being held there and even to associate current information with information that has previously been stored in a repository of more nearly permanent memory known as long-term memory.

Unlike STM, LTM is considered to have a limitless capacity for the storage of information. Moreover, once the information to be retained has been transferred to this large-capacity store, it is believed to remain there for an almost indefinite period of time. You will recall that the control process Atkinson and Shiffrin identified as instrumental in the transfer of information from short-term to long-term memory is rehearsal.

Long-term memory has been described as a relatively permanent storage area for memories, but it is not uncommon for us to be unable to remember an event witnessed many years ago or to find ourselves unable to perform a skill we had learned as a child. Although some researchers attribute the tendency to forget information already stored in long-term memory to the natural decay of the memory trace over time, others argue that forgetting is caused by different types of interference. Still more recently, a number of researchers have begun to turn to alternative explanations of forgetting that focus on the larger issue of retrieval failure. These contemporary theorists acknowledge that interference plays a role in forgetting, but they consider it only one explanation for our inability to retrieve information from memory. More will be said about theories of forgetting later in this chapter.

## Declarative and Procedural Memory

Declarative memory assists us in knowing "what to do," whereas procedural memory assists in knowing "how to do" a particular skill.

A second way of categorizing memory has been proposed by a number of researchers (J. R. Anderson, 1981, 1987; Tulving, 1985) interested in distinguishing among different types of memory on the basis of the types of knowledge stored there. Although Tulving originally proposed three types of memory (episodic, procedural, and semantic), there has been a tendency to describe only two types of memory: declarative memory and **procedural memory** (Anderson, 1987).

"Knowing *what* to do" in any movement situation is an important part of the learning process and appears to be subserved by declarative memory. Information stored in this area of memory may include the rules of a game, the components of a skill, or the facts of a particular situation. In contrast, procedural memory assists us in "knowing *how* to do" a particular skill.

# The Relationship Between Learning and Memory

Gordon (1989) has characterized the relationship between learning and memory as one where learning acts as the trigger or catalyst for the formation of memories and/or knowledge about a particular action. In light of the importance of this relationship between memory and learning, we will examine it more closely in this section.

In attempting to describe the way the role of memory changes during the acquisition of cognitive skills, Anderson (1982) has developed a theoretical framework that is highly reminiscent of Fitts' (1964) three-stage model of motor skill acquisition (see Chapter 6). According to Anderson, during the first stage of learning a cognitive task, information about the skill is encoded as factual or **declarative knowledge.** This type of knowledge can be interpreted and then used to generate a solution. In this stage, a learner may continually rehearse the information presented in order to hold it in working memory for later interpretation. The overt signs of this rehearsal may include mutterings or visible lip movements.

As the learner enters the second stage of learning, the existing knowledge is gradually converted from a declarative to a procedural form. This process of **knowledge compilation** not only vastly reduces the burden placed on working memory's small capacity, but also enables the learner to apply the knowledge directly to the task at hand. There is no longer a need for intermediary interpretation of the factual information, which tends to be slow and prone to error. Recall that Fitts described a similar transition stage at the behavioral level. He characterized the second associative stage of learning as one in which performers begin to blend individual components of a motor skill into a smooth sequence of movements.

During the final stage of learning, which Anderson called the procedural stage, learners continue to fine-tune their **procedural knowledge** to a level where it can be quickly and appropriately applied to a specific problem. The sequence of productions that are performed can be likened to a set of cognitive steps one might use to structure a geometry proof or perhaps to move a chess piece into a "checkmate" position. Anderson's three-stage description has been applied primarily to the acquisition of cognitive skills, but it can be useful in describing the role of memory in the learning of many different types of motor skills.

> The process of knowledge compilation is used to convert knowledge from a declarative to a procedural form.

# How Memory and Forgetting Are Studied

Memory and forgetting of motor learning are processes that are studied by directly observing and measuring motor performance not only in acquisition, but also on a retention test following an RI. Based on the extent to which the most proficient level of motor performance achieved in acquisition is retained on the retention test following an RI, we draw our inferences about the memory or forgetting of motor learning. If the motor performance achieved in acquisition is retained, then it is reasonable to infer that it was learned. Conversely, if the motor performance in acquisition was not retained, then it is reasonable to infer that it was forgotten. Thus, inferences about the memory or forgetting of motor learning are based on retention performance. Of course,

> Inferences about memory and forgetting processes are based on retention performance.

for such inferences to be valid there must be experimental control over variables not being studied (manipulated) that could operate and temporally influence motor performance during acquisition, or over an RI, and even on a retention test. Two such variables that frequently seem to be operating to confound their effects with those due to memory and forgetting include conditions of warm-up and motivation. (These two variables will be discussed in more detail later on page 334.)

Often there is some confusion over the exact meaning of the terms *retention* and *transfer* of motor learning—and for good reason. Some of the experimental designs and procedures used to study them appear to be very similar. Moreover, learners cannot transfer motor performance that they have not retained, so there is a very close relationship between them. To avoid such confusion, we will use the term *retention* when performance on the motor task practiced during the acquisition phase is assessed in the retention phase under conditions that are essentially the *same* as those that existed in the acquisition phase. The term *transfer* is used when the motor task and/or conditions present in the retention phase *differ* from those that existed in the acquisition phase. A number of issues related to the transfer of motor skill learning will be discussed more fully in Chapter 12. It is important to understand the concept that retention, as defined above, is actually a special case of transfer.

Retention and transfer are related in the sense that the post-acquisition context can differ from the acquisition context along the dimensions of time and overall similarity. The RI acquisition and post-acquisition contexts tend to become less similar because the mechanisms that affect the emotional, physical, and cognitive states of the learner are operating. For instance, the mechanisms that produce forgetting or that change one's motivation to perform can operate during an RI. In this sense, a retention test can be interpreted as a test of the transfer of motor learning to contexts that appear to match the context of the acquisition phase.

## What Retention Test Performance Tells Us

When we study motor performance in the acquisition phase we are studying the learning of a defined motor performance. However, when we study motor performance on a retention test, we are studying the durability of that learned performance over time.

Retention performance tells us something about the durability of the motor performance learned in acquisition.

In other words, we are studying the retention of motor learning over some RI. It is easy to make the mistake of thinking that retention performance is a direct measure of the durability of motor learning when, in fact, it is a direct measure of retention performance from which we draw our inferences about the memory and forgetting of motor learning. Retention performance measures tell us something about the durability or reliability of motor performance that was learned in acquisition, and we use that information to make inferences about memory and forgetting processes.

Retention test measures are direct measures of the retention performance from which inferences can be made about how much motor learning was remembered (memory) or lost (forgotten) over an RI. Performance measures in *acquisition* (e.g., performance curves) are used to help us make inferences about mechanisms, processes, and outcomes of motor learning. Performance measures in *retention* are used to help us make inferences about memory and forgetting processes that operate over the RI to affect the durability of the motor performance that was learned in acquisition.

Generally, the level of motor performance achieved in acquisition is assessed in post-acquisition with a retention test for at least two major reasons:

- ▪ To determine if the performance observed is temporary and due to variables that do not qualify as evidence for motor learning (e.g., fatigue, drugs, level of motivation) or if it is durable and the result of variables that do qualify as evidence for motor learning (instruction, practice, augmented feedback, and experience)
- ▪ To study the extent to which the level of motor performance achieved in acquisition is retained as a function of variables manipulated before, during, and after acquisition, as well as during the RI in order to make inferences about memory and forgetting. For example, we might study the retention of movement skills as a function of variables such as (a) practice distribution in acquisition, (b) amount of practice in acquisition, (c) duration of RI, and (d) motor responses learned before acquisition of the motor response to-be-recalled (proactive interference) or after it (retroactive interference).

Explicit tests of motor retention can tell us something about **recall memory** and **recognition memory.** Recall tests require a learner to retrieve the criterion movement from memory and perform it when the appropriate stimulus is presented. For example, we might ask a right-handed golfer to recall and perform the swing with a five iron that will move the ball from left to right with a high trajectory. On the other hand, recognition tests require a learner to indicate with an identification response whether the criterion movement was experienced before. For instance, we might ask a learner to try gripping the tennis racquet in different ways prior to executing a particular serve to see if he or she recognizes any of them as ones experienced before when serving well. Typically, explicit motor retention tests are more tests of recall than recognition. However, the relative roles of recall and recognition probably interact quite often. For instance, a criterion movement (e.g., a golf putting stroke or a particular tennis serve) that cannot be recalled at one moment can be recalled at a later time with the appropriate cueing (stimulus) from a teacher or coach.

Frequently, individuals have information stored in memory from implicit learning, but they have difficulty retrieving it on explicit retention tests because they are unaware of the information that was learned. For example, in motor learning, **implicit learning** could refer to improvements that occur in learners' capability to perform a movement skill as a result of practice and without their being aware of the parts of the movement skill that led to the improvements. **Explicit retention tests** are those that directly ask people to consciously remember (recall or recognize) what was learned. Asking a learner to perform a previously learned movement skill would be an example of an explicit retention test. The retention tests we discussed in the previous paragraph and earlier in this chapter are examples of explicit tests of memory. **Implicit retention tests** are ones in which people are asked in different ways

Retention tests that ask learners to retrieve the criterion movement and perform it are assessing recall memory.

Retention tests that ask learners to identify whether the criterion movement was experienced before are assessing recognition memory.

Implicit retention tests ask learners in different ways to demonstrate or report whether they have something in stored memory of which they are unaware.

to demonstrate or report whether they have something stored in memory of which they are unaware and, therefore, have difficulty retrieving for an explicit test.

A study by McPherson and Thomas (1989) provides a nice example of explicit and implicit retention tests in the movement domain of sport. They asked young male basketball players to complete a paper-and-pencil test by indicating what they would do in various game situations (explicit test). Thus, this explicit test was trying to find out if they remembered what to do (declarative knowledge). For their implicit test, they observed what the players actually did in the various game situations to determine if they possessed the procedural knowledge needed to do what they reported they should do on the explicit test. Their findings indicated that many of the players knew what to do in various game situations (declarative knowledge) but couldn't perform accordingly (procedural knowledge).

Retention tests also can provide us with useful information about intentional and incidental memory. When people know in advance that the movement skills presented to them or practiced by them will have to be recalled and performed later on a retention test, we are studying **intentional memory.** Conversely, if they do not know in advance that the movement skills presented to them or practiced by them would have to be recalled and performed later on a retention test, we are studying **incidental memory.** Essentially, these two types of retention test situations are used to investigate memory as a function of one's *intention* to remember.

Comparing the retention findings of the two situations can answer questions about the intention to remember and encoding of movement information processes. For instance, do we retain more of or perhaps only the information to which we consciously attend, as in the case of intentional memory? To what extent do we retain information to which we do not consciously attend? Questions such as these have been the focus of very little research in movement skills. However, the research that is available reveals that the intention to remember produces better retention than no intention to remember and that no intention to remember results in better retention than if no previous experience with the movement skills had occurred. (For a review, see Crocker & Dickinson, 1984.) One instructional implication from this research is that the retention (memory) of motor learning can be enhanced by telling participants at the outset of acquisition exactly what type of information they will be tested on and how they will be tested at a later time.

## Example of How the Retention of Motor Learning Is Studied

When studying motor retention, traditionally a distinction is made between the acquisition and retention phases of an experiment as shown in the example in Table 11.1. In this example, we are studying how well movement A is retained as a function of different retention intervals (RIs). The acquisition phase could consist of a set number of performance trials for all three groups, or it could involve the time or trials required for the groups to achieve a criterion level of proficiency in performing movement A. The retention phase follows the acquisition phase and consists of an RI and a retention test. The

**Table 11.1**
**Experimental Design to Study the Retention of Motor Learning**

|           | Acquisition Phase | Retention Phase      |                |
| --------- | ----------------- | -------------------- | -------------- |
| Group     | Learn             | Retention Interval (RI) | Retention Test |
| I         | Movement A        | 3 months             | Movement A     |
| II        | Movement A        | 6 months             | Movement A     |
| III       | Movement A        | 12 months            | Movement A     |

RI is a time period of nonuse or no practice of movement A; it can vary from being short (e.g., seconds or minutes) to long (e.g., weeks, months, or years) in duration. The retention test is used to determine how much of the movement A proficiency achieved in acquisition is retained when it is performed again after an RI or, alternatively, how many trials are saved in relearning the movement (known as a *savings score*, which is discussed on page 338).

Let's describe a published experiment as an actual example of how retention of motor learning is studied. Ryan (1965) studied the retention of stabilometer performance (a novel dynamic balancing task) over the three RIs shown in the preceding experimental design to study motor learning. The swinging motion of the stabilometer board was recorded by a counter, which produced a performance score that served as the outcome, or dependent measure of interest. The less the movement of the stabilometer board, the better the total body balance and the lower the performance score. A three-trial pretest was administered to provide a basis for matching and assigning participants to groups on the acquisition trials, familiarize participants with the stabilometer, answer questions related to performance of the task, and establish a basic relationship with the participants. After three days of no practice, the three groups returned for the acquisition phase and performed eleven 30-second trials on the stabilometer with a 30-second rest between trials. Following RIs of 3, 6, and 12 months, the groups performed a retention and relearning test in the retention phase of the study. Relearning consisted of the groups performing eight 30-second trials with a 30-second rest between trials. The results are shown in Figure 11.2. Essentially, this figure reveals considerable decrements in stabilometer performance over the RIs, with the longest RI resulting in the greatest decrement. All three groups demonstrated a significant decrement in performance on the first trial of the retention phase, with the group having the 12-month RI experiencing the greatest reduction in performance proficiency. Stabilometer performance was quickly relearned for the groups that had 3- and 6-month RIs, but the group that had the 12-month RI took longer to relearn than either the 3- or 6-month group and never acquired the level of performance achieved in acquisition. Thus, a savings score could not be calculated for the 12-month RI group.

It is worth pointing out that the results may have been different if more acquisition trials had been administered. Acquisition performance on the stabilometer has been shown to improve after as many as 60 trials. Thus, it may be that the retention decrements observed in Ryan's study were the result of incomplete learning and that, if more acquisition trials had been provided,

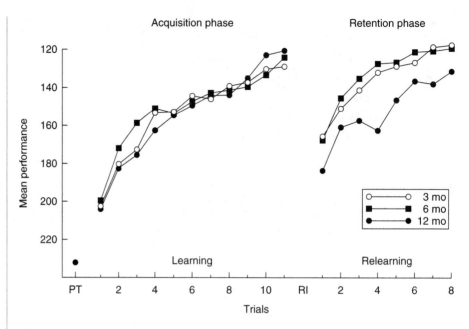

**Figure 11.2**   Mean stabilometer performance for learning and relearning following three different retention intervals of 3, 6, and 12 months

PT = pretest; RI = retention interval

*Source:* Adapted from E. D. Ryan (1965). Retention of stabilometer performance over extended periods of time. *Research Quarterly, 36,* 46–51.)

then the losses might have been less. Further, it is likely that in relearning the 12-month RI group would have returned to the level of performance achieved in acquisition, thereby making it possible to calculate a savings score.

## Controlling for Variables That Produce Contaminating Effects

If certain variables are allowed to operate uncontrolled, their effects will be confounded with those due to memory and forgetting.

As was pointed out previously in this chapter and in Chapters 6 and 7, when we assess the reliability or durability of motor learning that occurred in the acquisition phase, care must be taken through our experimental design and procedures to control or account for the temporary effects due to variables such as warm-up conditions, level of motivation, distribution of practice, reminiscence, and common daily variations in motor performance that could operate during an RI to affect retention test performance. The effects on acquisition and retention performance produced by these variables do not qualify as evidence for motor learning or the memory or forgetting of motor learning and thus are considered contaminating effects. If these variables are allowed to operate uncontrolled, their temporary effects on performance will be confounded with the effects on performance due to motor learning, memory, and forgetting. Let's look at some examples of how such confounding could occur and what can be done to avoid it.

***Example 1: Inappropriate RI.***   It is well known that massed practice (continued practice with little or no rest between trials) can depress performance in acquisition, which is a temporary effect. Longer RIs would allow more time for the massed practice effect to dissipate and thus make retention test performance less contaminated by this temporary effect. However, longer RIs could produce a more proficient level of performance on the retention test for the massed practice group than was ever achieved in acquisition. This improvement in retention performance over an RI has been called **reminiscence.** A reminiscence effect reveals that a more proficient level of motor performance was retained after the RI than was ever achieved in acquisition, whereas we would expect less to be retained if forgetting was operating.

The effect due to reminiscence is the opposite of the effect caused by forgetting, which makes these opposing effects somewhat challenging to interpret. A similar effect could occur for longer RIs as a result of a change in motivation. For instance, suppose a massed practice schedule led to increased physical fatigue and boredom as practice of a gross motor task (e.g., stabilometer or Bachman ladder) continued in acquisition. As a result, acquisition performance was depressed for the massed practice group because they gradually lost some motivation to perform as practice continued. A short RI (e.g., 1 minute) would not provide enough rest for much of the physical fatigue and boredom to dissipate and appreciably increase the group's motivation to perform on the retention test. However, a sufficiently long RI (e.g., 15 minutes) would allow these negative effects to dissipate, resulting in an increased motivation to perform on the retention test. The result would be a reminiscence effect, that is, a more proficient level of performance on the retention test than was achieved in acquisition.

In order to interpret a reminiscence effect of a massed practice group, it must be compared to the acquisition and retention test performance of a distributed practice group. For example, suppose a longer RI results in retention test performance of the massed practice group being about the same as the distributed practice group. This finding suggests that the massing of practice depressed performance in acquisition but had no effect on learning as evidenced by the retention test performance. Thus, reminiscence effects due to massed practice or changes in motivation can be interpreted if the temporary effects of these two variables are controlled and accounted for with complete experimental designs that include all the necessary control groups and procedures to effectively manage the distribution of practice and level of motivation of the participants.

Of course, longer RIs would also allow other variables to affect performance. For example, inappropriately warming up or motivating participants to perform could cause a decrement in retention test performance. At the same time, longer RIs could result in increased levels of forgetting, but it would be difficult to determine how much of the retention performance decrement was due to forgetting because it would be confounded with the effects caused by inappropriately warming up and motivating participants to perform. Thus, the use of retention tests to assess the reliability or durability of motor learning or to study memory and forgetting of motor learning could confound the amount learned in acquisition with warm-up and motivation if they operate over the RI and if our experimental design and procedures do not control or account for their effects (for a more detailed discussion, see Christina & Shea, 1988, 1993).

*Example 2: Contaminated Retention Test Measures.*    Retention test measures (discussed on page 338) that do (relative retention scores) and do not (absolute retention scores) make use of acquisition performance measures also could be contaminated with temporary effects caused by independent variables being manipulated in acquisition (e.g., massed practice, lack of motivation) such that they might not reflect motor learning. Some researchers have assumed that these effects are present only when the independent variables are present. However, temporary performance effects (e.g., due to massed practice) can persist and be present on the retention test well after the independent variables are removed in acquisition. For example, suppose we were studying stabilometer performance as a function of practice distribution. Certainly, it is reasonable to expect practice distributions with shorter intertrial rest intervals (more massed practice conditions) to require longer RIs of rest for the temporary performance effects (e.g., physical fatigue) to dissipate than will practice distributions with longer intertrial intervals (more distributed practice conditions). Further, if shorter RIs of rest are not long enough for all of the temporary effects to dissipate, then retention test performance (usually measured by an absolute retention score, discussed on page 338) would contain different amounts of temporary effect contamination, depending on the practice distributions used in acquisition. In other words, retention test performance resulting from the more distributed practice conditions probably would have less contamination than retention test performance resulting from the more massed practice conditions. Moreover, if we compared retention test performances of the different practice distributions, we would be taking the risk of comparing performances that not only could have different amounts of learning and forgetting, but different amounts of temporary effect contamination as well.

Appropriate experimental designs and procedures can control variables that cause contaminating effects.

Clearly, retention test performance can be easily contaminated by variables that cause temporary performance effects not only when they are present, but also after they are removed if their effects persist over the RI and into the retention test. One way to control these variables that cause temporary effects on performance is through the careful development of the experimental design and procedures to be used in the study. Certainly, one important design feature would be to include an RI of sufficient length. A single RI can be justified if there is evidence from other studies and/or your own pilot studies that all the temporary effects due to variables such as massed practice, warm-up, and level of motivation have dissipated over that RI.

Without this evidence, you may have to use more than one RI. In some situations, the presence of temporary performance effects can by assessed reasonably well by the administration of both immediate and delayed retention tests (Christina & Shea, 1993). In the case of an immediate retention test, the retention interval should be the same as the intertrial interval during the acquisition phase of the experiment. For both the immediate and delayed retention tests, the acquisition groups should be tested under the same experimental conditions.

A more definitive description of temporary performance effects might be obtained if conditions were included in the experimental design in which the independent variable (e.g., KR) was left intact for the retention tests. Presumably, temporary performance effects would still be present for the immediate retention test for all conditions but would have the opportunity to dissipate by the time of the delayed retention test. This would especially be the case for the conditions in which the independent variable of interest was removed for the retention tests.

***Example 3: Inappropriate Warm-Up.***   All retention performance decrements are not due to memory losses or forgetting. As has been pointed out previously, some are due to variables such as warm-up and motivation. Warm-up is a unique variable that deserves some special attention. It is not uncommon to observe a decrement in retention performance following acquisition and an RI. If the experiment is properly designed, we would interpret this decrement to memory loss or forgetting. However, some scholars have argued that this decrement is due to the lack of properly warming up and thus it is a **warm-up decrement** (Adams, 1952, 1961).

The decrement in retention performance may be due to forgetting or to inappropriately warming up.

Two hypotheses have emerged to explain warm-up decrement. The **forgetting hypothesis** proposes that the loss in retention performance is, in fact, due to forgetting. It is just another form of forgetting or loss of memory for performing the motor skill. The rest over an RI allows certain forgetting processes to operate, with the beginning stages of these processes being relatively rapid, which accounts for the rather sizable decrements in retention performance observed with only a few minutes of rest. The initial improvements in performance with practice during the retention phase that erase the warm-up decrement are thought to be due to relearning of the aspects of the motor skill that were forgotten.

In contrast to the forgetting hypothesis, the **set hypothesis** holds that the decrement in retention performance is due to a loss of set, which is a relatively temporary loss of bodily adjustments or internal states that support the memory of the capability for performing the motor skill at a proficient level as it was performed in later stages of acquisition. The set hypothesis argues that little or no forgetting has occurred over the RI and that the memory of the capability for performing the motor skill is largely intact. What initial practice in the retention phase (which could be considered warm-up practice) does for the learner is to reinstate the lost set, causing performance to rapidly improve and erase the decrement. Evidence from Schmidt and colleagues (Nacson & Schmidt, 1971; Schmidt & Nacson, 1971; Schmidt & Wrisberg, 1971) supports the set hypothesis. Moreover, evidence from imagery practice involving mental performance of the motor skill immediately before actual performance is resumed appears to reduce the warm-up decrement, but the nature of the reduction seems to be skill specific (Ainscoe & Hardy, 1987; Anshel & Wrisberg, 1988, 1993; Wrisberg & Anshel, 1993).

In summary, there may be some slight losses of memory or forgetting of the capability to perform a motor skill over short RIs (e.g., minutes), but the existing evidence largely favors the loss of set (internal adjustments) over the RI. The implication for studying memory or forgetting processes is that warm-up must be controlled, manipulated, or accounted for in the design and procedures of the experiment. One way to do this is to have participants in experimental and control groups perform an unrelated movement task during the RI just prior to the retention test. This sounds easy, but often it is difficult to find an appropriate movement task that is unrelated to the movement task to be recalled and performed on the retention test and can serve to eliminate warm-up decrement. If warm-up is not controlled, the decrement in retention performance that is due to not warming up properly will be confounded with the decrement that is due to forgetting. Such uncertainty about the cause of the decrement in retention performance severely limits the inference that can be made about the decrement being due to memory loss or forgetting.

## Retention Test Measures

Several measures have been used to assess performance on the retention test following acquisition and an RI. The most frequently used measures include an absolute retention score, savings score, and relative retention score. Each of these three measures is briefly discussed below.

*Absolute Retention Score.*   This score is the first-trial recall score or the actual performance on the initial trial of the retention test. Using the data shown in Figure 11.2 on page 334, we can estimate the absolute retention scores on the first trial of the retention phase to be approximately 165, 167, and 183 for the 3-month, 6-month, and 12-month RI groups, respectively. If all variables that cause temporary performance effects are controlled through the study design and procedures, the **absolute retention score** reflects the amount retained of what was originally learned in acquisition.

The absolute retention score represents the amount of acquisition performance retained after the RI.

We would like to point out that, although one expects absolute retention scores to indicate the amount retained and relative retention scores to reveal the amount of performance lost over an RI, there are a few times when they do not. For instance, under certain practice conditions (e.g., massed practice), absolute retention scores can reveal more retained than what was learned in acquisition and relative retention scores can show improvement or gain rather than loss in performance over the RI. This reminiscence effect was discussed on page 335.

Compared to a distributed practice schedule, a massed practice schedule temporarily depresses performance in acquisition but appears to have little or no effect on learning. When this temporary effect dissipates with rest over the RI (if it is long enough), retention test performance of the massed practice group usually improves and is equal to or approaches the performance of the distributed practice group. More importantly for our discussion, retention test performance of the massed practice group is better than it was at any time in acquisition. Consequently, when one calculates an absolute retention score, the massed practice group actually retains a higher performance level than was achieved in acquisition. Similarly, when one calculates either of the relative retention scores, the massed practice group actually shows a gain rather than a loss in performance over the RI from the end of acquisition.

The savings score is the number of trials or time saved in relearning a skill.

*Savings Score.*   The **savings score** is the number of trials or time saved in *relearning* a motor task that was originally learned in the acquisition phase. To calculate this score, you simply count the number of trials in the retention phase required for learners to reach the level of proficiency in performance that they achieved in acquisition. This number is then subtracted from the number of trials needed to originally learn the task in acquisition. The difference between the two scores constitutes the savings score. For example, using the data in Figure 11.2, it appears that it took the 3-month RI group 5 trials and the 6-month RI group 6 trials to relearn the stabilometer task. It also took both groups 11 trials in acquisition to reach the highest level of proficiency in performance in acquisition. Subtracting 5 from 11 results in a savings score of 6 trials for the 3-month RI group, while subtracting 6 from 11 produces a savings score of 5 for the 6-month RI group. A savings score could not be calculated for the 12-month group because they were not given enough trials in relearning to reach the level of performance they achieved in acquisition. However, it is clear that the 12-month group would have needed more relearning trials than the other two groups to reach the level they achieved in acquisition.

It is also possible to express a savings score as a percent retention score simply by dividing the savings score by the number of trials needed in acquisition to achieve the criterion level of performance, and then multiply by 100 to convert to a percentage. For example, using the 3-month RI group, simply divide 6 (savings score) by 11 (acquisition trials needed) and multiply by 100 to obtain the retention score of 55%. In this case the savings score of 6 trials, otherwise known as the retention score, is 55%. Conversely, the amount not retained (forgotten) would be 45%.

Christina and Shea (1993) encouraged the study of relearning in the retention phase by using the savings score in conjunction with the absolute retention score. By doing this, a more comprehensive assessment of retention performance could be performed and inferences about memory and forgetting processes more confidently made. Clearly, these two measures, used in combination, can tell us more about retention performance than only one of them. For example, based on an extensive literature review, Adams (1987) concluded that the "forgetting of procedural responses can be complete in about a year, although there are savings because relearning is rapid" (p. 54). Thus, learners might show little or no retention based on their absolute retention score on the first relearning trial but demonstrate a substantial savings in the number of trials required to relearn the skill (their savings score). In this situation, the absolute retention score tells us that nothing was retained of what was originally learned, but the savings score indicates that at least some skill-related information was retained. It is clear that if only the absolute retention score is used, the conclusion reached might be very different from the one reached when both scores are used.

*Relative Retention Score.*   Another way to assess retention is with a **relative retention score,** which actually reflects how much performance achieved (learned) in acquisition was lost or not retained over the RI. Two relative retention scores often used are a difference score and percent relative retention score. A **difference score** is the difference between performance achieved on the last trial or block of trials of acquisition and performance obtained on the first trial or block of trials of the retention test. For example, let's assume from the data in Figure 11.2 that the performance score on the last trial in acquisition for the 3-month RI group was 130 and that it was 165 on the first trial of retention. The difference between these two scores is 35, which represents the amount of balance performance that was lost or not retained (forgotten) over the 3-month RI. Thus, the difference score actually measures how much performance declined over the RI from the end of acquisition to the retention test.

A **percent relative retention score** is the difference score divided by the amount of change in performance during acquisition, which is then multiplied by 100 to convert it into a percentage. For example, let's estimate from the

The difference score and the percent relative retention score indicate the amount of performance lost over the RI.

data in Figure 11.2 that the first trial performance score in acquisition for the 3-month RI group was 204 and that it was 130 on the eleventh trial of acquisition. Subtract 130 from 204 to get the amount gained in acquisition (74) and then divide the difference score (35) by the amount gained in acquisition (74), which results in a quotient of 0.47. Lastly, multiply 0.47 by 100 to convert it into a score of 47%. This percent relative retention score represents the decline in performance over the RI relative to the amount of improvement in performance achieved during the acquisition phase. Thus, it assesses the amount of improvement in performance observed in acquisition that was not retained over the RI.

*Contrasting Retention Test Measures.* Obviously, the retention test measures discussed in the previous section are based on performance and are used to draw inferences about forgetting. These measures are subject to the same difficulties as performance measures obtained in acquisition (e.g., performance/learning curves) that are used to draw inferences about motor learning. You will recall that these types of measures were discussed in Chapters 6 and 7. We must always be mindful that performance in acquisition is no more a perfect index of motor learning than it is in retention for memory or forgetting—performance in acquisition and retention can be temporarily affected by variables such as a massed practice schedule, fatigue, level of motivation, and drugs that do not reflect motor learning, memory, and forgetting processes. Performance scores taken in acquisition and retention also can be affected by measurement limitations such as scoring sensitivity and ceiling and floor effects that were discussed in Chapter 7. Armed with an understanding of the limitations of performance measures as indicators of motor learning, memory, and forgetting, our inferences about these processes are likely to be made on solid ground.

It is not uncommon to find results from studies based on different retention measures that appear to be in conflict and lead to divergent inferences about motor learning, memory, or forgetting. For example, retention can be measured using an absolute retention score or a relative retention score. If forgetting is measured with an absolute retention score, we find that absolute retention increases with increases in the amount of original learning. However, if forgetting is measured by either of the relative retention scores, we find that relative retention decreases with increases in the amount of original learning (that is, amount of practice in acquisition).

At first glance, these results appear to be in conflict, but they are not because absolute retention scores and relative retention scores actually measure different aspects of performance (see Christina & Shea, 1988, for a detailed discussion of this issue). Absolute retention scores measure the *amount of performance retained* after the RI, whereas both relative retention scores measure the *amount of performance lost* relative to acquisition performance. Thus, absolute retention scores and relative retention scores are measuring opposite aspects of retention performance. Once this is understood, it becomes clear from the example that the amount of performance retained (absolute retention score) should increase with increases in the amount of original learning, and the amount of performance lost (relative retention scores) should decrease with increases in the amount of original learning. In other words, the more one practices in acquisition (original learning), the more performance should be retained and the less it should be lost over the RI. Taken together, these scores convey a similar idea and are therefore not in conflict. They actually provide converging lines of evidence to support the inference that the more one practices in acquisition the more one remembers, or, conversely, the less one forgets over the RI.

Clearly, each of these scores provides information about a particular aspect of retention performance that the other scores are incapable of providing. The keys to the successful use of these and other scores are:

■ Knowing what aspect of performance each of the scores reflects
■ Having a thorough understanding of the interrelations among the different scores
■ Understanding the methodological and measurement problems inherent in each of the scores

Such understanding will lead to more meaningful selection among the scores for a particular study and provide a basis for interpreting the results obtained in various studies that have used different scores to study retention.

# Theories of Forgetting

Trace decay, interference, and retrieval are three theories of forgetting that have concerned psychologists for a long time and all three apply to the forgetting of motor learning, which largely depends on the type of movement task that is learned. These theories of forgetting and forgetting as a function of type of movement task are discussed next.

## Trace Decay Theory

**Trace decay theory** proposes that forgetting is due to the passage of time, which causes degeneration of the memory trace, or engram, of the learned capability for producing a movement performance. The passage of time alone, in the absence of any other factors, is sufficient to cause forgetting. For instance, if over several months (retention interval) you do not play golf or practice hitting tee shots with your driver, trace decay theory predicts that you would, to some extent, forget your learned capability for hitting balls as proficiently as you did when you were playing and practicing regularly. Trace decay theory holds that the longer the period of time you do not play or practice, the more the memory trace of the learned capability for driving the golf ball will be eroded and the greater the forgetting. The fundamental experimental design used to study trace decay theory is shown in Table 11.2. Assume that both groups had the same number of acquisition trials in learning and that group I had a shorter RI than group II. If the longer RI causes a greater decrement in performance of movement A for group II when compared to the performance of movement A for group I, then evidence for motor memory trace decay may be claimed.

The pioneering evidence supporting trace decay theory in short-term motor memory was produced in a study by Adams and Dijkstra (1966), who had blindfolded participants perform a linear positioning task. They varied both

Trace decay theory holds that forgetting is due to the passage of time.

**Table 11.2**
**Experimental Design to Study Trace Decay Theory**

| Acquisition Phase | | Retention Phase | |
|---|---|---|---|
| Group | Learn | Retention Interval (RI) | Retention Test |
| I | Movement A | Period of nonuse (short RI) | Movement A |
| II | Movement A | Period of nonuse (long RI) | Movement A |

the amount of practice (repetitions) in learning and the duration of the RI and reported two main findings. First, absolute error was less on the retention test for groups that had more practice in learning, which was expected. Second, the absolute error rate increased steadily on the retention test as the RI increased up to 80 seconds, and then leveled off over RIs of 80 to 120 seconds, which they interpreted as support for trace decay theory.

Since the Adams and Dijkstra study, additional support for trace decay theory has been found by others (e.g., Adams, Marshall, & Goetz, 1972; Burwitz, 1974). Tests of trace decay theory for long-term motor memory are virtually nonexistent because it is very difficult, if not impossible, to conduct studies in which (a) competing movement responses do not occur during long RIs (e.g., weeks, months, or years) and (b) the only thing operating is the passage of time. However, evidence for trace decay in short-term motor memory suggests that it also could be operating in long-term motor memory.

## Interference Theory

Interference theory holds that forgetting is due to competing responses.

Conversely, **interference theory** attributes forgetting to competing movement responses that occur during the RI, not to the passage of time itself. Forgetting may or may not take place over the RI, depending on the nature and frequency of the competing movement responses that intrude. Competing responses experienced or acquired before learning of the criterion response (**proactive interference**) or after its learning (**retroactive interference**) induce the decrement in criterion performance on the retention test that we call forgetting.

An example of proactive interference would be learning an incorrect golf swing *before* learning a correct one (criterion response). The competing movement(s) between the two swings could cause interference with the memory trace of the capability for performing the correct swing and lead to forgetting over the RI. Evidence for this forgetting would be a decrement in performance of the correct swing following a period of no practice or play, which is the RI. The basic experimental design used to study proactive interference is presented in Table 11.3.

If the prior learning of movement B causes inferior retention test performance of movement A for the experimental group when compared to the retention test performance of movement A of the control group, then evidence for proactive interference may be claimed. There is some support for proactive

**Table 11.3**
**Experimental Design to Study Proactive Interference**

| Group | Acquisition Phase | | Retention Phase | |
|---|---|---|---|---|
| | Prior Learning | Learn | Retention Interval (RI) | Retention Test |
| Experimental | Movement B | Movement A | Period of nonuse (RI same as control group) | Movement A |
| Control | Nothing | Movement A | Period of nonuse (RI same as experimental group) | Movement A |

**Table 11.4**
**Experimental Design to Study Retroactive Interference**

| Group | Acquisition Phase | | Retention Phase | |
|---|---|---|---|---|
| | Prior Learning | Learn | Retention Interval (RI) | Retention Test |
| Experimental | Movement A | Movement B | Period of nonuse (RI same as control group) | Movement A |
| Control | Movement A | Nothing | Period of nonuse (RI same as experimental group) | Movement A |

interference in short-term motor memory (e.g., Ascoli & Schmidt, 1969; Stelmach, 1969b), but no research evidence was found for it in long-term motor memory. Proactive interference appears to occur in short-term motor memory when there is similarity between the movement to be remembered (movement A) and the interfering movement (movement B). It appears that proactive interference increases as the number of similar movements (B movements) preceding the movement to be remembered (movement A) increases.

An example of retroactive interference would be learning a golf swing change (movement B) *after* the initial golf swing (movement A) was learned. The competing movement(s) between the two swings could cause interference with the memory trace of the capability for performing the initial swing and lead to forgetting. Evidence for such forgetting would be a decrement in performance of the initial golf swing (movement A) on the retention test after a period of no practice or play (RI). The experimental design for retroactive interference is shown in Table 11.4.

If movement B causes a decrement in the performance of movement A on the retention test for the experimental group, relative to the performance of movement A on the retention test for the control group, then evidence for retroactive interference has been found. Movement B may not always interfere; it can be neutral or even transfer positively to the performance of movement A on the retention test. There is evidence of retroactive interference in short-term motor memory (e.g., Milone, 1971; Patrick, 1971; Pepper & Herman, 1970; Smyth & Pendleton, 1990), but it seems that forgetting effects in long-term motor memory are also a function of the type of motor task or skill (discrete, serial, continuous, or procedural) and the degree of organizational complexity of the task or skill, which will be discussed in more detail on page 346.

## Retrieval Theory

Retrieval theory holds that forgetting occurs because the memory trace cannot be found and recalled.

The **retrieval theory** of forgetting has its roots in psychology of verbal learning and memory that could apply to motor forgetting. Retrieval theory holds that the memory trace of the capability for producing a learned movement performance is not forgotten or eroded due to the passage of time or interference from competing movements. The memory trace resides at full strength in memory over the RI, and a recovery operation is required to recall it on the retention test. Failure to retrieve as a theory of motor forgetting says that the memory trace of the capability for producing a learned movement performance exists at full strength, but it cannot be found and so cannot be recalled.

Most of the psychological research of retrieval theory has used a stimulus at recall as a means of arousing forgotten verbal responses to recall (e.g., Bahrick, 1969; Tulving & Pearlstone, 1966; Thomson & Tulving, 1970; Tulving & Thomson, 1973). This method is referred to as *prompting* and the reminder stimulus is called the *prompter.* The study of retrieval using a prompting approach is a relatively new undertaking in psychology and is even newer in motor learning. Thus, there is little basis for choosing among the various explanations of retrieval theory, but three of them appear to have attracted researchers: mental search, generation-recognition, and encoding specificity.

The **mental search explanation** holds that, when the memory trace of the capability for producing a particular movement response needs to be recalled, a search process through a finite set of memory traces begins. Preferably, the finite set of memory traces being searched contains not only memory traces of capabilities for generating movement responses similar to the one that needs to be recalled, but also the memory trace for the particular movement response needed. Very likely, the prompter narrows the set of memory traces and makes the search more efficient. The more effective the prompter, the smaller the set and the more easily the memory trace needed is retrieved.

The **generation-recognition explanation** argues against mental searching as the process by which the memory trace is retrieved. It proposes that the prompter is a stimulus for generating a hierarchy of memory traces from past learning that are close to the memory trace needed; if the needed memory trace is among them, the learner will recognize it and recall it. The **encoding specificity explanation** argues that, for the prompter to be effective, it must be encoded along with the memory trace of the capability to produce the movement response at the time of learning. This explanation emphasizes the importance of encoding at the time of learning, which is intuitively appealing. However, there are some verbal learning results by Bahrick (1969) that are difficult to account for in terms of the encoding specificity explanation because prompters were present only at the time of recall and were quite effective. Bahrick's findings are best accounted for by the generation-recognition explanation.

Clearly, support can be found in research on verbal memory and forgetting for these three explanations of retrieval. The extent to which these or some other explanation of retrieval of verbal information can account for the retrieval of motor responses has yet to be determined by research.

## Which Theory Is Correct?

It would be simple and convenient if one of the three theories of forgetting (trace decay, interference, or retrieval) accounted for all of the circumstances of motor forgetting of which we are aware, and the other two did not. Unfortunately, simplicity and convenience do not prevail. There is evidence for all three theories in the verbal literature, but there is more evidence in the motor literature for trace decay and interference theories than for retrieval theory. However, there also has been less research testing retrieval theory than the other two theories of motor forgetting, so one would expect to find less evidence for retrieval explanations. The situation is further complicated when trying to apply these theories in the motor domain because there has been very little research testing these theories of forgetting in relation to the type of movement task. There is a greater amount of research for these theories over short rather than long retention intervals; and, consequently, the majority of the evidence supporting the theories does so more for short-term than for long-term motor forgetting. It is more difficult and often unrealistic to experimentally control what learners experience over longer retention intervals (e.g., months to years), hence less research has tested the validity of these theories for long-term motor forgetting. Nonetheless, all three theories appear to be viable explanations, and future research will have to determine the extent to which they or some other explanation can account for motor forgetting relative to type of movement task not only in the short term, but in the long term as well.

## Factors That Influence Memory Skill

Now that we have described the various changes in how knowledge is represented in memory as a learner progresses through the various stages of skill acquisition, let us consider the factors that are most likely to influence how well a particular skill is retained for later recall. It is possible to identify many of these factors by examining three important components of any learning situation: the characteristics of the movement skill to be learned, the environmental context in which the skill is to be learned, and the learner. The interaction among all of these components significantly influences how well a particular skill is learned. For example, we can expect a young child who is introduced to a new skill in an unfamiliar skill setting to operate very differently from an older child who is familiar with both the skill to be learned and the environment in which it is to be learned. Similarly, we will find that some skills are just inherently easier to remember than others.

# Characteristics of the Movement Skill

Continuous movement skills are better retained than are discrete, serial, and procedural skills.

*Type of Movement Skill.*    As indicated earlier (page 344), the type of movement task or skill to be learned has been shown to strongly influence retention. Continuous movement tasks appear to be more resistant to forgetting than are discrete, serial, and procedural movement tasks (e.g., Bell, 1950; Fleishman & Parker, 1962; Meyers, 1967; Ryan, 1965), but much more research is needed on this topic, especially studies that include relatively long retention intervals (e.g., months to years). Continuous tasks require us to respond to sensory information that is presented continuously, such as in a visual tracking task, riding a bicycle, or other repetitive motor task like swimming.

Procedural and serial tasks seem to be the most easily forgotten (for reviews see Christina & Bjork, 1991; Schendel & Hagman, 1991). Procedural tasks consist of a particular sequence of operations executed in the same way each time that the task is performed, such as disassembling and assembling a rifle or changing a tire. The technique of administering cardiopulmonary resuscitation is another example of a procedural skill that is easily forgotten (see highlight, The Skill of Resuscitation). Serial tasks are the same as procedural tasks except that the steps must be performed in rapid succession; they are self-paced in procedural tasks. If we asked someone to assemble and disassemble a rifle as fast as possible, it would become a serial task. The sequence of skills contained within a gymnastics floor exercise routine is another example of a serial task.

Discrete tasks appear to be forgotten more easily than continuous tasks but seem to be better retained than procedural or serial tasks (e.g., Lee & Genovese, 1988, 1989; Lersten, 1969; Neumann & Ammons, 1957; Shea, Lai, Black, & Park, 2000). Discrete tasks are characterized by having a clearly defined beginning and end such as responding to a signal by pressing the appropriate button or serving a volleyball after a whistle is blown by the referee. Although there are a number of investigations that have studied the forgetting of discrete motor tasks after relatively short RIs (e.g., minutes to days), very few have studied forgetting of discrete motor tasks after relatively long retention intervals (e.g., months to years).

*Degree of Task Organizational Complexity.*    Several hypotheses have been offered to explain why forgetting seems to be a function of task type. Some have argued that discrete and procedural/serial tasks are easily forgotten because they have a considerable verbal-cognitive component, which appears to be more difficult to retain over time than a motor component for a task (e.g., Adams, 1987). Also, some have proposed that continuous tasks are more readily retained because the inherent repetitive nature involved in performing them leads them to be more easily over-practiced and over-learned than discrete tasks. For instance, a practice trial for a discrete task might involve pressing the correct lever when the appropriate signal is heard, whereas a practice trial for a continuous task such as swimming might involve swimming one or more lengths of a pool.

Clearly, much more practice and repetition of the movements that make up the continuous task (swimming) are experienced than in the discrete task. Some scholars (e.g., Adams, 1967) have argued that retention differences as a

# HIGHLIGHT

## The Skill of Resuscitation

Have you ever wondered why you are required to renew your cardiopulmonary resuscitation (CPR) certificate every one to two years? The reason lies in the inherent organization and cohesion of the skill itself, which consists of a number of operations that must be carefully timed if the technique is to be administered correctly. Although cardiopulmonary resuscitation has been shown to enhance by as much as 40% a person's chances of surviving a serious accident, skill in CPR is difficult to retain for a long period of time.

In order to determine just how quickly the technique is forgotten, Glendon, McKenna, Blaylock, and Hunt (1985) tested a group of individuals who had successfully mastered the resuscitation skill and received their certificate of mastery some three months earlier. Four aspects of their performance were measured:

1. The *performance* and timing of the heart compression component
2. The *technique* used to inflate the lungs and depress the chest in the correct area
3. The quality of the initial *diagnosis* in which the level of consciousness, breathing, and pulse were checked
4. The outcome of the performance as measured by a *total score* representing the predicted survival rate of the patient

As the graph below indicates, the likelihood that Resusci® Annie, the mannequin used to teach resuscitation skills, will survive drops within a year from a level of 100% immediately following training to a low of 15%. After 36 months, the likelihood of survival is zero. It is clear that regular practice in administering this technique is critical if the skill is to be retained. When was the last time you renewed your own certification?

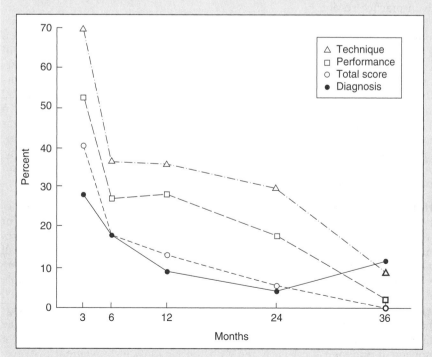

Techniques associated with CPR are quickly forgotten in the 36 months following certification.

function of task type are the result of the way trials and errors are scored. For instance, procedural and discrete motor tasks may be "relatively more sensitive to slight performance deviations than methods used to score the retention of continuous responses" (Schendel & Hagman, 1991, p. 58).

A third hypothesis holds that continuous tasks may be more *inherently organized* (coherent and integrated) than discrete motor tasks (Prophet, 1976; Van Dusen & Schlosberg, 1948), making them more meaningful to the learner. A number of scholars have hypothesized that the more meaningful the task, the more it enables the learner to use principles and relationships from past experiences to help store and retrieve the capability for producing the continuous task performance (Naylor & Briggs, 1961; Schmidt, 1972; Stelmach, 1974).

Among the criteria for determining organizational complexity for procedural tasks or skills are (a) the number of steps involved, (b) whether the order of the sequence can be varied in any way, (c) the extent of planning required to perform the skill, and (d) the degree to which one operation or part of the skill cues the next part. Prophet (1976) has shown that the procedures involved in piloting a plane are particularly susceptible to forgetting, especially when pilots are required to fly a plane using instruments only. The inherent *lack* of internal organization associated with piloting skills has been offered as the primary reason for the poor recall. It has also been suggested that continuous skills are much easier to over-learn because it is impossible to determine when one trial of the skill ends and the next begins (Schendel, Shields, & Katz, 1978). Considerably larger amounts of practice are therefore possible in any given practice session.

Regardless of the type of task, it appears that the degree of organizational complexity, whether inherent in the movement skill or imposed by the learner, is a major determinant of the level of original learning achieved and the amount retained long term (Annett, 1979; Gardlin & Sitterly, 1972; Hagman & Rose, 1983; Hurlock & Montague, 1982; Naylor & Briggs, 1961; Prophet, 1976). Unfortunately, there is no satisfactory way of operationally defining organizational complexity, which makes this factor somewhat difficult to study scientifically. In spite of this limitation, Annett (1979) proposed that variations in the organizational complexity of a task might be conceptualized as being equivalent to variations of task difficulty. As such, to learn a more difficult task successfully, its components may have to be intensively processed, which could lead to an increase in the level of over-learning and thereby promote retention.

*Movement Location.*   Movements can have many features such as velocity, distance moved, force produced, duration, timing, and spatial locations or positions that have the potential to be stored in memory: For instance, movement skills such as a golf swing, tennis serve, basketball shot, and baseball swing have all of these features. The question central to memory is, are some of these features more easily remembered than others? Based on the available basic research, it appears that movement location is remembered quite well relative to the other features (e.g., Diewert, 1975; Diewert & Roy, 1978; Hagman, 1978; Laabs, 1973). Much of this research has been done using simple limb position movements in which participants are blindfolded and found that movement endpoint location is remembered better than movement distance. When participants cannot rely on movement endpoint location and have only

*Movement skills that are more inherently organized and meaningful tend to be retained better.*

distance cues available, they tend to use a cognitive strategy (e.g., counting) to remember the target movement distance rather than some kinesthetic approach. This finding has been demonstrated in people older than nine years of age (Thomas, Thomas, Lee, Testerman, & Ashy, 1983).

It also appears that movement information about endpoint location is better remembered when it is within the participant's own body space (e.g., Chieffi, Allport, & Woodfin, 1999; Larish & Stelmach, 1982). Typically, people remember a target movement distance by associating the end location of the movement with one of their body parts. For instance, I moved my right hand and arm across my body from opposite my right shoulder to a position opposite my nose. Participants also seem to relate endpoint location of movements to external objects such as a clock face to help them remember. For example, I will move the golf club back to three o'clock and forward to nine o'clock for this short shot. Thus, the implication for teaching and learning is that if you want someone to learn a movement skill involving limb positions, instructional emphasis should be placed on these positions, especially the endpoints of each position to be learned.

*Movement endpoint location tends to be remembered quite well, especially within a person's own body space.*

### *Meaningfulness of the Movement.*
Some movements are more meaningful to a learner than others, and the ones that are more meaningful tend to be better remembered (e.g., Laugier & Cadpoli, 1996). For example, a movement skill or pattern that can be related to a previously learned skill or pattern is more meaningful to learn than a skill that does not resemble anything the learner has in memory. For instance, when teaching a tennis serve we might tell and show the learner how many elements of the tennis serve are like many elements of the overhand throw in baseball or softball, which was previously learned. Or when teaching a new defensive play in basketball, we might explain and show how it is similar to the defensive play that was previously learned in soccer. The "switching" strategy in man-to-man defense wherein two defensive players switch and guard each other's offensive player would be an example. Thus, it appears that the more meaningful the skill and patterns are, the better the chance that they will be remembered.

*Movements that are more meaningful tend to be better remembered.*

The degree of task organization also could contribute to the meaningfulness of a movement task. For instance, it has been proposed that continuous movement tasks are more resistant to forgetting because they are more inherently organized (coherent and integrated) than discrete tasks (Prophet, 1976), making them more meaningful to learners. Perhaps the more meaningful the task, the more it enables learners to use relevant past experiences in memory to help store and retrieve the capability for producing continuous movement task performance. Clearly, more research is needed before the validity of this explanation can be ascertained.

### *Length of a Series of Movements.*
When the length of a series of movements is greater than five movements, as it is in many procedural tasks (e.g., steps in changing a flat tire or shutting down a nuclear power plant), movements at the beginning and end of the series tend to be recalled better than movements in the middle (e.g., Craik, 1970; Magill & Dowell, 1977; Wrisberg, 1975; Wrisberg & Gerard, 1977). Traditionally, this finding has been referred to as the **primacy-recency effect.** It has been consistently obtained in the verbal research literature and to some extent in the motor skills literature with blindfolded participants trying to recall a series of linear positioning movements.

*The beginning and end of a series of movements tend to be recalled better than those in the middle.*

The amount of research validating this finding for real-world movement skills such as those found in sport or everyday life is also somewhat limited. Nonetheless, to facilitate retention it would be advisable for teachers or coaches to place more emphasis on the movements in the middle of serial routines such as those found in dance, synchronized swimming, or gymnastics. Furthermore, the routine may have to be broken down into smaller segments, with individual practice on these segments. Care should be taken not to overload the learner's memory span, however, which appears to have a limit of about eight movements, when dividing a whole routine into a series of components.

## The Level of Original Learning

A number of authors interested in the long-term retention of tasks (Annett, 1979; Hurlock & Montague, 1982; Prophet, 1976; Schendel, Shields, & Katz, 1978) strongly argue that how well a particular task is learned during original learning constitutes the most potent variable determining whether a skill is forgotten over time. This conclusion is echoed in the writings of Christina and Bjork (1991), who, in addition to providing a comprehensive review of the related literature, also discuss a number of strategies designed to optimize the level of original learning and thereby positively influence retention.

*The level of original learning for a task is the best single predictor of its long-term retention.*

The level of original learning is believed to be completed when a predetermined criterion of mastery has been reached. For example, a baseball coach might regard mastery of the skill of bunting as having been achieved when a player is able to bunt successfully on eight of every ten attempts. How automatically a learner is able to perform a particular skill has also been used as an indicator of learning. One very important way of determining the degree to which a skill has become automatic is to introduce a second skill and observe whether the learner has a sufficient reserve of attention to allocate to performance of the second skill while continuing to perform the first. How well the learner performs the two skills concurrently is a measure of the degree to which the primary skill has been learned.

## The Learner

*Ability level and past experiences affect how well a skill is remembered.*

An instructor has only to watch a class of students trying to recall a motor skill presented in a previous class to see that certain students are better able to recall the skill than are their classmates. Despite the fact that the instructor gave the same verbal instructions, demonstrated the skill in the same way, and provided the same amount of practice opportunities to everyone, some students are simply better able to recall the information necessary for performing the skill accurately. Why do these individual differences exist? More often than not, the ability level and past experiences of the learner affect how well a particular skill is remembered. Farr (1987) suggests that these characteristics of learners "have equipped them with a larger and more varied repertoire of memory-enhancing strategies" (p. 95).

The existence of a greater repertoire of memory strategies can therefore be expected to not only influence how long information can be retained, but also how quickly it can be retrieved from memory at the appropriate time (see highlight, The Structure of Skilled Memory). These memory differences

# HIGHLIGHT

## The Structure of Skilled Memory

How is it that certain people are capable of memorizing entire books, the days of the week associated with dates several thousand years ago, or the entire multiplication table for numbers between 1 and 100? Some researchers have been so fascinated by the abilities of these individuals that they have spent many years attempting to discover the underlying structure of what they refer to as skilled memory. Ericsson and Polson (1984), for example, studied J.C., a waiter who could memorize as many as 20 complete dinner orders. How was he able to accomplish this impressive feat? A review of the detailed observation notes compiled by these authors over a two-year study period reveals just how J.C. was able to remember such a large amount of information.

Instead of trying to recall each individual order in sequence, J.C. categorized the information into salad dressings that were encoded as a list of first letters corresponding to their names. For example if bleu cheese, oil and vinegar, oil and vinegar, and thousand island dressings were ordered by the first four members of the party, they were remembered as the word BOOT. In order to remember those items that were to accompany the entrée, J.C. used a different mnemonic strategy that involved encoding the food items into patterns (e.g., baked potato, rice, rice, baked potato = abba). Meat temperatures were encoded by first spatially associating them with a linear increase from rare to well-done and then expressing them with numbers from 1 to 4. J.C. finally associated each of the entrées ordered with the position of the person who was ordering it. What is perhaps most interesting about J.C.'s memory ability is that it was not limited to the recall of dinner orders. When asked to recall a new category of items, such as time intervals ranging from 1 second to 1 week, J.C. exhibited the same level of recall within two practice sessions. Apparently, the retrieval strategies he had developed for use in one situation were readily transferable to another.

The study of J.C. and many other skilled mnemonists led Chase and Ericsson (1982) to propose a theory of skilled memory that is predicated on three important principles: meaningful encoding, retrieval structure, and speed-up of memorization. They persuasively argue that individuals with skilled memory not only are capable of rapidly storing information in long-term memory (LTM) and then associating it with existing knowledge in a more meaningful way, but also can retrieve the information using a special set of retrieval cues that are explicitly associated with the information presented. The speed-up of memorization is a function of practice and can lead to storage rates in LTM that are equal to those of short-term memory (STM). The fact that the average individual can be trained to improve his or her memory skill significantly is an especially promising aspect of the theory.

were highlighted in a study conducted by Anderson and Reder (1979), who were able to distinguish between individuals who could recall historical facts well and those who could not. Those individuals with the better memory strategies were able to elaborate the information far beyond the content presented to them in a fictitious history passage during a free-recall test.

Although the instructor has little control over the abilities and past experiences an individual brings to a learning situation, it is important that individual differences be considered when designing the curriculum and instructing the class. It is clear that instructor-dominated approaches do little to capitalize on the strengths of the learner. In contrast, programs that emphasize self-paced learning or that place the responsibility for learning squarely in the hands and minds of the learner foster superior learning and long-term retention of skill-related knowledge.

## Disorders of Memory

Disorders of memory can result in anterograde and retrograde amnesia.

Disorders of memory may result from cerebral traumas that are either acute in nature (e.g., head trauma, hypoxia or ischemia, and transient global amnesia) or more gradual in onset (e.g., alcoholic amnestic (Korsakoff's) syndrome, brain tumor, and viral encephalitis). Selective memory loss is also observed: Some patients are unable to recall recent memories (**anterograde amnesia**), and others have difficulty retrieving more remote memories (**retrograde amnesia**). In some cases, these disruptions to memory are temporary; in others, they may be much longer lasting. In either case, the rehabilitation process is negatively affected. For example, recovering stroke patients are often unable to remember a set of instructions given as little as 30 seconds earlier even though they remain able to remember the minute details of events experienced some 30 years before. On some occasions, patients recall only a few bits of information from a series of commands, making it almost impossible for them to perform the activity correctly. The generalization of information is also problematic for these patients. It is most often observed when they are asked to perform an activity learned in one setting in a different setting. For example, a patient may learn to transfer from a hospital bed to a chair but may be unable to perform the same set of movements in the home. This inability to apply what has been learned in a practice situation to similar situations arising in daily life significantly slows the patient's return to independent functioning.

Mills (1988) provides a number of strategies for improving the memory of patients involved in a rehabilitation program. When a skill is first being presented to a recovering patient, for example, it is important to keep to a minimum any verbal descriptions and instructions related to how the task is to be performed. By this means, the therapist minimizes the confusion that can result from the overloading of working memory. One might even dispense with verbal instructions when introducing a skill, particularly when working with patients who have experienced damage to the right hemisphere following a stroke. Because these patients have difficulty remembering language, visual demonstrations may prove much more effective than verbal descriptions in conveying how best to perform a particular skill or exercise.

When verbal instructions *are* used to present a skill, the speed with which they are delivered should be carefully controlled. Speaking slowly and clearly will do much to enhance the amount of information understood. How effective the instructor has been in providing verbal instructions will soon be evident in the patient's or learner's response. The nature of the response should therefore be carefully monitored; where confusion is evident, subsequent instructions or demonstrations should be modified.

Self-paced practice should be encouraged so that the patient has adequate time to process the presented information and translate it into action.

Once the skill to be learned has been introduced, it is important that the patient be provided with an immediate opportunity to practice. Active rehearsal boosts the likelihood that the information will be transferred to long-term memory. Self-paced practice should also be encouraged so that the patient has enough time to process the information presented and then translate it into action. Imposing time constraints on action denies the patient sufficient time to rehearse and organize the information in a manner that is optimal for later retrieval and translation into action. Various part-task training methods are also useful for individuals with memory disorders or as-yet-undeveloped memory functions. These practice methods were discussed in greater depth in Chapter 9. The "Keep It Simple (KIS)" principle certainly should not be overlooked in these types of learning situations.

Mnemonic strategies and devices can enhance the learning process. These are most often provided in the form of verbal cues that the instructor uses to supplement a demonstration of the skill and highlight the important aspects of the task. These cues can then be repeated by the instructor as the learner practices the skill and can even be repeated by the learner as she or he prepares to practice. Encouraging learners to engage in self-talk, or verbal rehearsal, while they practice has been shown to increase how well a particular skill is recalled at a later time (Weiss, 1983; Weiss & Klint, 1987). This instructional technique was discussed further in Chapter 8. Mnemonic devices in the form of memory boards and logs are also frequently used in clinical facilities to help a patient remember a set of exercises or simply maintain a schedule. Skill-related cues written on sheets posted at activity stations set up in gymnasiums are also valuable for learners engaged in practicing many different types of skills at once.

> Mnemonic strategies and devices can enhance remembering and the learning process.

## Summary

One purpose of this chapter is to familiarize the reader with the construct of human memory and the nature of the operations involved in the acquisition, rehearsal, organization, and recall of skill-related information. Memory is generally divided into two components: short-term and long-term memory. Terms used to differentiate the various types of memory include recall, recognition, intentional, nondeclarative (implicit), declarative, and procedural memory. Whatever labels are used, it is the type of memory function that largely differentiates one kind from the other.

Another purpose was to introduce the reader to how memory and forgetting are studied. The storage and retrieval of the learned capability for producing a movement performance is the process of memory. The loss of the ability to store and/or retrieve the information needed for producing a movement performance is the process of forgetting. The durability of the learned changes in movement performance can be demonstrated over time without practice (that is, following a retention interval, or RI) and is referred to as retention. Memory and forgetting are processes that operate within the learner and hence cannot be directly observed and measured. What can be directly observed and measured is a learner's motor performance in acquisition and on a retention test following an RI, which can be used as evidence from which to draw inferences about memory and forgetting of motor learning.

Care must be taken in our experimental design and procedures to control for contaminating effects due to variables (e.g., changes in motivation, inappropriate warm-up, and reminiscence) that could operate during acquisition and over an RI to confound the effects due to learning, memory, and forgetting, and could seriously limit the inferences that can be made about these processes.

The trace decay, interference, and retrieval theories of memory were discussed. The trace decay theory holds that forgetting is simply due to the passage of time. Interference theory proposes that forgetting is due to competing responses that occur during the RI. Competing responses learned before learning the criterion response (proactive interference) or after learning it (retroactive interference) are the cause of forgetting. Retrieval theory contends that the memory trace of the capability for producing a learned movement performance is not forgotten and that forgetting occurs because the memory trace cannot be found and so it cannot be recalled. Retention also has been found to be a function of the type of movement skill. Continuous tasks are more resistant to forgetting than are discrete, serial, and procedural tasks, but much more research is needed, especially studies on long-term retention. Research also is needed that examines the three theories of forgetting in relation to the type of movement skill to be learned.

Several variables have been demonstrated to influence the learning and retention of verbal and motor skills. They include the level of original learning, the characteristics of the skill to be learned, the nature of the learning conditions, and the inherent abilities and past experiences of the learner. Research in this area has yielded several strategies that are recommended for the teacher and clinician whose goal is to optimize the learning and long-term retention of cognitive and motor skills. Integral to all of these strategies is the idea that the learner must be actively involved in the learning process.

## IMPORTANT TERMINOLOGY

After completing this chapter, readers should be familiar with the following terms and concepts.

absolute retention score
anterograde amnesia
consolidation theory
declarative knowledge
declarative (explicit) memory
difference score
encoding specificity explanation
equipotentiality
explicit retention test
forgetting
forgetting hypothesis
generation-recognition explanation
implicit learning
implicit retention test
incidental memory
intentional memory
interference theory
knowledge compilation
levels-of-processing framework

long-term memory (LTM)
memory
mental search explanation
mnemonic strategies
multistore model of stages of
    memory consolidation
nondeclarative (implicit) memory
percent relative retention score
primacy-recency effect
proactive interference
procedural knowledge
procedural memory
recall memory
recognition memory
rehearsal
relative retention score
reminiscence
retention
retention interval (RI)

retrieval theory
retroactive interference
retrograde amnesia
savings score
set hypothesis

short-term memory (STM)
short-term sensory stage (STSS)
trace decay theory
warm-up decrement

## SUGGESTED FURTHER READING

Awh, E., Jonides, J., Smith, E. E., Buxton, R. B., Frank, L. R., Love, T. E. C., & Gmeindl, L. (1999). Rehearsal in spatial working memory: Evidence from neuroimaging. *Psychological Science, 10,* 433–437.

Baxter, M. F., & Baxter, D. A. (1999). Neural mechanisms of learning and memory. In H. Cohen (Ed.), *Neuroscience for Rehabilitation* (2nd ed.). Philadelphia, PA: Lippincott, Williams & Wilkins.

Imanaka, K., & Abernethy, B. (1992). Interference between location and distance information in motor short-term memory: The respective roles of direct kinesthetic signals and abstract codes. *Journal of Motor Behavior, 24,* 274–280.

Kimberg, D. Y., D'Esposito, M., & Farah, M. J. (1998). Cognitive functions in the prefrontal cortex: Working memory and executive control. *Current Directions in Psychological Science, 6,* 185–192.

Roediger, H. L. (1990). Implicit memory: Retention without remembering. *American Psychologist, 45,* 1043–1056.

## TEST YOUR UNDERSTANDING

1. Cite the major features of the multistore model of memory. How does this view of memory differ from the levels-of-processing framework proposed by Craik and Lockhart (1972)?

2. What is the memory principle of equipotentiality? What types of measurement were used to provide support for this principle?

3. Identify the areas of the central nervous system that have been shown to play a role in memory.

4. Briefly describe the condition known as anterograde amnesia.

5. How does declarative memory differ from procedural memory?

6. According to Anderson, how does the role of memory change as a new cognitive skill is acquired?

7. Cite three factors that have been shown to influence how well a skill is retained for later recall.

8. Differentiate among the terms *memory, forgetting, retention,* and *learning.*

9. Explain the theories of forgetting, including warm-up decrement, and provide an example of how each works.

10. Prepare an experimental design and procedures to study the retention of motor learning, proactive interference, and retroactive interference.

11. Provide numerical examples of how the following retention measures are calculated: absolute retention score, savings score, difference score, and percent relative retention score. Also, explain what each score is measuring.

12. Identify several variables that can contaminate temporary performance effects with the performance effects due to the retention (memory or forgetting) of motor learning, and explain how this contamination occurs and how to control for it.

13. Give movement examples of the following terms: *recall memory, recognition memory, implicit learning, implicit retention, explicit retention,* and *reminiscence.*

# 12

# TRANSFER OF
# MOTOR LEARNING

*Transfer of motor learning is the process by which learning a movement task under one set of conditions influences the performance of a subsequent task under the same or different conditions.*

After studying this chapter, you should be able to:

- Explain the nature and types of transfer of learning and performance, especially as they relate to movement skills.

- Describe how transfer depends on similarity between the training (practice) task/conditions and the real-world (transfer) task/conditions and what the implications are for designing training conditions to facilitate transfer of learning for movement skills.

- Describe what general factors are thought to transfer and what the implications are for structuring training conditions to facilitate transfer of learning for movement skills.

- Explain (a) how level of original learning, background knowledge (expertise), perceived similarity, and transfer-appropriate processing

operate to influence the transfer of learning and performance and (b) what the implications are for designing training conditions to facilitate transfer of learning for movement skills.

- Explain how transfer of learning and performance is studied, especially with respect to the experimental designs and procedures used to study bilateral, proactive, and retroactive transfer.

- Demonstrate how transfer of learning and performance is measured, especially in terms of percentage of transfer and savings score methods.

- Explain why it is important to know how transfer was measured when interpreting transfer of learning effects.

In developing children and adults, **transfer of learning** (also called transfer of training) is pervasive in everyday life. For example, the learning students acquire at one grade level in school is expected to transfer to the new learning that takes place at the next grade level, and the learning that takes place in school and college is expected, to some extent, to transfer to work and everyday living tasks in the nonacademic world. How well athletes perform in game situations greatly depends on how well they are able to transfer what was practiced and learned in training. Similarly, how effective stroke patients are at walking again in various real-world settings greatly depends on how well they are able to transfer what was learned in the clinical training setting. Thus, our educational system and virtually all training or practice programs such as those used in clinical rehabilitation, sport, military, or occupational settings are based on the assumption that much of what was learned in one situation can be transferred to another situation.

Many things learned in one situation can be transferred, including knowledge or expertise, cognitive and movement skills, strategies, attitudes, emotions, concepts, and perceptions. However, in this chapter the focus is mainly on the transfer of movement task learning and performance and on the conditions that affect it. With each passing year of life, learning how to perform new movement patterns or skills under previously experienced or new conditions becomes more and more a matter of transfer of learning rather than original learning. New movement patterns and skills largely are learned on the foundation of previously acquired patterns and skills. Based on the movement focus of this chapter, we define the **transfer of motor learning** as the process by which learning a movement task under one set of conditions influences the performance of a subsequent movement task under the same or different conditions.

Clearly, transfer of motor learning is widespread in everyday life in people of all ages. But, what are the principles regarding effective transfer? What variables and conditions optimize transfer? How should training or practice programs be structured to facilitate transfer? The answers to these and other related questions are essential if practitioners expect to design training (practice) programs that promote effective transfer of motor learning and performance. Practitioners are in a position to either facilitate or interfere with the transfer of a person's motor learning and performance, depending on what they know about transfer and how they apply that knowledge. Consequently, this chapter focuses on that knowledge and its applications.

## Transfer of Motor Learning Depends on Similarity

The idea that transfer of motor learning depends on the structural similarity between the training and transfer tasks emanated from the **identical elements theory** (Thorndike, 1903; Thorndike & Woodworth, 1901). This theory held that transfer depended on the extent to which the training and transfer tasks shared identical elements. The more shared elements the more similar the two tasks, and the more the transfer of learning from the training to the transfer task. One difficulty with the identical elements theory was that it was unclear exactly what defined identical elements. Some thought identical elements referred to mental elements, but typically they have been interpreted to mean stimulus-response connections. Let's look more closely at how stimulus-response connections have been used to explain and predict the direction and amount of transfer.

*To a large extent, new movement patterns and skills are learned on the foundation of previously acquired movement patterns and skills.*

*Transfer of motor learning is a process by which learning a movement task under one set of conditions influences the performance of a subsequent movement task under the same or different conditions.*

*The identical elements theory proposes that transfer depends on the extent to which the training and transfer tasks shared identical elements.*

# Direction and Amount of Transfer

The **direction of transfer** from one task to another can be positive, negative, or zero. It is (a) **positive transfer** when the training task enhances performance of the transfer task; (b) **negative transfer** when the training task interferes with performance of the transfer task; and (c) **zero transfer** when the training task has no effect on the transfer task. The **amount of transfer** refers to the quantity or magnitude of what was transferred. Although an abundance of empirical findings related to predicting the direction and amount of transfer has accumulated over the years, the theoretical picture is still not completely clear. Consequently, it is still not possible to accurately predict the direction and amount of transfer in all situations mainly because of incomplete knowledge of *what* is actually learned in training and *how* the transfer task is represented (Cormier & Hagman, 1987).

In spite of this limitation there is much that is known, which can be very helpful in predicting transfer in many situations. For instance, the amount and direction of transfer is a function of the similarity of the relationship between the structure of the training and transfer tasks (Osgood, 1949; Ellis, 1965; Holding, 1965). Essentially, the greater the similarity between task structures in terms of stimulus and response requirements, the greater the positive transfer between them. Moreover, **stimulus generalization** can occur when a particular response is learned to a stimulus and similar stimuli evoke the same response. Similarly, **response generalization** can occur when a response has been learned to a specific stimulus and the stimulus elicits similar responses. Thus, we can learn to associate the same response to a given range of stimuli as well as a range of responses to a particular stimulus.

> Stimulus generalization occurs when a particular response is learned to a stimulus and similar stimuli evoke the same response.

Osgood (1949) attempted to diagram the relationship of stimulus-response similarity and amount and direction of transfer using a **transfer surface** that allows for different degrees of similarity. Osgood's transfer surface was originally intended to make predictions about the transfer of verbal learning, and many of his predictions have been verified in the learning of pairs of words (Bugelski & Cadwallader, 1956; Dallett, 1962). However, Osgood's transfer surface also has been the target of motor skills research because of its apparent relevance for explaining and predicting the transfer of motor learning. Osgood's transfer surface also may be expressed in a simplified summary table (see Table 12.1), and the six examples below provide further detail.

> Response generalization occurs when a response has been learned to a specific stimulus and the stimulus elicits similar responses.

*Example 1: Highly Positive Transfer.*   The stimuli and responses of the training task and conditions are the same as or highly similar to those of the transfer task and conditions, and the direction and amount of transfer should be highly positive. For instance, if we have learned to use a particular golf, tennis, or basketball shot (response) under certain stimulus conditions, using it the next time those or similar conditions appear is simply a continuation of the same learning process.

*Example 2: Slightly Positive Transfer.*   The stimuli between the training task and conditions are the same as or highly similar to those in the transfer task and conditions; but, because the responses required are similar but not the same, we would predict the direction and amount of transfer to be slightly rather than highly positive at the beginning of learning the transfer task. For instance, if we have learned to use a particular golf, tennis, or basketball shot

> The greater the similarity between stimulus conditions and responses of the training and transfer tasks, the greater the positive transfer.

**Table 12.1**
**Direction and Amount of Transfer Depends on the Stimulus-Response Similarity of Training and Transfer Tasks**

| Example | Stimuli | Responses | Transfer Tendency |
|---|---|---|---|
| 1 | Same or highly similar | Same | High positive |
| 2 | Same or highly similar in critical ways | Similar and do not differ | Slightly positive |
| 3 | Same or highly similar discernable | Dissimilar and easily | None (zero) |
| 4 | Same or highly similar critical ways | Similar, but differ in | Negative |
| 5 | Dissimilar | Same | Slightly positive |
| 6 | Dissimilar | Dissimilar | None (zero) |

(response) under certain stimulus conditions, we should find it somewhat easy to learn to use a slight variation of the shot under the same conditions provided the similar shot does not differ in any critical way from the way the shot was originally learned. Essentially, the greater the similarity between the stimulus conditions and responses of the training and transfer tasks, the greater the positive transfer from the training task to the transfer task (Ammons, Ammons, & Morgan, 1956; Gagne, Baker, & Foster, 1950; Leonard, Karnes, Oxendine, & Hesson, 1970; Nelson, 1957b).

***Example 3: Zero Transfer.***   The stimuli between the training task and conditions are the same as or highly similar to the transfer task and conditions; but, because the responses are dissimilar, we would expect little or no transfer at the outset of learning the transfer task. Sometimes negative transfer occurs over which a response is appropriate to make to the same stimulus, but this typically does not occur when the training and transfer tasks are dissimilar and easily discernible (Gagne, Baker, & Foster, 1950).

***Example 4: Negative Transfer.***   Negative transfer is more likely to occur when the stimuli between training and transfer task and conditions are the same or highly similar, and the movement responses between tasks are similar, but differ enough in critical ways to cause some interference (Siipola, 1941). For instance, if we have learned to perform a particular golf, tennis, or basketball shot in a certain way under one set of stimulus conditions, we are likely to have some difficulty (especially at the outset) in learning to perform it using similar movements in a different way under the same stimulus conditions. Negative transfer is likely to occur when movements of the same length, duration, and force are made in one direction in the training task (e.g., to the left) and in the other direction in the transfer task (e.g., to the right) or when the difference between upward and downward movement is all that matters (Adams, 1954; Holding, 1965).

An example of the negative transfer effect produced by such a reversal of movement responses is evident when someone who learned to drive a car in

Negative transfer tends to occur when movement responses learned to be made in one direction now must be made in the opposite (reverse) direction.

the United States now has to drive a car in Australia, because some of the movement responses are reversed (opposite). For instance, (a) one drives on the right-hand side of the road in the United States, but on the left-hand side in Australia; (b) a left-hand turn in the United States is the same as a right-hand turn in Australia and vice versa; and (c) traffic circles ("roundabouts") are driven in a counter-clockwise direction in the United States, but in a clockwise direction in Australia. In this situation the stimulus conditions are essentially the same or highly similar, but the responses are reversed, which can easily lead to confusion about what to do in the transfer situation. A similar situation has been shown to lead to negative transfer under controlled conditions in the laboratory using a piloting-type task called a Mashburn task (Lewis, McAllister, & Adams, 1951; McAllister, 1953). However, the negative transfer produced in situations in which responses are reversed is likely to have been due to cognitive confusion about what to do, which in turn prompted incorrect responses to be selected and performed. In other words, the negative transfer produced probably was due to more cognitive confusion than to motor interference (Ross, 1974).

> Negative transfer produced by the reversal of responses is probably due to cognitive confusion about what to do rather than to motor interference.

An example that illustrates more motor than cognitive interference was evident during the evolution of the butterfly stroke in swimming (Fischman, Christina, & Vercruyssen, 1982). Prior to the 1960s the butterfly stroke was swum using a breaststroke kick. The introduction of the dolphin kick caused some negative transfer among butterfly swimmers because of the pairing of the new kick with the traditional butterfly arm stroke. Apparently, the breaststroke kick competed somewhat with the dolphin kick when the latter was being learned to be performed with the butterfly arm stroke. This type of negative transfer is often seen in sports such as golf or baseball where a player is trying to learn to make major changes in swing technique to improve performance.

Another situation that has been applied to Example 4 is that of *bilateral transfer,* where training is transferred from the right hand to the left hand, arm to arm, leg to leg, or arm to opposite leg. These combinations often yield positive rather than negative transfer at the outset of learning the transfer task because the responses are not different. The response is the same in the training and transfer tasks, but it is performed with different limbs. Thus, applying bilateral transfer to the fourth example is not really appropriate. (More will be said about bilateral transfer on page 376.)

### *Example 5: Slightly Positive Transfer.*

If the stimulus conditions are dissimilar and the responses are the same between the training and transfer tasks and conditions, we would predict the direction of transfer to be slightly positive early in learning the transfer task. For instance, if we have learned to use a particular offensive play (response) under certain stimulus conditions of the game of soccer, we should find it somewhat easy at the outset to learn to use the same play under dissimilar stimulus conditions such as those found in basketball. The pass-and-go play is an example of such a play in which we would expect to have slightly positive transfer from soccer to basketball. Another example would be having to respond by stopping your car or bicycle at a traffic intersection to a green (rather than a red) light and driving through the intersection to a red (rather than a green) light. There is a good chance of the transfer being slightly positive at the outset of learning in such situations.

# HIGHLIGHT

### Generalizability of Learning:
### How Early Does It Begin?

In the motor development laboratory at Indiana University, infants as young as 12 months of age have demonstrated the ability to generalize their learning in one movement context to vastly different movement contexts (Titzer, Smith & Thelen, 1995). This rather surprising finding emerged when young infants who had participated in an earlier study designed to investigate whether infants could learn the perceptual properties associated with opaque and transparent surfaces were subsequently able to perform a very different movement task not usually observed at such a young age.

In the first of the two studies, 8-month-old infants were provided with an assortment of either transparent or opaque containers with which they played for 10 minutes per day over a two-month training period. The researchers were primarily interested in knowing whether increasing an infant's exploratory experience with the different types of containers would enhance her or his ability to retrieve objects placed within the different types of containers.

Not only did the two months of playing experience with the containers lead to greatly improved performance on an object retrieval task performed by the trained infants, but it also facilitated their performance on a second, very different developmental task: crawling across the well-known "visual cliff." After watching four of the infants who had participated in the earlier container study cross the transparent cliff surface with little hesitation in a later study, the researchers decided to test whether playing with transparent containers, in particular, contributed to the infants' ability to cross the visual cliff. The now 12-month-old infants who had played with transparent containers between 8 and 10 months of age were brought back into the laboratory, and their performance on the visual cliff task was compared to that of the infants who had played with opaque containers.

The results indicated that 71.4% of the infants in the transparent container group crossed the visual cliff, whereas only 30% of the infants in the opaque container group could perform the task. A second observation of special note was

---

Zero transfer would be expected when stimuli and responses between training and transfer tasks and conditions are dissimilar.

*Example 6: Zero Transfer.*    If the stimuli and responses are dissimilar between the training and transfer tasks and conditions, we would predict no (zero) transfer from the training tasks to the transfer task (Burdenshaw, Spragens, & Weis, 1970; Lindberg, 1949; Nelson 1957a). For instance, if we have learned to use a particular golf, tennis, or basketball shot (response) under certain conditions, we should find that such learning has no effect on learning to do the crawl stroke in swimming.

## Extent of Transfer

Generalization of transfer refers to the extent to which original task training will transfer to other tasks.

Being able to predict the **generalization of transfer** (see highlight, above), that is, the extent to which the original task training will transfer to other tasks is as important as being able to predict the direction and amount of transfer. It appears that the **extent of transfer** is influenced by the nature of the intertask relationships and the amount as well as variety of previous training experienced by the learner. Also, it seems that the inability to accurately pre-

HIGHLIGHT, CONTINUED

that all the infants in the transparent container group patted the cliff's transparent Plexiglas surface before crossing. None of the infants who crossed the cliff in the opaque container group patted the surface prior to crossing.

The researchers concluded that the activity of playing with transparent containers, in particular, assisted the infants in deriving haptic, visual, and auditory information that could be used to develop a perceptual category for transparency. They further reasoned that touching the visual cliff's surface prior to crossing reinforced the infant's decision that the surface was navigable.

Results such as these clearly illustrate the importance of enriching young infants' environments as a means of developing their knowledge of different perceptual properties that can then be applied to performance in future movement contexts. The study also illustrates just how early we can begin to generalize global perceptual knowledge acquired in one movement context to other, quite different settings.

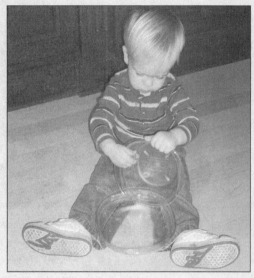

Playing with transparent containers helped the infants derive important haptic, visual, and auditory information that could be used to develop a perceptual category for transparency.

dict the extent of transfer in various situations is largely due to an incomplete understanding of *what* is learned in training, and *how* the transfer task itself is represented.

***Transfer-Appropriate Processing.***   In an attempt to better understand the generalization of transfer, researchers have placed more emphasis on studying *how* rather than *what* knowledge and skills are used. The former emphasis focuses on studying transfer as a function of the similarity of the goals between the training and transfer tasks and how the knowledge and skills of the training and transfer tasks are processed in relation to (a) the abilities underlying learning and performance, (b) the contextual conditions in which the learning and performance occurs, and (c) sensory feedback available for improving and controlling performance. In contrast, the latter emphasis focuses on what knowledge, skills, abilities, contextual conditions and sensory feedback conditions are the same or similar between the training and transfer tasks. The "what" emphasis, which was discussed in Chapter 9, emanates largely from identical elements theory (Thorndike, 1903; Thorndike & Woodworth, 1901)

The inability to accurately predict direction, amount, and extent of transfer in many situations is probably due to an incomplete understanding of what is learned and how the transfer task is represented.

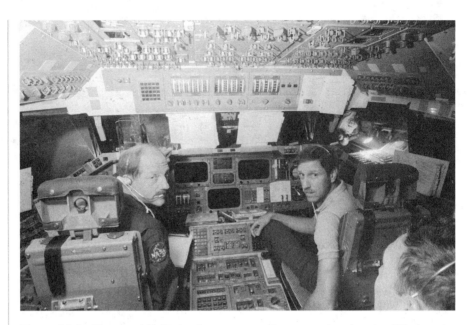

**Figure 12.1**   The use of flight simulators rests on the assumption that the skills, knowledge, and processing acquired in training will transfer to the real-world setting in which an aircraft is actually flown.

*Source:* National Aeronautics and Space Administration (2002).
http://spaceflight.nasa.gov/gallery/images/shuttle/sts-98/html/jsc2000-04775.html

TAP holds that transfer is not merely a function of the similarity between the training and transfer tasks and conditions, but also the similarity of the goals and cognitive processing between them.

and in the motor domain from the specificity of practice (learning) principle. (For reviews see Fleishman, 1972, 1978; Henry, 1958.) The "how" emphasis, also mentioned in Chapter 9, does not view transfer as being guaranteed merely because the same knowledge and skills are present in the training task as are needed to successfully perform the transfer task.

The knowledge and skills must not only be the same in both tasks, but the way in which they are used (processed) must be the same in both tasks as illustrated in Figure 12.1 (e.g., Anderson, 1987; Battig, 1979; Bransford & Franks, 1976; Bransford, Franks, Morris, & Stein, 1979; Morris, et al., 1977, 1979). For example, transfer would be predicted when the same knowledge and skills are used in the same way across training and transfer tasks. However, less or no transfer would be predicted when the same knowledge and skills are used in different ways across training and transfer tasks. This research approach, referred to as **transfer-appropriate processing (TAP),** studies transfer of learning as a function of the similarity of goals and processing between training and transfer tasks. Essentially, TAP holds that it is not merely the similarity between the training and transfer tasks and conditions, but also the *similarity of the goals and cognitive processing* between them that determines the transfer of movement learning.

The TAP concept also has penetrated the motor domain (e.g., Coull, et al., 2001; Lee, 1988; Schmidt, 1988b, pp. 401–402; Shea & Morgan, 1979; Tremblay & Proteau, 2001; Wright & Shea, 1991, 1994) and extended the traditional specificity of practice (learning) hypothesis. This hypothesis simply held that transfer of learning and performance was largely a function of the similarity of the movement task and conditions between training and transfer (e.g., Barnett et al., 1973; Henry, 1958). Thus, according to the specificity hypothesis, all one had to do to optimize transfer was simply match training task and conditions to transfer task and conditions. However, the TAP concept clearly argues that transfer is not as simple as the specificity hypothesis would have us believe. Instead, it holds that not only must the movement task and conditions be the same or similar as proposed by the specificity hypothesis, but the way in which they are processed must be the same or similar to maximize transfer of learning and performance. In fact, one might introduce conditions in training (e.g., contextual interference) that simulate those anticipated in the real world under which the task will have to be performed so that the processing needed to successfully learn and perform the task is acquired (see Figure 8.5). In this sense, TAP extends the specificity hypothesis by adding cognitive processing to the mix of movement task and conditions. Although much more research is needed before the role of TAP in the transfer of movement learning and performance is completely understood, the concept is intuitively appealing and appears to hold considerable promise. Unfortunately, at the present time little is known about the exact nature of the appropriate processes acquired in movement task training and the capability of these processes transferring to dissimilar movement tasks and conditions. Clearly, much more research is needed to enhance our knowledge in these areas.

*Practical Implication.*   What is the practical implication of the TAP concept? Practitioners who want to structure a learning environment based on the TAP concept would try to match the type of processing activities in which the learner engaged during training to those that would be required or expected in future transfer settings. Positive transfer is thought to be enhanced by making the processing activities the same or similar between the training and transfer tasks and conditions (such as different movement conditions or the performance of a new but similar movement pattern). For example, suppose a coach structures a practice environment in which a gymnast is learning a new and more difficult somersault while suspended in a harness above a trampoline. Although the practice conditions are unlike the competitive conditions in which the skill will ultimately be performed, the coach has the performer practice the somersault exactly the way it would be performed in competition. Thus, the gymnast is not only learning to perform the *same skill* in training (practice) and transfer (competition), but also is learning to perform the skill in the *same way* in training and transfer. This insures not only that the movement task is the same, but the cognitive processing that is necessary for successfully performing the skill on a floor exercise mat in competition is the same.

A case study that provides some evidence supporting the TAP concept in a sport setting was conducted by Christina, Barresi, and Shaffner (1990). Essentially, they structured the practice (training) conditions to develop one type of cognitive processing appropriate for playing an outside linebacker's position in football. The linebacker's problem was that he was responding quickly enough in game situations but all too often was selecting the incorrect defensive response to execute. Thus, practice conditions were designed to

The TAP concept extends the traditional specificity of practice (learning) hypothesis by proposing that transfer not only depends on the similarity of tasks and conditions between training and transfer, but also the similarity of goals and processing activities.

The TAP concept suggests that practitioners structure practice conditions so that the person learns to perform the same movement skills in the same ways in training as will be required in transfer (real-world setting).

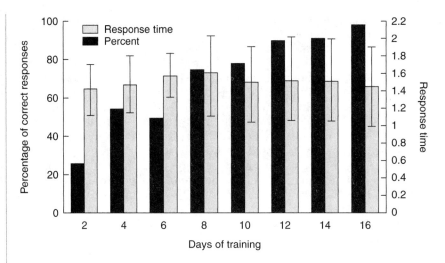

**Figure 12.2** Percentage of correct responses and mean response time (including standard deviations) as a function of days of video training in which responses were made by a football linebacker as quickly and accurately as possible to a series of offensive plays.

*Source:* Christina, R. W., Barresi, J. V., & Shaffner, P. (1990). The development of response selection accuracy in a football linebacker using video training. *The Sport Psychologist, 4,* 11–17.

develop cognitive processing appropriate for selecting the correct defensive response as quickly as possible. The task required the linebacker to view 40 offensive plays that were displayed on a video monitor and presented in a random order. The plays were similar to those an outside linebacker would ordinarily experience in a game situation, and they were seen from about the same viewing angle. The linebacker, who was seated in front of a video monitor, was instructed to view the videotape simulation of each play and to respond as quickly and accurately as possible to the cues of the play by moving a joystick in the direction in which he would ordinarily move in a game situation. He trained four days a week for four weeks. The 16 sessions consisted of eight practice and eight test days that were alternated such that the first day was practice, the second day was test, and so forth. The results, shown in Figure 12.2, clearly revealed that there was an improvement in response selection accuracy without sacrificing response selection speed (time). Based on two coaches' evaluations, this improvement transferred from the training setting to practice and game situations. Thus, the linebacker's movement responses and training conditions were very different than they were in actual practices and games, but the goals and cognitive processing involved in selecting the correct responses was the same.

Similarly, if the rehabilitation setting can be structured so that the patient, while performing various rehabilitation exercises, engages in processing activities that are the same or similar to those required to perform various activities of daily life, then positive transfer is expected. Support for the idea that such an approach fosters positive transfer was provided in a study involving a group of older adults who were experiencing balance problems (Rose & Clark, 1995). These adults participated in a two-month training program and performed a wide variety of dynamic balance activities in a seated and standing position on specialized balance training equipment. In order to investigate whether the adults could transfer what they had learned during training to the performance of daily activities, including gait, the adults were tested prior to and following the training intervention on their ability to perform functional tasks that required balance and again included gait. Significant improvements were observed in their ability to perform balance-related skills (e.g., transfer between chairs, turn in a circle, retrieve an object from the floor) and to walk more quickly.

## Additional Factors Influencing Transfer

At least three additional factors have been found to affect the direction, amount, and/or extent of transfer. These factors include the (a) level of original learning of the task to be transferred, (b) background knowledge or expertise of the learner, and (c) perceived similarity between the training task and setting and those of the real-world (transfer) task and setting. Each of these factors is discussed next.

*Level of Original Learning.*    It has been known for some time that increasing the amount of quality practice can increase the **level of original learning** (level of performance achieved in acquisition or training), which is likely to enhance long-term retention and transfer of that learning and performance to real-world settings. (For reviews see Christina & Bjork, 1991; Ericsson, 2001.) Indeed, positive transfer can be expected to increase with the level of original learning, provided that structurally similar responses are required in training and transfer tasks (Ellis, 1965). In addition to increasing the amount of quality practice, any variable (e.g., manipulation of practice variability, augmented feedback, and contextual interference) that can help people achieve a higher or more complete level of original learning of the task is capable of enhancing its long-term retention and transfer (Farr, 1987; Hurlock & Montague, 1982). For instance, delaying or giving less frequent augmented feedback during practice, using variable practice within and among movement skills, or increasing the amount of contextual interference during practice by simulating real-world conditions may be conceptualized as being functionally equivalent to increasing the amount of quality practice.

Positive transfer of learning can be expected to increase with the level of original learning, provided structurally similar responses are demanded in training and transfer.

In other words, the level of original learning during practice is being indirectly increased by appropriately manipulating such variables and hence may be conceived as an analog to directly increasing the level of original learning by increasing the amount of quality practice. In golf, for example, appropriate manipulation of these variables would actually create transfer-training conditions that would make practice more like actual play and learning more specific to the way one plays (Christina & Alpenfels, 2002). One resulting effect would be that golf skills would be more difficult to learn to perform under these transfer-training conditions. Appropriate manipulation of these variables also would encourage players to be more cognitively engaged in the learning and performing process, which should produce a higher or more complete level of learning and thus facilitate positive transfer to actual playing conditions. While intuitively appealing, this proposal is based on a limited amount of research from contexts other than golf. Further research is needed within a golf context before the validity can be ascertained.

*Background Knowledge.*   The influence of a learner's **background knowledge,** or expertise, on the learning of new knowledge and its transfer also has been a target of some research. For instance, Bransford and Franks (1976) studied how prior knowledge about baseball transferred to a novel task involving the classification of visual patterns into two categories. They found that providing a baseball framework in training based on prior knowledge had a positive influence on transfer. However, providing a framework in training based on prior knowledge is not likely to enhance transfer unless it can be used to improve one's understanding of concepts and formulas that permit proficient application of the learned knowledge (Mayer, 1975, 1985; Mayer & Greeno, 1972). Further, providing such a framework will only result in positive transfer if it is structurally similar to the transfer subject matter (Burstein, 1986; Gentner & Gentner, 1983).

Also related to background knowledge is the influence of expertise in a subject area (e.g., physics) on transfer. There is evidence that experts alter their basis for classifying problems from surface to more abstract structural characteristics of problems that cue principles pertinent to the solution (Chi et al., 1981). The experts' altered classifications or categories may change their perceived similarity of problems and thus influence different kinds of transfer (Novick, 1986).

Much more research is needed on expertise and transfer—especially to determine the conditions that enable experts to transfer strategies to more complex problems not only in their domain of expertise, but outside of that domain as well. (Of course, the problems outside their domain of expertise would be related to it to some extent.) Research with the same focus would also be useful in the motor domain to better understand the influence of expertise on transfer. There has been some research looking at expertise in the motor domain, but much more is needed. (For reviews see Abernethy, Thomas, & Thomas, 1993; Housner & French, 1994.)

*Perceived Similarity.*   Whether transfer of task learning from the training setting to the real-world setting is even attempted depends on the extent to which the two settings are perceived as being similar (Gick & Holyoak, 1987; Holyoak, 1985). If the performer does not recognize that the movement task or strategy (e.g., offensive or defensive play) is appropriate to use in the real-world setting, the task or strategy will not be attempted. For example, a young basketball player who recently learned how to perform a bounce pass in practice may not perceive when to use it in game situations and so not even attempt to use it.

**Perceived similarity** between two settings depends, in part, on any salient shared component (surface or structural). Components of a setting are structural if they are causally or functionally related in goal attainment, and they are surface when they are not. For example, learning the various game situations in which the bounce pass is most appropriate to use in practice is a structural component because this learning is likely to transfer and result

*(margin notes)* Whether transfer of training-task learning is even attempted depends on the extent to which the two settings are perceived as similar.

Perceived similarity between two settings depends on any salient shared surface or structural component.

in the bounce pass being used effectively in actual games (goal attainment). Further, learning to perform the bounce pass under competitive pressure in practice that attempts to simulate pressure likely to be experienced in games also is a structural component because learning is likely to result in the bounce pass being used appropriately in games.

In addition to structural components, practice and game settings also will have surface features that may be the same or different. For instance, the height of the basket, the dimensions of the basketball court, and the size of the basketball will be the same between practice and game settings, but in actual games the opposing team players against whom the bounce pass will be performed will be different than they were in practice. These examples constitute surface features because they are functionally unrelated to the situations in which the bounce pass is most appropriate to use.

Perceived similarity between training and the real-world tasks and settings is a function of shared surface or structural components and of several other factors such as knowledge or expertise and context of the two settings. A person's knowledge or expertise of the task, to a great extent, determines whether salient similarities observed are surface or structural. The context of the real-world setting (transfer setting) is specified by the events that take place near it in time or that are retrieved from memory during performance of the task in the real-world setting (transfer task). Whether the direction of the actual transfer is positive or negative depends on the objective structural similarity (e.g., as shown in Table 12.1 on page 360) between the training and real-world tasks and settings. Transfer is positive when the training and transfer responses are highly similar, that is, they contain many shared structural components and few distinctive ones. Transfer is negative when the training and real-world responses are less similar, that is, they contain few shared components and many distinctive ones. The amount of transfer obtained between settings, however, is a function of perceived similarity. The greater the perceived similarity of the two settings, the greater the amount of transfer. Of course, no transfer would be expected to occur when the two settings are perceived as unrelated, regardless of the degree of objective structural response similarity.

> The greater the perceived similarity between training and transfer settings, the greater the amount of transfer.

Perceived similarity has been the target of research investigating the cognitive basis of knowledge transfer. The topic is intuitively appealing and does contribute to our understanding of how the transfer of knowledge takes place. Moreover, it is relevant to the transfer of motor learning because every learned movement task (a) has a perceptual–cognitive component and demands decision making to some extent and (b) can be influenced by a person's previously acquired knowledge. For instance, having well-learned batting skills in baseball (e.g., *how* to control and coordinate movements to hit a baseball) is a prerequisite for successful hitting performance, but so too is deciding *what to do*, which involves deciding what pitch to swing at and knowing what type of swing to make in relation to the type of pitch thrown and the game situation. The batter's capability to appropriately make use of the previously acquired knowledge that is specific to deciding what to do is essential to successful performance. Clearly, the topic of perceived similarity is relevant to our understanding the transfer of motor learning, especially the perceptual cognitive component. In spite of its relevance, however, it has not been the target of very much research in the motor domain.

# Transfer of General Factors

Identical elements theory can account for some of the transfer that is observed, but it cannot account for all of it. Moreover, there is research evidence indicating that some transfer can be accounted for by general factors such as principles of problem solving, strategies, laws, rules, and learning to learn. **Transfer of general factors** will be discussed next.

## Transfer of Principles

In addition to identical elements, general principles have been shown to transfer from training to transfer settings.

Another explanation for transfer of learning was first proposed by Judd (1908), who took exception to the extent and nature of Thorndike's theory of identical elements. He and others (Hendrickson & Schroeder, 1941) presented evidence that learners could use or apply *general* principles to transfer learning from one task to another. Judd's view was quite different than that of Thorndike, who held that transfer could be accounted for by identical elements, that is, elements that were the same in both the training and the transfer tasks.

Other studies involving motor skills have shown that knowledge of principles, strategies, and relationships can transfer from the training task to the transfer task (e.g., Broer, 1958; Mohr & Barrett, 1962; Papcsy, 1968). Werner (1972) demonstrated that teaching four science concepts involving levers, Newton's first and third laws of motion, and work to fourth, fifth, and sixth grade students transferred to a variety of gross movement tasks. Taken together, the findings from these studies involving motor skills show that biomechanical principles can be transferred from the training task to the transfer task.

Mechanical principles have been shown to transfer from the training task to the transfer task in the motor domain.

There are, however, instances in which the use of mechanical principles failed to show a transfer effect (e.g., Burack & Moss, 1956; Colville, 1957). Simply because, in training, the learners have been taught general principles that have the potential for application to learning to perform a movement skill in transfer does not guarantee their application. Teaching general principles in training is one thing, and learning to transfer them to the acquisition of other movement skills is very much another. Nonetheless, there is enough research evidence demonstrating the transfer of general principles for practitioners to seriously consider their use when teaching movement skills. One way to facilitate the transfer potential of a general principle and bridge the gap between knowledge and application is to provide a variety of examples when teaching a concept or principle and to specifically show how it is applied or works across different movement skills (Gallahue et al., 1975). Once learners have the idea of how a principle is applied from one movement task to another, they are likely to have a better chance of transferring it to the learning of a new movement task. For example, having learned the principle that lowering your center of gravity (by squatting more) when starting to lose your balance can help you maintain your balance when walking or skiing downhill, you are now in a position to transfer and use that same principle when starting to lose your balance while walking on a balance beam.

## Learning to Learn

Another general factor that has been shown to transfer from one task to another as a function of the similarity between tasks is **learning to learn.** The transfer produced by this general factor depends on the gross-similarity relationships between training and transfer tasks even though the specific dimensions of similarity may not have been analyzed as Osgood (1949) and others have done in terms of stimulus-response similarity between tasks.

Early research reported that people improve their ability to learn new verbal tasks (e.g., lists of nonsense syllables, words, numbers) when they have previously learned a series of similar verbal tasks (e.g., Ward, 1937; Melton & von Lackum, 1941). Subsequent work by Harlow (1949, 1951, 1959) revealed that this learning-to-learn phenomenon also was observed for discrimination problems and other problem solving tasks that were similar. He proposed that people who have learned how to solve certain problems quickly have learned how to learn problems of this type; that is, they have previously acquired a **learning set** for this group or category of problems. However, each learning set must be well learned so that it is reliable enough to transfer to solving new or more complex problems. Harlow's work appears to provide a basis for explaining the often observed phenomenon referred to as **insight,** a term used to explain how someone rapidly solved a problem. For Harlow, insight is a phenomenon that occurs as a consequence of learning to learn or acquiring a learning set for that class of problems.

People who know how to solve various problems of a particular type have acquired a learning set for this group or category of problems and have learned how to learn.

Harlow's work is related to motor learning in at least two ways. First, it could explain, in part, how certain individuals are able to learn new motor skills much faster than most others. It is possible that these individuals have learned how to learn a class of motor skills such as ball-striking skills involved in racket sports (e.g., tennis, racquetball), which makes it easier to learn a new skill in this group. For example, having previously acquired a learning set for the hand–eye coordination involved in the ball-striking skills of tennis and racquetball could make it is easier to learn the new skills of badminton and squash. Second, most movement skills have a perceptual–cognitive component that involves problem solving and decision making to some extent. For instance, having well-learned batting skills in baseball (e.g., *how* to control and coordinate movements to hit a baseball) are a prerequisite for successful hitting performance, but so too is solving the problem of *what* to do. Solving this problem is perceptual and cognitive in nature because it involves deciding whether to swing at a pitch and, if the decision is made to swing, knowing what type of swing to make in relation to the type of pitch thrown and the game situation. It does little good to have learned the appropriate motor skills but not know how to solve problems in order to appropriately use them.

Movement skills of the same type (e.g., racket sports) have a perceptual–cognitive component that involves problem solving and decision making about what to do for which a learning set could be developed.

## Two-Factor Theory

Essentially, the **two-factor theory** of transfer of learning holds that transfer of learning and performance can take place by both identical elements and general factors. People not only transfer identical stimulus-response elements from training task to transfer task, but they also transfer general factors. Based on this fact, Munn (1932) advanced the two-factor theory that transfer effects

Transfer effects are best explained as a result of a combination of identical elements and general factors.

are best explained in terms of a combination of identical elements and general factors. He studied the bilateral transfer of mirror tracing and concluded that the formulation of method (general factors) and discrete movements of the opposite hand (identical elements) were responsible for the transfer effects observed. Further support for the two-factor theory was found by Wieg (1932) when, after studying bilateral transfer in adults and children learning cul-de-sac mazes, he found that attention to the task and attention to discrete cues facilitated transfer from one maze to another. Duncan (1953) also found support for the two-factor theory when, after studying transfer in a lever-positioning skill, he concluded that learning-how-to-learn, as well as response generalization, had facilitated transfer. Based on such early evidence, psychologists proposed that people not only transfer identical stimulus-response elements from task to task, but they also transfer general factors, such as principles of problem solving, learning to learn, and insight. Thus, it is not surprising that the more contemporary view is to explain transfer effects as being due to a combination of identical stimulus-response elements and general factors.

## Types of Transfer

The transfer of learning literature contains terms that describe several types of transfer: vertical, lateral, near, and far. Each of these types of transfer is discussed next.

### Vertical Transfer

Vertical transfer is part-to-whole or within-task transfer.

**Vertical transfer,** also called **part-to-whole transfer,** is **within-task transfer** that involves a person first learning to perform one or more component parts of a movement task and then transferring that part learning to learn to perform the whole task. Vertical transfer of learning is especially useful when movement skills are too complex, difficult, and/or dangerous to perform as a whole. Examples of such skills include the crawl stroke in swimming, a handstand, a front or back handspring in gymnastics, a golf swing or tennis serve, and a head-first dive off a diving board into a swimming pool. Typically, learners are not able to perform complex skills successfully and safely at the outset of learning. Others may even resist attempting to perform the new skill because it involves or they perceive that it involves some danger and risk of injury.

Vertical transfer also is called for when a movement skill contains component parts that are prerequisites for learning to perform the whole skill. For example, before a person learns the proper way to perform a golf swing he or she should first learn the proper way to grip the golf club, next learn the proper stance, and finally the ball position in relation to that stance. Because the swing emanates from the grip, stance, and ball position, they are prerequisites to learning the golf swing.

There are at least three ways in which part learning and vertical transfer of that learning can take place: (a) part-to-whole learning, (b) progressive-part learning, and (c) repetitive-part learning. Each of these three ways of transferring part learning to the acquisition of the whole skill is discussed next.

***Part-to-Whole Learning.***   **Part-to-whole learning** involves having a person learn each of the parts before attempting to learn to perform the whole skill. This approach is especially useful when the parts do not seem to form a natural and meaningful sequence of actions and, therefore, do not need to be practiced together at the outset of learning. For example, if the game of basketball is defined as the whole task to be learned, several nonsequential parts can be easily identified such as the technique used to (a) execute a foul shot, (b) defensively guard an opponent, (c) pass a basketball, and (d) dribble a basketball. No apparent purpose is served by practicing these parts in sequential order. They can be practiced and learned separately, and the part learning that results can be transferred directly into playing the game.

***Progressive-Part Learning.***   Another way to transfer part learning to the learning of the whole skill is to learn one part, then another; when the two parts are acquired, they are combined and practiced together until learned. Next, the third part is practiced and learned by itself before the three parts are combined and practiced together until learned. This procedure is followed for each of the remaining parts until all of them can be practiced as a whole. This **progressive-part learning** approach is appropriate to use when the parts form a natural and meaningful sequence of actions and thus need to be practiced and learned together. For example, if this method was being used to learn a lay-up shot in basketball, the learner would first learn how to dribble the basketball while moving toward the basket. Next, the learner would learn the proper leg action to perform the take-off and would practice this skill alone (without dribbling). Then, the learner would combine dribbling and take-off, practicing them together until they are acquired. Third, the learner would learn how to use his or her arms and hands to shoot the lay-up and practice until it is learned. Finally, the learner would combine dribbling, take-off, and shooting and practice them together as a whole until learned.

***Repetitive-Part Learning.***   A third way of transferring part learning to the learning of the whole skill involves practicing a part until it is learned, and then *combining* it with a new part and practicing them together until they are learned. These two parts are then combined with a third part and practiced together until they are learned. This procedure is followed for each of the remaining parts until all of the parts can be practiced as a whole. **Repetitive-part learning** is a variation of progressive-part learning and would be used in similar situations. For example, if this method was being used to learn a lay-up shot in basketball the learner would learn how to dribble the basketball toward the basket. Next, the learner would combine dribbling with the take-off and practice them together until learned. And finally, the learner would combine dribbling, take-off, and shooting and practice them together until learned.

***Part versus Whole Learning.***   Whether a part-to-whole method should be used rather than the whole method to learn a motor skill is a question that needs to be asked. Several scholars have suggested that when there is a high degree of interaction and integration among component parts of the motor skill or task, it is likely that learning will proceed more effectively if it is practiced as a whole and not divided into parts for practice (Knapp & Dixon, 1952; Lersten, 1968; Lewellen, 1951; Niemeyer, 1959). It is the characteristic of

Part-to-whole learning is appropriate when the parts do not seem to form a natural and meaningful sequence of actions and hence do not have to be practiced together at the beginning of learning.

Progressive-part learning is appropriate to use when the parts form a natural and meaningful sequence of actions and thus need to be practiced together.

If there is a high degree of interaction and integration among component parts of the movement skill, it is likely that learning will proceed more effectively if it is practiced as a whole rather than divided into parts for practice.

wholeness that gives a motor skill its unique quality. When the parts of the skill are practiced by themselves, often it is difficult to perform the exact movements as they are performed in the whole skill. For instance, if the front crawl kick in swimming is practiced alone, the legs move up and down in the vertical plane and the body does not roll on its longitudinal axis. However, when the kick is used in the whole stroke the legs thrust diagonally sidewards when the body rolls on its longitudinal axis. Because transfer of learning depends (in part) on the similarity of the training and transfer movements (that is, the greater the similarity, the greater the transfer) and the kick and body movements in part practice are somewhat different than those used in whole practice, some vertical transfer of learning could be lost. Conversely, because plantar flexion of the ankle is the same or very similar in both part and whole training, vertical transfer of learning of that movement should be high.

Furthermore, whole-practice methods are often more efficient than part methods in that they permit the learner to reach the criterion of mastery in fewer trials. If the whole movement skill or task is complex or involves a number of separate and independently performed component parts, however, then it is recommended that the part rather than the whole method of training be used (Adams & Hufford, 1962; Bahrick, 1957; Seymore, 1954).

When using a part method of training for the purpose of vertical transfer of learning to the whole movement skill, the greatest transfer is likely to occur for the movements that are identical or highly similar between the component part(s) and whole skill. Thus, practice on isolated parts of a movement skill or task always should be done in relation to the whole skill.

## Lateral Transfer

*Lateral transfer, also referred to as horizontal transfer and intertask transfer, is task-to-task transfer, and the tasks do not contain any part-whole relationships as in vertical transfer.*

**Lateral transfer,** also referred to as **horizontal transfer** and **intertask transfer,** is **task-to-task transfer** and takes place between movement tasks. Often these movement tasks are similar in terms of their complexity or difficulty to perform, and they may vary in terms of **inclusion relation,** that is, the extent to which the movements in the training task are included in the transfer task. However, the inclusion relation of the movement tasks used to study lateral transfer does not contain any part-whole relationships as the tasks do in the study of vertical transfer. Gagne (1970) refers to lateral transfer as a "kind of generalization that spreads over a broad set of situations at roughly the same level of complexity" (p. 231). For instance, this kind of transfer occurs when a young athlete recognizes that the fundamental defensive positioning he or she has been learning to use to guard or defend against an opponent in soccer also pertains to playing defense in basketball, such as how to (a) assume the proper defensive stance, (b) position his or her body the appropriate distance from the opponent, and (c) position his or her body between the opponent and the basket.

Let's assume that the inclusion relation between the training and transfer tasks can be expressed along a continuum. At one end of the continuum are different or very dissimilar movement tasks in which none of the movements in the training task (e.g., crawl stroke in swimming) are included in the transfer task (e.g., free-throw shooting in basketball). At the other end of the continuum are identical movement tasks in which all of the movements in the training task (crawl stroke in swimming) are included in the transfer task (crawl stroke in swimming). Between these two ends are movement tasks that vary in the extent to which movements in the training task are included in the transfer task. For instance, some of the overhand throwing movements used in baseball or softball may be viewed as being similar to and included in the overhand serve in volleyball.

When the training and transfer tasks are different or dissimilar, little or no transfer is expected. For example, Nelson (1957a) studied the transfer effect of swimming on the learning of a volleyball tap and a high hurdle skill, and no transfer effect was found. Lindberg (1949) studied the transfer effect of practicing table tennis and "quickening exercises" (tasks demanding rapid movement and decision making) on reaction time and peg shifting (moving pegs from one place on a board as quickly as possible). No transfer effect was found. Other studies (e.g., Coleman, 1967; Burdenshaw, Spragens, & Weis, 1970; Toole & Arink, 1982) investigating lateral transfer between different tasks also found no effect. Thus, the evidence reviewed indicates that there are no appreciable lateral transfer effects between training and transfer tasks that do not have very much of an inclusion relation.

On the other hand, training and transfer tasks that do have more of an inclusion relation have movements in common and can be expected to show transfer effects. Generally, the greater the inclusion and similarity between two tasks, the greater the transfer between them. This relationship has been studied in terms of stimulus and response characteristics of the training and transfer tasks and was discussed in the section entitled "Transfer of Motor Learning Depends on Similarity" on page 358. Other headings under which this inclusion relation between training and transfer tasks has been studied have been referred to in the literature as *task difficulty, speed versus accuracy,* and *bilateral transfer.* Let's take a closer look at each of these.

***Task Difficulty.***    Transfer may be unequal between training and transfer tasks that are of different levels of difficulty to perform. There is some evidence for greater transfer from difficult to easy tasks than from easy to difficult tasks (e.g., Baker, Wylie, & Gagne, 1950; Gibbs, 1951; Szafran & Welford, 1950). There also is some evidence for greater transfer from easy to difficult tasks than from difficult to easy tasks (Ammons et al., 1956; Boswell & Irion, 1975; Lincoln & Smith, 1951; Livesey & Lazlo, 1979; Lordahl & Archer, 1958; Poulton, 1956). However, there is even more convincing evidence that direct practice on the transfer task rather than training first on easier or more difficult versions of the transfer task leads to the greatest transfer (Holding, 1962, 1965; Leonard, Karnes, Oxendine, & Hesson, 1970; Scannell, 1968; Singer, 1966). Thus, if one wants to optimize transfer of learning from a training task to a transfer task, it is recommended that the transfer task be practiced in training at the same **task difficulty** level that will be demanded in transfer.

Although the complete answer explaining why unequal transfer has been found between training and transfer tasks of unequal difficulty is still a matter of some uncertainty, Holding (1962, 1965) proposed one possible explanation. He reasoned that difficult versions of training tasks include all aspects of their easier versions (which he referred to as *inclusion*), which could explain why high positive transfer is usually found when going from difficult to easy versions of a task. However, inclusion is not a viable explanation for transfer from

Inclusion relation refers to the extent to which the movements in the training task are included in the transfer task.

Training and transfer tasks that have more of an inclusion relation have more movements in common, and the greater the inclusion and similarity between the two tasks, the greater the transfer between them.

easy to difficult task versions because easy versions do not include all aspects of their difficult versions. To explain positive transfer from easy to difficult task versions, he proposed the transfer of **performance standards.** If training on an easier version of a task results in learning to make performance errors that are small in size, and if they are transferred to the more difficult version of the task in which an error of the same real size is proportionately smaller, there could be a positive transfer effect when changing from the easy to the difficult version. Further, if training on the easier task version results in learning to prefer accuracy over speed, the transfer of that learning could elevate standards of performance when changing to the difficult task version.

*Speed versus Accuracy.*    Some movement tasks, such as serving a tennis ball to a certain location on the court (target), require both speed and accuracy for successful performance. What is the best way to train for transfer of learning with such tasks? Should people emphasize movement speed and sacrifice accuracy during original learning? Should they emphasize movement accuracy and sacrifice speed? Or, should the same emphasis be placed on both movement speed and accuracy during learning as will be required during transfer? These questions are central to the **speed versus accuracy** training issue.

Transfer of learning to a movement task requiring both speed and accuracy is best facilitated by emphasizing the same speed and accuracy during training that will be required when the task is performed during transfer as long as it is safe to do so.

Research suggests that transfer of learning to a movement task requiring both speed and accuracy is best facilitated by emphasizing the same speed and accuracy during learning (training) that will be required when the task is performed during transfer, provided it can be performed safely and with an acceptable degree of accuracy (e.g., Hornak, 1971; Jensen, 1975; Lordahl & Archer, 1958; Namikas & Archer, 1960; Nixon & Locke, 1973; Woods, 1967). Of course, early in learning, performance of a task may have to be slowed down until a reasonable degree of accuracy is achieved. For instance, when trying to serve a tennis ball, it does little good to repeatedly swing a tennis racket fast using a totally inappropriate technique and completely miss the ball. Performance of the task may have to be slowed down early in learning until an acceptable level of accuracy is achieved.

Moreover, a progressive practice schedule of gradual increases in speed may have to be used, which has been shown to have about the same transfer benefits as practicing the movement task at the speed it is ordinarily performed (Baker et al., 1950; Sage & Hornak, 1978). However, if there is no reason to slow down the speed to achieve a reasonable degree of accuracy or safety, it is recommended that the movement task be practiced at "game speed" as soon as possible in order to facilitate optimum transfer of learning. Lastly, if the performance of the transfer task will demand movement at different speeds, training under variable speed conditions is likely to provide more beneficial transfer effects than practice at a single speed (Siegel & Davis, 1980).

Transfer of learning to perform a movement skill from one limb on one side of the body to a limb on the opposite side is referred to as *bilateral transfer.*

*Bilateral Transfer.*    Transfer of learning to perform a movement skill from a limb on one side of the body to a limb on the opposite side is referred to as **bilateral transfer** (also referred to as *cross-education*). For instance, when people practice a movement skill, such as kicking or juggling a soccer ball with their preferred leg, there is usually some positive transfer of that learning to their nonpreferred leg even though they have not practiced the kick or juggling with their nonpreferred leg.

Studies investigating bilateral transfer have typically used the experimental design shown in Table 12.2.

**Table 12.2**
**Experimental Design to Study Bilateral Transfer**

| Limb | Training Phase | | Transfer Phase |
| | Pretest | Training | Transfer Test |
| --- | --- | --- | --- |
| Preferred | Movement A | Movement A | Movement A |
| Nonpreferred | Movement A | Rests | Movement A |

This design enables the researcher to determine if bilateral transfer to the non-trained (nonpreferred limb) limb occurred because of training with the other limb (preferred limb). If training on movement task A with the preferred limb facilitates transfer test performance of movement task A with the nonpreferred limb as compared to pretest performance, then evidence for positive, bilateral transfer of learning may be claimed. Of course, one would expect preferred-limb performance on the transfer test to be better than the pretest because of training. However, because the nonpreferred limb received no training, one would not expect its performance on the transfer test to be better than the pretest unless training with the preferred limb transferred to cause it to improve. In the example, experimental design training was given to the pre-ferred limb, but this need not be the case. It could be given to the nonpre-ferred limb instead to determine bilateral transfer of learning effects from non-preferred to preferred limb.

One of the earliest studies of bilateral transfer using a movement skill (jug-gling) was conducted by Swift (1903). Participants in his study were asked to keep two balls going with one hand, receiving and throwing one while the other was in the air. He found clear evidence that training with one hand transferred to the other. Cook (1936) systematically determined the bilateral transfer relations between hands and feet showing that it was greater between corresponding limbs (arm to arm or hand to hand). He also revealed that trans-fer was least between incongruous limbs (diagonally between hand and foot). Cook claimed that there was sufficient evidence to conclude that bilateral transfer of learning does, in fact, occur for movement skills. In an extensive review of the research literature, Ammons (1958) also concluded that there was consistent evidence indicating that movement skill learned in training with one limb transfers to the untrained limb. Moreover, Ammons reported that this transfer occurs from hand to foot, hand to hand, or foot to foot, but the greatest transfer was between corresponding limbs. Lastly, there appears to be sufficient evidence to recommend that the greatest amount of bilateral trans-fer occurs from the preferred limb to the nonpreferred limb, although some controversy still continues regarding this recommendation.

Several explanations have been proposed to explain bilateral transfer effects, but perhaps the most notable are cognitive learning, motor program, and motor outflow. The **cognitive learning explanation** is based on the idea that the early phase of learning a movement skill involves cognitive activities such as understanding the goal of the skill, thinking about which movements to perform to achieve the goal, and cognitively formulating the techniques that will work best to produce successful movements. In fact, Kohl and Roenker (1980) found that bilateral transfer occurs when people mentally imagine

The cognitive learning explanation holds that when the skill that was first learned with one limb has to be learned with the opposite limb, the learner already knows what to do to successfully per-form the skill and does not have to reacquire it when practice begins.

themselves performing a movement with one limb. Taken together, these cognitive activities are essentially focused on learning what to do to successfully perform the skill. When the skill that was first learned with one limb has to be learned with the opposite limb, the learner already cognitively knows what to do to successfully perform the skill and therefore does not have to reacquire it when practice begins.

The **motor program explanation** is based on the idea of a generalized motor program proposed by Schmidt (1976) and previously discussed in Chapter 6. Essentially, this explanation holds that there is only one general motor program for a movement skill or movement skills that fall into the same response class. Muscles needed to produce the movements that make up the skill are a parameter or variant characteristic of the motor program that the learner is free to adjust in order to adapt the program so that the skill can be performed by either limb. Once the skill has been learned with one limb, the generalized motor program that controls it also has been learned and is now available for use to produce the skill with the other limb (Shapiro, 1977). Additional evidence supporting the hypothesis that in performing a particular movement the two hands can be controlled by the same generalized motor program has been provided by several researchers (e.g., Kelso, Southard, & Goodman, 1979; McGown & Schmidt, 1981).

This explanation would predict that performance would be better at the outset of learning the skill with the nonpracticed limb than it would be if the skill was not previously learned at all because there would be no generalized program in memory to call upon to perform the skill. Thus, there could be no bilateral transfer between limbs because there would be no generalized program for the skill in memory. This explanation also would predict that the rate of learning the skill with the nonpracticed limb would be faster than it was for the practiced limb because of the presence of the generalized program in memory. One could ask that if there is one generalized program controlling the production of the movement skill regardless of the muscles and limbs involved, why doesn't the nonpracticed limb perform the skill at the outset of acquisition as well as the practiced limb did at the end of acquisition? One possible reason is that practice is needed to learn to effectively adjust the parameters of the generalized motor program so that the muscles of the nonpracticed limb can effectively produce the movements that make up the skill. In other words, practice specific to the parameterization of the generalized motor program is needed to learn to proficiently generate the skill movements with the nonpracticed limb. This is yet another example of how specificity of practice operates in the learning and bilateral transfer of movement skills.

The **motor outflow explanation** has its roots in neuroanatomical and neurophysiological evidence of the transmission of neural signals to the muscles that produce movement. Although neural signals to the muscles sent via the corticospinal (pyramidal) and indirect (extrapyramidal) tracts are mainly contralateral, there is substantial ipsilateral transmission. Neural signals sent from the left motor cortex have their first effect on the spinal motoneurons controlling limbs on the right side of the body, but there is some overflow of these neural signals ipsilaterally that stimulates spinal motoneurons controlling the limbs on the left side of the body (Davis, 1942).

One effect of motor outflow that has been found in exercise physiology is a gain in strength and endurance in an untrained limb as a consequence of

The motor program explanation holds that once the skill has been learned with one limb, the generalized motor program that controls it also has been learned and is now available for use to produce the skill with the other limb.

training in the contralateral muscle group (deVries, 1980; Moritani & deVries, 1979). Clearly, this gain is the result of neural signals being sent to the untrained *and* trained limb. Extending this notion to the learning of a movement skill, it is possible that bilateral transfer effects are the result of the neural signals being sent to the unpracticed limb (perhaps to a lesser degree) as well as to the practiced limb. One line of support for this notion can be found in evidence indicating that some bilateral transfer of skill is negotiated in the brain by transfer of movement components of the task between cerebral hemispheres (Hicks, Gualtieri, & Schroeder, 1983). This negotiation was demonstrated by recording electromyographic (EMG) activity in all four limbs when one limb performs a movement. When EMG activity occurs in a limb that is not performing the movement, it indicates that the central nervous system has forwarded neural signals to the muscles of the nonperforming limb as well. This same effect was demonstrated many years ago by Davis (1942), who found that more EMG activity occurred in the two arms (contralateral limbs), less activity occurred in the arm and leg on the same side (ipsilateral limbs), and the least activity for the diagonal limbs.

> The motor outflow explanation holds that neural signals sent to the practiced limb are also sent (perhaps to a lesser extent) to the unpracticed limb, which facilitates some learning in the unpracticed limb and makes it available for transfer when it is time to learn the skill with the unpracticed limb.

Which of the three explanations provides the best account of bilateral transfer? Evidence can be found to support each one. Presently, one cannot be ruled out in favor of another based on the lack of evidence supporting its possibility. Further, all three explanations are intuitively appealing and each one provides us with a different account of how bilateral transfer occurs. In a sense, the explanations appear to complement rather than detract from or oppose each other. Until research provides evidence that advances one of these explanations over the others or supports an entirely new explanation, bilateral transfer is perhaps best accounted for as a result of a combination of the three explanations.

## Near and Far Transfer

The training task and the conditions can be near or far from the transfer task and conditions in terms of *time* and *overall similarity*. These two dimensions are closely connected in the sense that the passage of time will tend to decrease the similarity of the training and transfer contexts and allow other mechanisms that produce forgetting or changes in motivation to operate. Thus, **near transfer** is learning that is transferred from one movement task and/or set of conditions in training after a relatively brief time delay to the same or a very similar movement task and/or set of conditions. Examples of near transfer include (a) transfer of learning to perform a new basketball skill or a new basic offensive play from the training environment after several days to game conditions; (b) transfer of learning to walk again (recovery of function) following a stroke from the training (clinical) environment as soon as possible to the real-world; (c) transfer of learning to perform a golf swing from the training environment immediately to a variation of that swing in the same training environment. In all three examples the time delays are relatively short, which minimizes the effect of mechanisms (e.g., forgetting, motivation) that could operate over time to decrease the similarity of the training and transfer contexts. Moreover, in all three examples there is a great deal of overall similarity between the training task and/or conditions and the transfer task and/ or conditions. In examples (a) and (b) the same movement skills are being

> Near transfer is learning that is transferred from one task and/or set of conditions in training after a relatively brief time delay to the same or a very similar task and/or set of conditions.

transferred to different environments, whereas in example (c) a variation of a movement skill is being transferred to the same environment.

**Far transfer** of learning can occur from one movement task and/or set of conditions in training after a relatively long time delay to the same or very similar movement task and/or set of conditions if the passage of time decreases the similarity of the training and transfer contexts. It also can occur from one movement task and/or set of conditions in training to another less similar movement task and/or set of conditions. Examples of far transfer include (a) transfer of learning to perform golf shots from the training environment after a three-month lay-off back to the training environment; (b) transfer of learning to walk again (recovery function) after a stroke from the training (clinical) environment to real-world terrains (e.g., uneven, sidehill, downhill, and uphill) not experienced in training; and (c) transfer of learning to perform tennis skills from training to learning to perform badminton skills in training. In example (a), the movement task and conditions are the same in training and transfer, but the relatively long time delay could reduce the similarity between the training and transfer contexts. In example (b), the training and transfer task are the same, but the conditions are different; and, in example (c), the training and transfer tasks and the conditions are different.

> Far transfer of learning occurs from one task and/or set of conditions in training after a relatively long time delay to the same or a very similar task and/or set of conditions, provided the passage of time decreases the similarity of the training and transfer contexts.

## How Transfer Is Studied

What is known about transfer of motor learning is very much a function of the way in which it has been studied, especially in terms of the experimental designs, procedures, and measures used. Traditionally, when studying transfer a distinction is made between the training phase (also called the acquisition, or learning, phase), which involves the time or trials required to reach a criterion level of task proficiency, and the transfer phase, which follows the training phase either immediately or after a delay (retention interval). Essentially, the transfer phase consists of a test to determine how the task learned under one set of conditions in the training phase (training task) influences performance on some subsequent task (transfer task) under the same or another set of conditions. A variety of experimental designs have been used to study transfer, but it is beyond the scope of this chapter to discuss all of them. The two basic ones that will be presented are called proactive and retroactive transfer designs.

> What is known about transfer is very much a function of the way in which it has been studied, especially in terms of the experimental designs, procedures, and measures used.

### Experimental Design to Study Proactive Transfer

The **proactive transfer** design can be used to study lateral transfer of motor learning. For example, it can be used to study the immediate or delayed effect that the prior learning of a movement task (e.g., overhand throw in baseball or softball) has on the subsequent learning of another task (e.g., overhand serve in volleyball). The proactive design also can be used to study vertical transfer of motor learning. For instance, it can be used to study the immediate or delayed effect that prior learning of a component part of a movement task (e.g., leg kick or arm stroke) has on the subsequent learning of the whole movement task (e.g., the side stroke in swimming).

**Table 12.3**
**Experimental Design to Study Proactive Transfer**

| Training Phase | | Transfer Phase | |
|---|---|---|---|
| Group | Learn | Retention Interval (RI) | Transfer Test |
| Experimental | Movement A | Immediate or delayed | Movement B |
| Control | Rests or performs an unrelated movement task | (RI same as experimental group) | Movement B |

In both of the previous examples, the longer the time delay or retention interval between training and the transfer test, the more far transfer is being studied, whereas the shorter the time delay, the more near transfer is being investigated. This assumes that the passage of time will decrease the similarity between the training and transfer contexts. If it does, then any transfer effects found may be due to the passage of time as well as overall similarity between the training and transfer tasks and conditions. Of course, the proactive transfer design could be used to investigate both near and far transfer in terms of the passage of time separately from overall similarity between training and transfer contexts. The basic proactive design is illustrated in Table 12.3.

If the prior learning of movement task A in the training phase facilitates the performance of movement task B for the experimental group when compared to the performance of movement task B of the control group on the transfer test, then evidence for positive, proactive transfer of learning may be claimed. Conversely, if the transfer test performance of the experimental group is inferior to that of the control group on movement task B, evidence for negative, proactive transfer may be claimed. Finally, if both groups perform the same on movement task B on the transfer test, no evidence for transfer (zero transfer) has been found.

When using this design the experimenter must be certain that the two groups are equivalent with respect to variables critical to learning both movement tasks (e.g., developmental level, previous motor learning experiences). Also, the experimenter must be cognizant of what the control group does during the training phase in which the experimental group learns movement task A; typically, the control group either rests or performs some unrelated movement task. This is important to the interpretation of the transfer results because studies have shown that the learning of a task can be facilitated by an immediately preceding activity, known as a *warm-up increment* (Hamilton, 1950; Thune, 1950). Further, research has shown that the learning of a task can be facilitated by prior practice on similar tasks, which is referred to as a *learning-to-learn increment* (see page 371). If the control group rests and does nothing during the training phase, the superior performance on movement task B by the experimental group during the transfer phase as compared to the control group could have been due to warm-up and/or learning-to-learn effects rather than proactive transfer from having learned task A. Of course, it also could have been due to a summation of all three of these effects. If one wishes to know the specific proactive transfer effects of learning movement task A before learning to perform movement task B, it is necessary to control for both

The basic proactive transfer design is used to study the effect (either immediate or delayed) that prior learning of a task has on the subsequent learning of another task.

**Table 12.4**
**Experimental Design to Study Retroactive Transfer**

| | Training Phase | | | Transfer Phase | |
|---|---|---|---|---|---|
| Group | Prior Learning | Learn | | Retention Interval | Transfer Test |
| Experimental | Movement A | Movement B | | Immediate or delayed | Movement A |
| Control | Movement A | Rests or performs an unrelated movement task | | (RI same as experimental group) | Movement A |

warm-up and learning-to-learn effects. Warm-up effects can be controlled by having the control group perform the same number of practice trials on an unrelated movement task as were used by the experimental group to learn movement task A during the training phase. Learning-to-learn effects can be controlled by ensuring that the participants in each group have similar backgrounds, especially in terms of prior learning of movement tasks that are similar to movement task B.

## Experimental Design to Study Retroactive Transfer

The basic retroactive transfer design is used to study how subsequent learning of a task (training task) affects the performance of a previously learned task (transfer task).

Another type of design is used to study **retroactive transfer.** It is called *retroactive* because the subsequent learning of a task (training task) affects the performance of a previously learned task (transfer task). Thus, the transfer task is familiar to the learner and *backward* transfer is being studied, whereas in the proactive transfer design, the transfer task is new to the learner and *forward* transfer is being studied. Essentially, the retroactive transfer design simply involves transfer to a familiar rather than a new task; and, as Osgood (1949) has pointed out, it produces no major differences in empirical results from the proactive transfer design. The basic retroactive design is illustrated in Table 12.4.

If learning movement task B in the training phase facilitates the performance of movement task A on the transfer test for the experimental group when compared to the performance of movement task A of the control group, then evidence for positive, retroactive transfer of learning may be claimed. Conversely, if the performance of the experimental group is inferior to the control group on movement task A during the transfer test, evidence for negative, retroactive transfer may be claimed. Lastly, if both groups perform the same on movement task A on the transfer test, no evidence for transfer (zero transfer) has been found. When using this design, the experimenter must be sure that (a) the two groups are essentially the same in terms of their learning performance on movement task A during the training phase, and (b) they are equivalent with respect to factors that are critical to learning both movement tasks (e.g., developmental level, prior motor learning experiences). Lastly, as with the proactive transfer design, the experimenter must be mindful of what the control group does during the training phase.

## Measuring Transfer

What is known about transfer is not only a function of the various experimental designs and procedures that have been used to study it, but also of the ways in which it has been measured. In this section we will discuss two basic ways of measuring the effects of transfer: percentage of transfer and savings score.

*Percentage of Transfer.*   A number of different transfer formulas have been used over the years to measure the direction and amount of transfer that have occurred in various experiments. The various formulas express transfer as a percentage, and it is important to note that different percentages are obtained when the formulas are calculated on the same performance measures. Moreover, the range of sensitivity in terms of **percentage of transfer** differs from one formula to another. For example, one formula can range from positive infinity to negative 100%; another formula can range from positive 100% to negative infinity; and the third can range from positive 100% to negative 100%. Thus, 47% transfer calculated by one formula will not be the same as 47% calculated by another formula. Because different formulas can produce (a) different percentages of transfer based on the same set of performance measures and (b) the same percentage based on a different set of performance measures, it is very important to know which transfer formula was used so that the percentage obtained can be accurately interpreted. Of course, it also is quite important to know the transfer formula used when we are comparing the percentages of transfer (for direction and amount) across studies. For more information about these formulas and the issues surrounding them, the reader is referred to Gagne, Foster, and Crowley (1948) and Murdock (1957).

It is important to know what formula was used to calculate percentage of transfer so that the percentage can be accurately interpreted.

One of these formulas, recommended by Murdock (1957), may be expressed as follows:

$$\text{Percentage of Transfer} = \frac{E - C}{E + C} \times 100$$

E = performance measure for the experimental group on the transfer movement task

C = performance measure for the control group on the transfer movement task

This formula is appropriate to use when the performance measure increases with better performance such that the higher the performance number, the better the performance. Examples of such performance measures include the number of correct responses to reach a criterion level of mastery, the number of shots made out of a certain number of attempts, and the amount of time on target in a tracking task or in balance on a stabilometer. This formula has a distinct advantage over the other formulas because the direction and amount of transfer expressed as a percentage by this formula range from +100% to −100%. Thus, the upper and lower limits are equal, and the percentage of transfer is symmetrical about zero.

Let's look at an example of how to calculate the percentage of transfer using this formula. Figure 12.3 shows the results from a hypothetical proactive

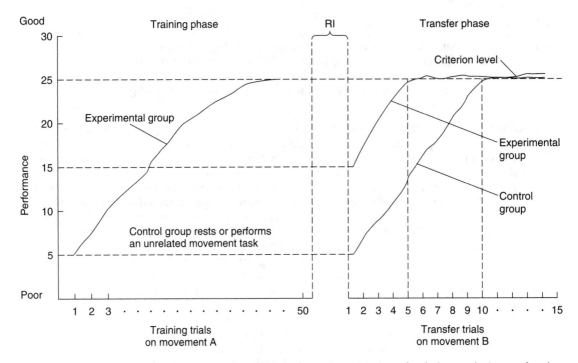

**Figure 12.3**  Hypothetical results from a proactive transfer design study. In transfer, the experimental (E) group began movement task B at a performance level of 15, whereas the control (C) group began at a performance level of 5, revealing that the E group had 50% transfer from movement task A to the initial performance of movement task B. Also, in transfer, it took the E group five trials to reach the performance level of 25, whereas the C group needed 10 trials to reach the same level. Thus, five trials were saved by the E group first learning to perform movement task A.

RI = retention interval

transfer study design in which the two groups were equivalent in terms of their prior movement learning experiences and ability to learn to perform movement task B. In training, the experimental (E) group experiences 50 practice trials in learning to perform movement task A, while the control (C) group either rests or experiences 50 practice trials learning to perform a movement task that is unrelated to movement task A. The C group performs an unrelated task if it is important to control for amount of practice in training and learning-to-learn and warm-up effects. It took the E group 50 training trials to reach the criterion level of 25 performances of movement A. In transfer, the E group began movement task B at a performance level of 15, whereas the C group began at a performance level of 5. To quantify the initial transfer effect of the E group training on movement task A before learning to perform movement task B, we would insert these transfer performance measures into the preceding formula as follows:

$$\text{Percentage of Transfer} = \frac{15 - 5}{15 + 5} \times 100 = 50\%$$

This percentage, which reveals the direction and amount of transfer, indicates that the E group had 50% transfer from movement task A to the initial performance of movement task B. This means that it performed 50% better on movement task B compared with the C group. Conversely, if the C group had initially performed better on the transfer task (movement B) than the E group such that the performance measures were reversed, then we would have a case of negative transfer. In this case the formula would produce –50% transfer, which means that the C group performed 50% better on movement task B compared with the E group.

In the preceding example, the performance measure increased with better performance. When the performance measure decreases with better performance such that the lower the performance number the better the performance, the formula should be modified as follows:

$$\text{Percentage of Transfer} = \frac{C - E}{E + C} \times 100$$

Performance measures that decrease with better performance include number of errors made in reaching a given criterion of mastery and number of trials or amount of time needed to reach some criterion level of mastery.

The percentage of transfer resulting from two formulas has a couple of unique characteristics. First, to obtain a large percentage of transfer the control group would have to achieve a very low score (performance measure) on the transfer movement task, and the experimental group would have to achieve a very high score. Second, a transfer of 100% can be obtained only when the control group scores zero or the experimental group scores zero on the transfer movement task.

***Savings Score.***  A **savings score** is used when it is important to determine how much practice time or how many practice trials in learning the transfer movement task are saved by having first learned the training movement task. Let's calculate a savings score based on the transfer trials and performance data shown in Figure 12.3. In transfer, it took the E group 5 trials to reach the criterion performance level of 25, whereas the C group needed 10 trials to reach the same performance level. Thus, 5 practice trials were saved by the E group by first learning to perform movement task A. Or the savings score could be expressed as a percentage by using the following formula:

$$\text{Percentage of Savings} = \frac{C - E}{C} \times 100$$

E = number of practice trials (or amount of time) needed for the E group to reach the performance level achieved by the C group on the transfer task

C = number of practice trials (or amount of time) for the C group to reach the criterion performance level or level of mastery on the transfer task

This formula is appropriate to use when fewer practice trials or amount of time reflect better performance. Inserting the transfer practice trials into the preceding formula, we have:

$$\text{Percentage of Savings} = \frac{10 - 5}{10} \times 100 = 50\%$$

A savings score is used when it is important to determine how much practice time or how many practice trials in learning the transfer task are saved by having first learned the training movement task.

Thus, the transfer effect of learning movement task A before learning movement task B amounts to a savings of five trials out of 10, or 50%. Of course, whether this savings amount is really any savings at all is another question because either the E group (if the C group rested) or both groups (if the C group practiced an unrelated task) had to practice in training and that took a considerable amount of time and effort. We might conclude that the amount of savings was not worth the effort, especially in many sport situations. On the other hand, it would be worth the effort in the case of learning to fly an airplane, especially in terms of safety and cost. Spending the extra training time on a flight simulator to obtain 50% savings when transferring to the actual plane would be worth the time and effort spent in training because there would be less chance of crashing the plane.

This savings method also can be employed to examine the transfer effect throughout the learning of the transfer movement task by using successive performance criteria. The practice trials needed to reach each performance criterion by the C group and the E group are counted, and the percent savings is calculated at each criterion level. Using the savings method in this way, the transfer effect can be traced throughout the entire process of learning the transfer task.

## Summary

Transfer of learning is a process by which learning acquired in one situation is used in another situation to learn to perform either the same (or a highly similar) or a different task under conditions that may be the same or different. The idea that transfer depends on the structural similarity between the training and transfer tasks emanated from Thorndike's identical elements theory. Essentially, this theory held that transfer depended on the extent to which the training and transfer tasks shared identical elements: the more similar the two tasks, the more the transfer of learning from the training to the transfer task. The direction of transfer is (a) positive when the training task facilitates performance of the transfer task; (b) negative when the training task interferes with performance on the transfer task; and (c) zero when the training task has no effect on the transfer task. Amount of transfer refers to its magnitude or quantity, whereas extent of transfer refers to its generalization, that is, the extent to which the original task training transfers to other tasks.

The difficulty, at times, of accurately predicting the amount, direction, and extent of transfer may be due to an incomplete understanding of *what* is learned in training and *how* the transfer task itself is represented. In an attempt to deal with this limitation, a number of scholars have directed their research efforts toward the concept of transfer-appropriate processing (TAP). This concept holds that it is not only the structural similarity between the training and transfer tasks and conditions, but also the similarity of the goals and cognitive processing between them that contributes to the transfer of learning. One practical implication emanating from this concept is that positive transfer should be facilitated by making the processing activities the same or similar between the training and transfer tasks and conditions. Additional factors influencing transfer include the level of original learning, background knowledge or expertise, and perceived similarity. Positive transfer increases with the level of original learning, providing that structurally similar responses are required in training and transfer tasks. Background knowledge or expertise appropriate to the transfer task also can facilitate transfer of learning and performance. It also plays an important role in perceived similarity, which has been found to influence the amount of transfer. Finally, not only are identical elements transferred between tasks, but so are general factors such as principles, strategies, laws, rules, and learning to learn.

Four types of transfer were discussed: vertical, lateral, near, and far. Vertical transfer, also called part-to-whole transfer, is within-task transfer. Lateral transfer, also referred to as horizontal transfer and intertask transfer, is task-to-task transfer. It appears that the best way to optimize lateral transfer of learning from a training task to a transfer task is to practice the transfer task in training at the same level of difficulty and the same speed and accuracy that will be demanded in transfer settings. Transfer of learning to perform a movement task from a limb on one side of the body to a limb on the opposite side is referred to as bilateral transfer. There is convincing evidence for bilateral transfer, especially between corresponding limbs and from the preferred to the nonpreferred limb. Near transfer is learning that is transferred from one task and/or set of conditions in training to the same or a very similar task and/or set of conditions after a relatively brief time delay. Far transfer is the same as near transfer except that it occurs after a relatively long time delay and is based on the assumption that the passage of time decreases the similarity of the training and transfer contexts.

What is known about transfer of learning is very much a function of the way in which it has been studied, especially in terms of experimental designs, procedures, and measures used. Traditionally when studying transfer, a distinction is made between the training phase and the transfer phase. The transfer phase consists of a test to determine how the task learned under one set of conditions in training (training task) influences performance on some subsequent task (transfer task) under the same or another set of conditions. Essentially, two types of basic experimental designs have been used to study proactive and retroactive transfer. The proactive transfer design studies the influence that prior learning has on the subsequent learning of a new task (transfer task), whereas the retroactive design studies the influence that subsequent learning of a task has on the performance of a previously learned task (transfer task). Thus, the transfer task is familiar to the learner in the retroactive transfer design but is new to the learner in the proactive transfer design.

What is known about transfer also is a function of ways in which it has been measured. A number of different transfer formulas have been used over the years to measure the direction and amount of transfer. The various formulas express transfer as a percentage, and different percentages are obtained when the formulas are calculated on the same performance measures. Further, the range of sensitivity in terms of percentage of transfer varies from one formula to another. Thus, it is important to know what transfer formula was used so that the percentage obtained can be accurately interpreted, especially when comparing percentages across studies. Another way to measure transfer is with a savings score, which is used to determine how much practice time or how many practice trials in learning the transfer task are saved by having first learned the training task.

## IMPORTANT TERMINOLOGY

After completing this chapter, readers should be familiar with the following terms and concepts.

amount of transfer
background knowledge (expertise)
bilateral transfer
cognitive learning explanation
direction of transfer
extent of transfer
far transfer
generalization of transfer
horizontal transfer
identical elements theory
inclusion relation
insight
intertask transfer
lateral transfer
learning set
learning to learn
level of original learning
motor outflow explanation
motor program explanation
near transfer
negative transfer
part-to-whole learning
part-to-whole transfer

perceived similarity
percentage of transfer
performance standards
positive transfer
proactive transfer
progressive-part learning
repetitive-part learning
response generalization
retroactive transfer
savings score
speed versus accuracy
stimulus generalization
task difficulty
task-to-task transfer
transfer-appropriate processing (TAP)
transfer of general factors
transfer of learning (training)
transfer of motor learning
transfer surface
two-factor theory
vertical transfer
within-task transfer
zero transfer

## SUGGESTED FURTHER READING

Christina, R. W., & Bjork, R. A. (1991). Optimizing long-term retention and transfer. In D. Druckman & R. A. Bjork (Eds.), *In the mind's eye: Enhancing human performance* (pp. 23–56). Washington, DC: National Academy Press.

Ferrari, M. (1999). Influence of expertise on the intentional transfer of motor skill. *Journal of Motor Behavior, 31*, 79–85.

Hesketh, B. (1997). Dilemmas in training for transfer and retention. *Applied Psychology: An International Review, 46*, 317–386.

Ma, H. I., Trombly, C. A., & Robinson-Podolski, C. (1999). The effect of context on skill acquisition and transfer. *American Journal of Occupational Therapy, 53*, 138–144.

Reder, M., & Klatzky, R. L. (1994). Transfer: Training for performance. In D. Druckman & R. A. Bjork (Eds.), *Learning, remembering, believing: Enhancing human performance* (pp. 25–56). Washington, DC: National Academy Press.

Schmidt, R. A., & Bjork, R. A. (1992). New conceptualizations of practice: Common principles in three paradigms suggest new concepts for training. *Psychological Science, 3,* 207–217.

Zanone, P. G., & Kelso, J. A. S. (1997). Coordination dynamics of learning and transfer: Collective and component levels. *Journal of Experimental Psychology: Human Perception and Performance, 23,* 1454–1480.

## Test Your Understanding

1. Provide a real-world motor learning and performance example of positive, negative, and zero transfer.

2. Distinguish among the following terms: *direction, amount, extent of transfer, stimulus generalization,* and *response generalization.*

3. How does the direction and amount of transfer depend on the stimulus-response similarity of training and transfer tasks? Provide examples to support your explanation.

4. How do identical elements theory and general factors theory differ in explaining transfer of learning?

5. What is transfer-appropriate processing? Provide a motor skills example of how you would structure training (practice) conditions to facilitate the transfer of this type of processing to a real-world setting.

6. Explain how level of original learning, background knowledge or expertise, and perceived similarity influence transfer of learning and performance.

7. Explain the meaning of vertical transfer, lateral transfer, near transfer, and far transfer. Provide an example of each one.

8. If you want to optimize the transfer of learning, is it better to train on an easier version of the transfer task, the same level of difficulty as the transfer task, or a more difficult version of the transfer task? Explain your answer.

9. If you want to optimize transfer of learning, is it better during training (practice) to emphasize movement speed and sacrifice accuracy, emphasize movement accuracy and sacrifice speed, or place the same emphasis on both speed and accuracy as will be required when the skill is performed in the real-world setting?

10. What does research tell us about why bilateral transfer occurs as it does? What are the implications for designing training (practice) conditions?

11. Provide an example of how you would study the proactive transfer of learning between two similar movement skills.

12. Provide an example of how you would study the retroactive transfer of learning between two movement skills.

13. Explain how direction and amount of transfer can be expressed as a percentage and as a savings score.

# REFERENCES

Abernethy, B., Burgess-Limerick, R., & Parks, S. (1994). Contrasting approaches to the study of motor expertise. *Quest, 46,* 186–198.

Abernethy, B., & Russell, D. G. (1984). Advance cue utilisation by skilled cricket batsmen. *The Australian Journal of Science and Medicine in Sport, 16*(2), 2–10.

Abernethy, B., & Russell, D. G. (1987a). Expert-novice differences in an applied selective attention task. *Journal of Sport Psychology, 9,* 326–345.

Abernethy, B., & Russell, D. G. (1987b). The relationship between expertise and visual search strategy in a racquet sport. *Human Movement Science, 6,* 283–319.

Abernethy, B., Thomas, K. T., & Thomas, J. R. (1993). Strategies for improving understanding of motor expertise (or mistakes we have made and things we have learned!!). In J. L. Starkes & F. Allard (Eds.), *Cognitive issues in motor expertise* (pp. 317–356). Amsterdam: Elsevier.

Abernethy, B., & Wood, J. M. (2001). Do generalized visual training programs for sport really work? An experimental investigation. *Journal of Sport Sciences, 19,* 203–222.

Adams, J. A. (1952). Warm-up decrement in performance on the pursuit-rotor. *American Journal of Psychology, 65,* 404–414.

Adams, J. A. (1954). Psychomotor response acquisition and transfer as a function of control-indicator relationships. *Journal of Experimental Psychology, 48,* 10–18.

Adams, J. A. (1961). The second facet of forgetting: A review of warm-up decrement. *Psychological Bulletin, 58,* 257–273.

Adams, J. A. (1966). Some mechanisms of motor responding: An examination of attention. In E. A. Bilodeau (Ed.), *Acquisition of skill* (pp. 169–200). New York: Academic Press.

Adams, J. A. (1967). *Human memory.* New York: McGraw-Hill.

Adams, J. A. (1971). A closed-loop theory of motor learning. *Journal of Motor Behavior, 3,* 111–149.

Adams, J. A. (1977). Feedback theory of how joint receptors regulate the timing and positioning of a limb. *Psychological Review, 84,* 504–523.

Adams, J. A. (1986). Use of the model's knowledge of results to increase the observer's performance. *Journal of Human Movement Studies, 12,* 89–98.

Adams, J. A. (1987). Historical review and appraisal of research on the learning, retention, and transfer of human motor skills. *Psychological Bulletin, 101,* 41–74.

Adams, J. A., & Creamer, L. R. (1962). Anticipatory timing of continuous and discrete responses. *Journal of Experimental Psychology, 63,* 84–90.

Adams, J. A., & Dijkstra, S. (1966). Short-term memory for motor responses. *Journal of Experimental Psychology, 71,* 314–318.

Adams, J. A. & Goetz, E. T. (1973). Feedback and practice as variables in errror detection and correction. *Journal of Motor Behavior, 5,* 217–224.

Adams. J. A., Goetz, E. T., & Marshall, P. H. (1972). Response produced feedback and motor learning. *Journal of Experimental Psychology, 92,* 391–397.

Adams, J. A., & Hufford, L. E. (1962). Contributions of a part-task trainer to the learning and relearning of a time-shared flight maneuver. *Human Factors, 4,* 159–170.

Adams, J. A., Marshall, P. H., & Goetz, E. T. (1972). Response feedback and short-term motor retention. *Journal of Experimental Psychology, 92,* 92–95.

Ainscoe, M., & Hardy, L. (1987). Cognitive warm-up in a cyclical gymnastics skill. International *Journal of Sport Psychology, 18,* 269–275.

Albus, J. S. (1971). A theory of cerebellar function. *Math and Bioscience, 10,* 25–61.

Alderson, G. J. K., Sully, D. J., & Sully, H. G. (1974). An operational analysis of a one-handed catching task using high speed photography. *Journal of Motor Behavior, 6,* 217–226.

Allard, F., Graham, S., & Paarsalu, M. E. (1980). Perception in sport: Basketball. *Journal of Sport Psychology, 2,* 14–21.

Allard, F., & Starkes, J. L. (1980). Perception in sport: Volleyball. *Journal of Sport Psychology, 2,* 22–33.

Allison, L., & Fuller, K. (2001). Balance and vestibular disorders. In D. A. Umphred (ed.), *Neurological rehabilitation* (4th ed.) (pp. 616–660). Philadelphia: Mosby.

Amaral, D. G. (2000). The anatomical organization of the central nervous system. In E. R. Kandel, J. H. Schwartz, & T. M. Jessell (Eds.), *Principles of neural science* (4th ed.) (pp. 653–673). New York: McGraw-Hill.

Ammons, R. B. (1958). Le mouvement. In G. H. Steward & J. P. Steward (Eds.), *Current psychological issues* (pp. 146–183). New York: Holt, Rinehart, & Winston.

Ammons, R. B., Ammons, C. H., & Morgan, R. L. (1956). Transfer of skill and decremental factors along the speed dimension in rotary pursuit. *Perceptual and Motor Skills, 6,* 43.

Anderson, D. I., & Sidaway, B. (1994). Coordination changes associated with practice of a soccer kick. *Research Quarterly for Exercise and Sport, 65,* 93–99.

Anderson, J. R. (1981). A theory of language based on general learning mechanisms. *Proceedings of the Seventh International Joint Conference on Artificial Intelligence.* pp. 97–103.

Anderson, J. R. (1982). Acquisition of cognitive skill. *Psychological Review, 89, 4,* 369–406.

Anderson, J. R. (1987). Skill acquisition: Compilation of weak-method problem solutions. *Psychological Review, 94,* 192–210.

Anderson, J. R., & Reder, L. M. (1979). An elaborative processing explanation of depth of processing. In L. S. Cermak & F. I. M. Craik (Eds.), *Levels of processing in human memory* (pp. 385–403). Hillsdale, NJ: Erlbaum.

Anderson, M. P. (1981). Assessment and imaginal processes: Approaches and issues. In T. V. Merluzzi, C. R. Glass, & M. Genst (Eds.), *Cognitive assessment* (pp. 149–187). New York: Guilford Press.

Annett, J. (1959). Learning a pressure under conditions of immediate and delayed knowledge of results. *Quarterly Journal of Experimental Psychology, 11,* 3–15.

Annett, J. (1979). Memory for skill. In M. Gruneberg & P. Morris (Eds.), *Applied problems in memory* (pp. 215–247). London: Academic Press.

Anshel, M. H., & Wrisberg, C. A. (1988). The effect of arousal and focused attention on warm-up decrement. *Journal of Sport Behavior, 11,* 18–31.

Anshel, M. H., & Wrisberg, C. A. (1993). Reducing warm-up decrement in the performance of the tennis serve. *Journal of Sport and Exercise Psychology, 15,* 290–303.

Anson, J. G. (1982). Memory drum theory: Alternative tests and explanations for the complexity effects on simple reaction time. *Journal of Motor Behavior, 14,* 228–246.

Anson, J. G. (1989). Effects of moment of inertia on simple reaction time. *Journal of Motor Behavior, 21,* 60–71.

Arbib, M. A., Erdi, P., & Szentagothai, J. (1998). *Neural organization: Structure, function and dynamics.* Cambridge, MA: MIT Press.

Ascoli, K. M., & Schmidt, R. A. (1969). Proactive interference in short-term motor retention. *Journal of Motor Behavior, 1,* 29–35.

Atkinson, J. W., & Birch, D. (1978). *An introduction to motivation* (Rev. ed.). New York: Van Nostrand Reinhold.

Atkinson, R. C., & Shiffrin, R. M. (1968). Human memory: A proposed system and its control processes. In K. W. Spence & J. T. Spence (Eds.), *The psychology of learning and motivation: Advances in research and theory* (Vol. 2, pp. 90–196). New York: Academic Press.

Atkinson, R. C., & Shiffrin, R. M. (1971). The control of short-term memory. *Scientific American, 225,* 82–90.

Baddeley, A. D. (1978). The trouble with levels: A reexamination of Craik and Lockhart's framework for memory research. *Psychological Review, 85,* 139–152.

Baddeley, A. D. (1981). The concept of working memory: A view of its current state and probable future development. Cognition, *10,* 17–23.

Bahill, A. T., & LaRitz, T. (1984). Why can't batters keep their eyes on the ball? *American Scientist, 72,* 249–252.

Bahrick, H. P. (1957). An analysis of stimulus variables influencing the proprioceptive control of movement. *Psychological Review, 64,* 324–328.

Bahrick, H. P. (1969). Measurement of memory by prompted recall. *Journal of Experimental Psychology, 79,* 213–219.

Bahrick, H. P., Fitts, P. M., & Briggs, G. E. (1957). Learning curves—facts or artifacts? *Psychological Bulletin, 54,* 256–268.

Bahrick, H. P., & Noble, M. E. (1966). Motor behavior. In J. B. Sidowski (Ed.), *Experimental methods and instrumentation in psychology* (pp. 645–675). New York: McGraw-Hill.

Baker, K. E., Wylie, R. C., & Gagne, R. M. (1950). Transfer of training to a motor skill as a function of variation in rate of response. *Journal of Experimental Psychology, 40,* 721–732.

Bakker, F. C., Boschker, M. S. J., & Chung, T. (1996). Changes in muscular activity while imagining weight lifting using stimulus response propositions. *Journal of Sport and Exercise Psychology, 18,* 313–324.

Balko Perry, S. (1998). Clinical implications of a dynamic systems theory. *Neurology Report, 22,* 4–10.

Baloh, R. W., & Hornrubia, V. (1990). *Clinical neurophysiology of the vestibular system* (2nd ed.). Philadelphia: F. A. Davis.

Bandura, A. (1977). Self-efficacy: Toward a unifying theory of behavioral change. *Psychological Review, 84,* 191–215.

Bandura, A. (1986). *Social foundations of thought and action: A social cognitive theory.* Englewood Cliffs, NJ: Prentice-Hall.

Bandura, A., Jeffrey, R. W., & Bachica, D. L. (1974). Analysis of memory codes and cumulative rehearsal in observational learning. *Journal of Research in Personality, 7,* 295–305.

Barclay, C. D., Cutting, J. E., & Kozlowski, L. T. (1978). Temporal and spatial factors in gait perception that influence gender recognition. *Perception and Psychophysics, 23,* 145–152.

Bard, C., & Fleury, M. (1981). Considering eye movement as a prediction of attainment. In I. M. Cockerill & W. W. MacGillivray (Eds.), *Vision and sport* (pp. 28–41). Cheltenham, UK: Stanley Thornes Publishers.

Barela, J. A., Whitall, J., Black, P., & Clark, J. E. (2000). An examination of constraints affecting the intra-limb coordination of hemiparetic gait. *Human Movement Science, 19,* 251–273.

Barkow, A., & Barrett, D. (1998). *Golf legends of all time.* Lincolnwood, IL: Publications International.

Barnett, M. L., Ross, D., Schmidt, R. A., & Todd, B. (1973). Motor skills learning and the specificity of training principle. *Research Quarterly for Exercise and Sport, 44,* 440–447.

Baron, R. A. (1970). Attraction toward the model and model's competence as determinants of adult initiative behavior. *Journal of Personality and Social Psychology, 14,* 345–351.

Barrett, K., Clark, J., French, K., Langendorfer, S., Whitall, J., & Williams, K. (1995). *Looking at physical education from a developmental perspective: A guide to teaching.* Reston, VA: National Association for Sport and Physical Education.

Battig, W. F. (1972). Intratask interference as a source of facilitation in transfer and retention. In R. F. Thompson & J. F. Voss (Eds.), *Topics in learning and performance* (pp. 131–159). New York: Academic Press.

Battig, W. F. (1979). The flexibility of human memory. In L. S. Cermak & F. I. M. Craik (Eds.), *Levels of processing in human memory* (pp. 23–44). Hillsdale, NJ: Erlbaum.

Baxter, M. L., & Baxter, D. A. (1999). Neural mechanisms of learning and memory. In H. Cohen (Ed.), *Neuroscience for rehabilitation* (2nd ed.) (pp. 321–348). Philadelphia: Lippincott.

Beals, R. P., Mayyasi, A. M., Templeton, A. E., & Johnston, W. L. (1971). The relationship between basketball-shooting performance and certain visual attributes. *American Journal of Optometry and Archives of the American Academy of Optometry, 48,* 585–590.

Beek, P. J. (1989). Timing and phase locking in cascade juggling. *Ecological Psychology, 1,* 55–96.

Beek, P., & Meijer, O. (1988). On the nature of the motor-action controversy. In O. Meijer & K. Roth (Eds.). *Complex movement behavior: "The" motor-action controversy* (pp. 157–185). Amsterdam: Elsevier.

Behrman, A. L., & Harkema, S. J. (2000). Locomotor training after spinal cord injury: A series of case studies. *Physical Therapy, 80,* 688–700.

Bell, H. M. (1950). Retention of pursuit rotor task after one year. *Journal of Experimental Psychology, 40,* 648–649.

Benedetti, C., & McCullagh, P. (1987). Post-knowledge lof results delay: Effects of interpolated activity on learning and performance. *Research Quarterly for Exercise and Sport, 58,* 375–381.

Berardelli, A., Rona, S., Inghilleri, M., & Manfredi, M. (1996). Cortical inhibition in Parkinson's disease. A study with paired magnetic stimulation. *Brain, 119*(1), 71–77.

Berg, W. P., Wade, M. G., & Greer, N. L. (1994). Visual regulation of gait in bipedal locomotion: Revisiting Lee, Lishman, & Thomson (1952). *Journal of Experimental Psychology: Human Perception and Performance, 20,* 854–863.

Bernstein, N. (1967). *The co-ordination and regulation of movement.* London: Pergamon Press.

Bilodeau, E. A., & Bilodeau, I. M. (1958a). Variable frequency of knowledge of results and the learning of a simple skill. *Journal of Experimental Psychology, 55,* 379–383.

Bilodeau, E. A., & Bilodeau, I. M. (1958b). Variation of temporal intervals among critical events in five studies of knowledge of results. *Journal of Experimental Psychology, 55,* 603–612.

Bilodeau, E. A., Bilodeau, I. M., & Schumsky, D. A. (1959). Some effects of introducing and withdrawing knowledge of results early and late in practice. *Journal of Experimental Psychology, 58,* 142–144.

Bird, A. M., & Rikli, R. (1983). Observational-learning and practice variability. *Research Quarterly for Exercise and Sport, 54,* 1–4.

Bliss, C. B. (1892–1893). Investigations in reaction time and attention. *Studies from the Yale Psychological Laboratory, 1,* 1–55.

Blundell, N. L. (1984). Critical visual-perceptual attributes of championship level tennis players. In M. Howell & B. Wilson (Eds.), *Proceedings of the VII Commonwealth and International Conference on Sport, Physical Education, Recreation and Dance, Kinesiological Sciences, 7,* 51–61.

Blundell, N. L. (1985). The contribution of vision to the learning and performance of sport skills. Part I: The role of selected visual parameters. *Australian Journal of Science and Medicine in Sports, 17,* 3–11.

Bobath, B. (1965). *Abnormal postural reflex activity caused by brain lesions.* London: Heinemann Medical Books.

Bobath, B. (1978). *Adult hemiplegia: Evaluation and treatment* (2nd ed.). London: Heinemann Medical Books.

Bobath, K. A., & Bobath, B. (1984). Neuro-developmental treatment. In D. Scrutton (Ed) *Management of motor disorders in children with cerebral palsy* (2nd ed.). Philadelphia: J. B. Lippincott.

Boder, D. P. (1935). The influence of concomitant activity and fatigue upon certain forms of reciprocal hand movements and its fundamental components. *Comparative Psychology Monographs, 11* (No. 4).

Bonnet, M., Decety, J., Jeannerod, M., & Requin, J. (1997). Mental simulation of an action modulates the excitability of spinal reflex pathways in man. *Cognitive Brain Research, 5,* 221–228.

Bootsma, R. J., & van Wieringen, P. C. W. (1990). Timing an attacking forehand drive in table tennis. *Journal of Experimental Psychology: Human Perception and Performance, 16,* 21–29.

Borgeaud, P., & Abernethy, B. (1987). Skilled perception in volleyball defense. *Journal of Sport Psychology, 9,* 400–406.

Boswell, J. J., & Irion, A. L. (1975). Transfer of training as a function of target speed in pursuit-rotor performance: Proactive and retroactive effects. *Journal of Motor Behavior, 7,* 105–111.

Boyce, B. A. (1992). Effects of assigned versus participant-set goals on skill acquisition and retention of a selected shooting task. *Journal of Teaching in Physical Education, 11,* 220–234.

Bransford, J. D., & Franks, J. J. (1976). Toward a framework for understanding learning. In G. H. Bower (Ed.), *The psychology of learning and motivation: Vol. 10.* New York: Academic Press.

Bransford, J. D., Franks, J. J., Morris, C. D., & Stein, B. S. (1979). Some general constraints on learning and memory research. In L. S. Cermak & F. I. M. Craik (Eds.), *Levels of processing in human memory* (pp. 331–354). Hillsdale, NJ: Erlbaum.

Bridgman, C. F. (1980). Comparisons of structure of tendon organs in the rat, cat, and man. *Journal of Comparative Neurology, 138,* 369–372.

Broer, M. (1958). Effectiveness of a general basic skills curriculum for junior high school girls. *Research Quarterly for Exercise and Sport, 29,* 379–388.

Brooks, V. B. (1984). Cerebellar functions in motor control. *Human Neurobiology, 2,* 251–260.

Brooks, V. B. (1986). *The neural basis of motor control.* New York: Oxford University Press.

Brophy, J. E. (1981). Teacher praise: A functional analysis. *Review of Educational Research, 51,* 5–32.

Brown, T. G. (1911). The intrinsic factors in the act of progression in the mammal. Proceedings of the Royal Society of London. *Biological Sciences, 84,* 308–319.

Brown, L. A., Shumway-Cook, M. H., & Woollacott, M. H. (1999). Attentional demands and postural recovery: The effects of aging. *Journal of Gerontology: Medical Sciences, 54A,* M165–M171.

Bryan, W., & Harter, N. (1897). Studies in the physiology and psychology of telegraphic language. *Psychological Review, 4,* 27–53.

Buchanan, P. A. & Ulrich, B. D. (2001). The feldenkrais method: A dynamic approach to changing motor behavior. *Research Quarterly for Exercise and Sport, 72,* 315–323.

Buchtal, F., & Schmalbruch, H. (1980). Motor unit of mammalian muscle. *Physiological Review, 60,* 90–142.

Buchwald, N. A., Hull, C. D., Levine, M. S., & Villablanca, J. (1975). The basal ganglia and the regulation of response and cognitive sets. In M. A. B. Brazier (Ed.), *Growth and development of the brain* (pp. 171–190). New York: Raven Press.

Bugelski, B. R., & Cadwallader, T. C. (1956). A reappraisal of the transfer and retroaction surface. *Journal of Experimental Psychology, 52,* 360–366.

Bulsara, A. R., & Gammaitoni, L. (1996, March). Tuning into noise. *Physics Today,* 39.

Burack, B., & Moss, D. (1956). Effect of knowing the principle basic to solution of a problem. *Journal of Educational Research, 50,* 203–208.

Burdenshaw, D., Spragens, J. E., & Weis, P. A. (1970). Evaluation of general versus specific instruction of badminton skills to women of low motor ability. *Research Quarterly for Exercise and Sport, 41,* 472–477.

Burgess, P. R., & Clark, F. J. (1969). Characteristics of knee joint receptors in the cat. *Journal of Physiology, 203,* 317–335.

Burgess-Limerick, R., Shemmell, J., Barry, B. K., Carson, R. G., & Abernethy, B. (2001). Spontaneous transitions in the coordination of a whole-body task. *Human Movement Science, 20,* 549–562.

Burke, R. E. (1981). Motor units: Anatomy, physiology, and functional organization. In V. B. Brooks (Ed.), *Handbook of physiology: Section 1. The nervous system: Vol. II. Motor control* (Pt. 1, pp. 345–422). Bethesda, MD: American Physiological Society.

Burke, R. E., & Edgerton, V. R. (1975). Motor unit properties and selective involvement in movement. *Exercise and Sport Science Reviews, 3,* 31–81.

Burstein, M. K. (1986). Concept formation by incremental analogical reasoning and debugging. In R. S. Michalski, J. G. Carbonell, & T. M. Mitchell (Eds.), *Machine learning: An artificial intelligence approach* (Vol. 2, pp. 351–370). Los Altos, CA: Kaufmann.

Burton, D. (1993). Goal setting in sport. In R. N. Singer, M. Murphy, & L. K. Tennant (Eds.), *Handbook of research on sport psychology* (pp. 467–491). New York: Macmillan.

Burwitz, L. (1974). Short-term motor memory as a function of feedback and interpolated activity. *Journal of Experimental Psychology, 102,* 338–340.

Cafarelli, E. (1988). Force sensation in fresh and fatigued human skeletal muscle. *Exercise and Sport Sciences Reviews, 16,* 139–168.

Calancie, B., Needham-Shropshire, B., Jacobs, P., Willer, K., Zych, G., & Green, B. A. (1994). Involuntary stepping after chronic spinal cord injury? Evidence for a central rhythm generator for locomotion in man. *Brain, 117,* 1143–1159.

Carlton, L. G. (1981). Processing visual feedback information for movement control. *Journal of Experimental Psychology: Human Perception and Performance, 7,* 1019–1030.

Carnahan, H., Vandervoort, A. A., & Swanson, L. R. (1996). The influence of summary knowledge of results and aging on motor learning. *Research Quarterly for Exercise and Sport, 67,* 280–287.

Carr, J. H., & Shepherd, R. B. (1998). *Neurological rehabilitation: Optimizing performance.* Edinburgh: Butterworth and Heinemann.

Carr, J. & Shepherd, R. (2003). *Stroke rehabilitation: Guidelines for exercise and training to optimize motor skill.* Edinburgh: Butterworth and Heinemann.

Carroll, W. R., & Bandura, A. (1982). The role of visual monitoring in observational learning of action patterns: Making the unobservable observable. *Journal of Motor Behavior, 14,* 153–167.

Carroll, W. R., & Bandura, A. (1985). The role of visual monitoring and motor rehearsal in observational learning of action patterns. *Journal of Motor Behavior, 17,* 269–281.

Carroll, W. R., & Bandura, A. (1990). Representation guidance of action production in observational learning: A causal analysis. *Journal of Motor Behavior, 22,* 85–97.

Carron, A. V. (1969). Performance and learning in a discrete motor task under massed vs. distributed practice. *Research Quarterly for Exercise and Sport, 40,* 481–489.

Carson, L. M., & Wiegand, R. L. (1979). Motor schema formation and retention in young children: A test of Schmidt's schema theory. *Journal of Motor Behavior, 11,* 247–251.

Catalano, J. F., & Kleiner, B. M. (1984). Distant transfer in coincident timing as a function of practice variability. *Perceptual and Motor Skills, 58,* 851–856.

Cauraugh, J. H., Chen, D., & Radlo, S. (1993). Effects of traditional and reversed bandwidth knowledge of results on motor learning. *Research Quarterly for Exercise and Sport, 64*(4), 413–417.

Cermak, L. S., & Craik, F. I. M. (Eds.) (1979). *Levels of processing in human memory.* Hillsdale, NJ: Erlbaum.

Cesari, P., Formenti, F., & Olivato, P. (2003). A common perceptual parameter for stair climbing for children, young and old adults. *Human Movement Science, 22,* 111–124.

Chase, W. G., & Ericsson, K. A. (1982). Skill and working memory. In G. H. Bower (Ed.), *The psychology of learning and motivation* (Vol. 16, pp. 1–58). New York: Academic Press.

Chase, W. G., & Simon, H. A. (1973). Perception in chess. *Cognitive Psychology, 4,* 55–81.

Chen, H. C., Schultz, A. S., Ashton-Miller, J. A., Giordani, B., Alexander, N. B, & Guire, K. E. (1996). Stepping over obstacles: Dividing attention impairs performance of old more than young adults. *Journal of Gerontology, 51A,* M116–M122.

Chi, M. T. H. (1976). Short-term memory limitations in children: Capacity of processing deficits? *Memory and Cognition, 4,* 559–572.

Chi, M. T. H. (1977). Age differences in memory span. *Journal of Experimental Child Psychology, 23,* 266–281.

Chi, M. T. H., Feltovich, P. J., & Glaser, R. (1981). Categorization and representation of physics problems by experts and novices. *Cognitive Science, 5,* 121–152.

Chi, M. T. H., & Koeske, R. D. (1983). Network representation of a child's dinosaur knowledge. *Developmental Psychology, 19,* 29–39.

Chieffi, S., Allport, D. A., & Woodfin, M. (1999). Hand-centered coding of target location in visuo-spatial working memory. *Neuropsychologia, 37,* 495–502.

Christina, R. W. (1987). Motor learning: Future lines of research. In M. Safrit & H. Eckert (Eds.), *The academy papers: The cutting edge in physical education and exercise science research* (pp. 26–41). Champaign, IL: Human Kinetics.

Christina, R. W. (1989). Whatever happened to applied research in motor learning? In J. Skinner, C. Corbin, P. Martin, & C. Wells (Eds.), *Future directions in exercise and sport science research* (pp. 411–422). Champaign, IL: Human Kinetics.

Christina, R. W. (1992). Unraveling the mystery of the response complexity effect in skilled movements. *Research Quarterly for Exercise and Sport, 63,* 218–230.

Christina, R. W. (1997). Concerns and issues in studying and assessing motor learning. *Measurement in Physical Education and Exercise Science, 1,* 19–38.

Christina, R. W., & Alpenfels, E. (2002). Why does traditional training fail to optimize playing performance? In E. Thain (Ed.), *Science and golf IV: Proceedings of the world scientific congress of golf* (pp. 231–245). London: Routledge.

Christina, R. W., & Anson, J. G., (1981). The learning of programmed- and feedback-based processes controlling the production of a positioning response in two dimensions. *Journal of Motor Behavior, 13,* 48–64.

Christina, R. W., Barresi, J. V., & Shaffner, P. (1990). The development of response selection accuracy in a football linebacker using video training. *The Sport Psychologist, 4,* 11–17.

Christina, R. W., & Bjork, R. A. (1991). Optimizing long-term retention and transfer. In D. Druckman & R. A. Bjork (Eds.), *In the mind's eye: Enhancing human performance* (pp. 23–56). Washington, DC: National Academy Press.

Christina, R. W., & Corcos, D. M. (1988). *Coaches' guide to teaching sport skills.* Champaign, IL: Human Kinetics.

Christina, R. W., Fischman, M. G., Vercruyssen, M. J. P., & Anson, J. G. (1982). Simple reaction time as a function of response complexity: Memory drum theory revisited. *Journal of Motor Behavior, 14,* 301–321.

Christina, R. W., & Merriman, W. (1977). Learning the direction and extent of a movement. *Journal of Motor Behavior, 9,* 1–9.

Christina, R. W., & Rose, D. J. (1985). Premotor and motor reaction time as a function of response complexity. *Research Quarterly for Exercise and Sport, 56,* 306–315.

Christina, R. W., & Shea, J. B. (1988). The limitations of generalization based on restricted information. *Research Quarterly for Exercise and Sport, 59,* 291–297.

Christina, R. W., & Shea, J. B. (1993). More on assessing the retention of motor learning based on restricted information. *Research Quarterly for Exercise and Sport, 64*(2), 217–222.

Clark, F. J., & Burgess, P. R. (1975). Slowly adapting receptors in the cat knee joint: Can they signal joint angle? *Journal of Neurophysiology, 38,* 1448–1463.

Clark, F. J., Matthews, P. B. C., & Muir, (1979). Anesthetizing skin. The role of cutaneous receptors.

Clark, J. E., & Ewing, M. (1985). A meta-analysis of gender differences and similarities in the gross motor skill performances of prepubescent children. Paper presented at the annual meeting of the North American Society for the Psychology of Sport and Physical Activity. Gulf Port, MS.

Clark, J. E., & Phillips, S. J. (1993). A longitudinal study of intralimb coordination in the first year of independent walking: A dynamical systems analysis. *Child Development, 64,* 1143–1157.

Clark, J. E., Whitall, J., & Phillips, S. J. (1988). Human interlimb coordination: The first 6 months of independent walking. *Developmental Psychobiology, 21,* 445–456.

Cohen, H. (1999). Special senses 2: The vestibular system. In H. Cohen (Ed.), *Neuroscience for rehabilitation* (pp. 149–167). Philadelphia: Lippincott, Williams & Wilkins.

Cohen, M. S., & Bookheimer, S. Y. (1994). Localization of brain function using magnetic resonance imaging. *Techniques in Neuroscience, 17*(7), 268–277.

Coleman, D. M. (1967). The effect of a unit of movement education upon the level of achievement in the specialized skill of bowling. Unpublished doctoral dissertation, Texas Women's University, Denton, TX.

Colley, A. M. (1989). Learning motor skills: Integrating cognition and action. In A. M. Colley & J. R. Beech (Eds.), *Acquisition and performance of cognitive skills* (pp. 167–189). New York: Wiley.

Colley, A. M., & Beech, J. R. (1988). Grounds for reconciliation: Some preliminary thoughts on cognition and action. In A. M. Colley & J. R. Beech (Eds.), *Cognition and action in skilled behaviour* pp. 1–11). Amsterdam: North-Holland.

Colville, F. M. (1957). The learning of motor skills as influenced by knowledge of mechanical principles. *Journal of Educational Psychology, 48,* 321–327.

Connor, N. P., & Abbs, J. H. (1991). Sensorimotor contributions of the basal ganglia: Recent advances. In J. M. Rothstein (Ed.), *Movement science* (pp. 112–120). Alexandria, VA: American Physical Therapy Association.

Conrad, R. (1962). The design of information. *Occupational Psychology, 36,* 159–162.

Cook, T. (1936). Studies in cross education. V. Theoretical. *Psychological Review, 43,* 149–178.

Cooke, J. D. (1979). Dependence of human arm movements on limb mechanical properties. *Brain Research, 165,* 366–369.

Cooper, L. A. (1995). Varieties of visual representation: How are we to analyze the concept of mental images? *Neuropsychologia, 33,* 1575–1582.

Corcos, D. M., Gottlieb, G. L., & Agarwal, G. C. (1989). Organizing principles for single-joint movements. II. A speed-sensitive strategy. *Journal of Neurophysiology, 62,* 358–368.

Cormier, S. M., & Hagman, J. D. (1987). Introduction. In S. M. Cormier & J. D. Hagman (Eds.), *Transfer of learning: Contemporary research and applications* (pp.1–8). New York: Academic Press.

Coull, J., Tremblay, L., & Elliot, D. (2001). Examining the specificity of practice hypothesis: Is learning modality specific? *Research Quarterly for Exercise and Sport, 72,* 345–354.

Courneya, K. S., & Carron, A. V. (1992). The home advantage in sport competitions: A literature review. *Journal of Sport and Exercise Psychology, 14,* 13–27.

Covington, M. V., & Berry, R. G. (1976). *Self-worth and school learning.* New York: Holt, Rinehart & Winston.

Craik, F. I. M. (1970). The fate of primary items in free recall. *Journal of Verbal Learning and Verbal Behavior, 9,* 143–148.

Craik, F. I. M. (1977). Depth of processing in recall and recognition. In S. Dornic (Ed.), *Attention and performance VI.* Hillsdale, NJ: Erlbaum.

Craik, F. I. M., & Lockhart, R. (1972). Levels of processing: A framework for memory research. *Journal of Verbal Learning and Verbal Behavior, 11,* 671–676.

Craik, F. I. M., & Tulving, E. (1975). Depth of processing and the retention of words in episodic memory. *Journal of Experimental Psychology: General, 104,* 268–294.

Crocker, P. R. E., & Dickinson, J. (1984). Incidental psychomotor learning: The effects of number of movements, practice, and rehearsal. *Journal of Motor Behavior, 16*, 61–75.

Cuddy, L. J., & Jacoby, L. L. (1982). When forgetting helps memory: An analysis of repetition effects. *Journal of Verbal Learning and Verbal Behavior, 21*, 451–467.

Cutting, J. E. (1978). Generation of synthetic male and female walkers through manipulation of a biomechanical invariant. *Perception, 7*, 393–405.

Cutting, J. E., & Kozlowski, L. T. (1977). Recognising friends by their walk: Gait perception without familiarity cues. *Bulletin of the Psychonomic Society, 9*, 353–356.

Cutting J. E., & Proffitt, D. R. (1982). Gait perception as an example of how we may perceive events. In R. Walk & H. L. Pick, Jr. (Eds.), *Intersensory perception and sensory integration* (pp. 32–47). New York: Plenum Press.

Dail, T., & Christina, R. W. (2004). Distribution of practice and metacognition in the learning and long-term retention of a discrete motor task. *Research Quarterly for Exercise and Sport, 75*, 148–155.

Dallet, K. M. (1962). The transfer surface re-examined. *Journal of Verbal Learning and Verbal Behavior, 1*, 91–94.

Damarjian, N. M. (1997). *The short-term training effects of practice variability on posttraining performance of three golf skills with experienced golfers.* Unpublished doctoral dissertation, University of North Carolina at Greensboro, NC.

Davis, G. M., & Thomson, D. M. (1988). *Memory in context: Context in memory.* New York: Wiley.

Davis, R. C. (1942). The pattern of muscular action in simple voluntary movement. *Journal of Experimental Psychology, 31*, 347–366.

Decety, J., Jeannerod, M., Durozard, D., & Baverel, G. (1993). Central activation of autonomic effectors during mental simulation of motor actions. *Journal of Physiology, 461*, 549–563.

Decety, J., Jeannerod, M., Germain, M., & Pastene, J. (1991). Vegetative response during imagined movement is proportional to mental effort. *Behavioral Brain Research, 42*, 1–5.

Decety, J., Perani, D., Jeannerod, M., Bettinardi, V., Tadary, B., Woods, R., Mazziotta, J. C., & Fazio, F. (1994). Mapping motor representations with positron emission tomography. *Nature, 371*, 600–602.

DeGroot, A. D. (1966). Perception and memory vs. thought. In B. Kleinmuntz (Ed.), *Problem solving research methods and theory* (pp. 19–50). New York: Wiley.

Del Rey, P. (1989). Training and contextual interference effects on memory and transfer. *Research Quarterly for Exercise and Sport, 60*, 342–347.

Del Rey, P., Whitehurst, M., & Wood, J. (1983). Effects of experience and contextual interference on learning and transfer. *Perceptual and Motor Skills, 56*, 581–582.

Del Rey, P., Whitehurst, M., Wughalter, E., & Barnwell, J. (1983). Contextual interference and experience in acquisition and transfer. *Perceptual and Motor Skills, 57*, 241–242.

Del Rey, P., Wughalter, E., & Whitehurst, M. (1982). The effects of contextual interference on females with varied experience in open skills. *Research Quarterly for Exercise and Sport, 53*, 108–115.

deLeon, R. D., Hodgson, J. A., Roy, R. R., & Edgerton, V. R. (1998). Locomotor capacity attributable to step training versus spontaneous recovery after spinalization in adult cats. *Journal of Neurophysiology, 79*, 1329–1340.

Della Sala, S. D., Lorenzo, G. D., Giordano, A., & Spinnler, H. (1986). Is there a specific visuo-spatial impairment in parkinsonians? *Journal of Neurology, Neurosurgery, and Psychiatry, 49*, 1258–1265.

DeLong, M. R. (1972). Activity of basal ganglia neurons during movement. *Brain Research, 40*, 127–135.

DeLong, M. R. (2000). The basal ganglia. In E. R. Kandel, J. H. Schwartz, & T. M. Jessell (Eds.), *Principles of neural science* (4th ed.) (pp. 853–867). New York: McGraw-Hill.

DeLong, M. R., & Georgopoulos, A. P. (1981). Motor functions of the basal ganglia. In J. M. Brookhart (Ed.), *Handbook of physiology: The nervous system* (pp. 1017–1061). Bethesda, MD: American Physiological Society.

Denny-Brown, D. (1949). Interpretation of the electromyogram. *Archives of Neurology and Psychiatry, 61*, 99–128.

Denny-Brown, D. (1962). *The basal ganglia and their relation to disorders of movement.* Liverpool, UK: Liverpool University Press.

Denny-Brown, D., & Pennybacker, J. B. (1938). Fibrillation and fasciculation in voluntary muscle. *Brain, 61*, 311–334.

deVries, H. A. (1980). *Physiology of exercise.* Dubuque, IA: Wm. C. Brown.

Dewhurst, D. J. (1967). Neuromuscular control system. *IEEE Transactions on Biomedical Engineering, 14*, 167–171.

Diedrich, F. J., & Warren, W. H., Jr. (1995). Why change gaits? Dynamics of the walk-run transition. *Journal of Experimental Psychology: Human Perception and Performance, 21*, 183–202.

Diedrich, F. J., & Warren, W. H., Jr. (1998). The dynamics of gait transitions: Effects of grade and load. *Journal of Motor Behavior, 30*, 60–78.

Dietz, V., Nakazawa, K., Wirz, M., & Erni, Th. (1999). Level of spinal cord lesion determines locomotor activity in spinal man. *Experimental Brain Research, 128*(3), 405–409.

Diewert, G. L. (1975). Retention and coding in motor short-term memory: A comparison of storage codes for distance and location. *Journal of Motor Behavior, 7,* 183–190.

Diewert, G. L., & Roy, E. A. (1978). Coding strategy for memory of movement extent information. *Journal of Experimental Psychology: Human Learning and Memory, 4,* 666–675.

Dimitrijevic, M. R., Gerasimenko, Y., & Pinter, M. M. (1998). Evidence for a spinal central pattern generator in humans. *Annals of the New York Academy of Sciences, 860,* 360–376.

Dobkin, B. H., Harkema, S., Requejo, P., & Edgerton, V. R. (1995). Modulation of locomotor-like EMG activity in subjects with complete and incomplete spinal cord injury. *Journal of Neurological Rehabilitation, 9,* 183–190.

Doody, S. G., Bird, A. M., & Ross, D. (1985). The effect of auditory and visual models on acquisition of a timing task. *Human Movement Science, 4,* 271–281.

Doyon, J., & Ungerleider, L. G. (2002). Functional anatomy of motor skill learning. In L. R. Squire & D.L. Schacter (Eds.), *Neuropsychology of memory* (3rd ed.). New York: Guilford.

Driskell, J. E., Copper, C., & Moran, A. (1994). Does mental practice enhance performance? *Journal of Applied Psychology, 79,* 481–492.

Duchateau, J., & Enoka, R. M. (2002). Neural adaptations with chronic activity patterns in able-bodied humans. *American Journal of Physical Medicine and Rehabilitation, 81*(Suppl.), S17–S27.

Duncan, C. P. (1953). Transfer of motor learning as a function of first task learning and inter-task similarity. *Journal of Experimental Psychology, 45,* 1–11.

Dunham, P. (1976). Distribution of practice as a factor affecting learning and/or performance. *Journal of Motor Behavior, 8,* 305–307.

Dunn, A. J. (1980). Neurochemistry of learning and memory: An evaluation of recent data. *Annual Review of Psychology, 31,* 343–390.

Edwards, J. M., Elliott, D., & Lee, T. D. (1986). Contextual interference effects during skill acquisition and transfer in Down's syndrome adolescents. *Adapted Physical Activity Quarterly, 3,* 250–258.

Egeth, H. E., & Yantis, S. (1997). Visual attention: Control, representation, and time course. *Annual Review of Psychology, 48,* 269–297.

Elliot, D., Chua, R., Pollock, B. J., & Lyons, J. (1995). Optimizing the use of vision in manual aiming: The role of practice. *The Quarterly Journal of Experimental Psychology, 48,* 72–83.

Elliot, D., & Jaeger, M. (1988). Practice and the visual control of manual aiming movements. *Journal of Human Movement Studies, 14,* 279–291.

Elliot, D., Lyons, J., & Dyson, K. (1997). Rescaling an acquired discrete aiming movement: Specific or general motor learning? *Human Movement Science, 16,* 81–96.

Ellis, H. C. (1965). *The transfer of learning.* New York: Macmillan.

Emmon, H. H., Wesseling, L. G., Bootsma, R. J., Whiting, H. T. A., & van Wieringen, P. C. W. (1985). The effect of video-modelling and video-feedback on the learning of the tennis serve by novices. *Journal of Sport Sciences, 3,* 127–138.

Enoka, R. M. (1994). *Neuromechanical basis of kinesiology* (2nd ed.). Champaign, IL: Human Kinetics.

Enoka, R. M. (2002). *Neuromechanics of human movement* (3rd ed.). Champaign, IL: Human Kinetics.

Enoka, R. M., Miller, D. I., & Burgess, E. M. (1982). Below-knee amputee running gait. *American Journal of Physical Medicine, 61,* 66–84.

Ericsson, K. (2001). The path to expert golf performance: Insights from the masters on how to improve by deliberate practice. In P. Thomas (Ed.), *Optimising performance in golf* (pp. 1–58). Brisbane, Australia: Australian Academic Press.

Ericsson, K., Krampe, R. Th., & Tesch-Römer, C. (1993). The role of deliberate practice in the acquisition of expert performance. *Psychological Review, 100,* 363–406.

Ericsson, K. A., & Polson, P. G. (1984). A cognitive analysis of exceptional memory for restaurant orders. In M. Chi, R. Glaser, & M. Farr (Eds.), *The nature of expertise.* Hillsdale, NJ: Erlbaum.

Estes, W. K. (1956). The problem of inference from curves based on group data. *Psychological Bulletin, 53,* 134–140.

Etnier, J. L., & Landers, D. M. (1996). The influence of procedural variables on the efficacy of mental practice. *The Sport Psychologist, 10,* 48–57.

Eyzaguirre, C., & Fidone, S. J. (1975). *Physiology of the nervous system* (2nd ed.). Chicago: Year Book Medical Publishers.

Farr, M. J. (1987). *The long-term retention of knowledge and skills: A cognitive and instructional perspective.* New York: Springer-Verlag.

Feldman, A. G. (1966). Functional tuning of the nervous system with control of movement or maintenance of a steady posture. II. Controllable parameters of the muscle. *Biophysics, 11,* 565–578.

Feldman, A. G. (1986). Once more on the equilibrium-point hypothesis (lambda symbol model) for motor control. *Journal of Motor Behavior, 18,* 17–54.

Feltz, D. L. (1982). The effect of age and number of demonstrations on modeling form and performance. *Research Quarterly for Exercise and Sport, 53,* 291–296.

Feltz, D. L., & Landers, D. M. (1983). The effects of mental practice on motor skill learning and performance: A meta-analysis. *Journal of Sport Psychology, 5,* 25–57.

Feltz, D. L., Landers, D. M., & Becker, B. J. (1988). A revised meta-analysis of the mental practice literature on motor skill learning. In D. Druckman & J. Swets (Eds.), *Enhancing human performance: Issues, theories and techniques* (pp.19–88). Washington, DC: National Academy Press.

Fendrich, D. W., Healy, A. F., Meiskey, L., Crutcher, R. J., Little, W., & Bourne, L. E., Jr. (1988). Skill maintenance: Literature review and theoretical analysis (Tech. Rep. R30 AFHRL-TP-87-73). San Antonio, TX: Air Force Human Resources Laboratory, Brooks Air Force Base.

Field-Fote, E. C. (2000). Spinal cord control of movement: Implications for locomotor rehabilitation following spinal cord injury. *Physical Therapy, 80*(5), 477–484.

Fischman, M. G., Christina, R. W., & Vercruyssen, M. J. (1982). Retention and transfer of motor skills: A review for the practitioner. *Quest, 33,* 181–194.

Fischman, M. G., & Schneider, T. (1985). Skill level, vision, and proprioception in simple one-hand catching. *Journal of Motor Behavior, 17,* 219–229.

Fitch, H. L., & Turvey, M. T. (1977). On the control of activity: Some remarks from an ecological point of view. In D. Landers & R. Christina (Eds.), *Psychology of motor behavior and sport.* Champaign, IL: Human Kinetics.

Fitts, P. M. (1954). The information capacity of the human motor system in controlling the amplitude of movement. *Journal of Experimental Psychology, 47,* 381–391.

Fitts, P. M. (1964). Perceptual-motor skills learning. In A. W. Melton (Ed.), *Categories of human learning* (pp. 243–285). New York: Academic Press.

Fitts, P. M., & Peterson, J. R. (1964). Information capacity of discrete motor responses. *Journal of Experimental Psychology, 67,* 103–112.

Fleishman, E. A. (1964). *The structure and measurement of physical fitness.* Englewood Cliffs, NJ: Prentice-Hall.

Fleishman, E. A. (1972). On the relation between abilities, learning, and human performance. *American Psychologist, 27,* 1017–1032.

Fleishman, E. A. (1978). Relating individual differences to the dimensions of human tasks. *Ergonomics, 21,* 1007–1019.

Fleishman, E. A., & Hempel, W. E., Jr. (1954). Changes in factor structure of a complex psychomotor test as a function of practice. *Psychometrika, 19,* 239–254.

Fleishman, E. A., & Hempel, W. E., Jr. (1955). The relation between abilities and improvement with practice in a visual discrimination reaction task. *Journal of Experimental Psychology, 49,* 301–312.

Fleishman, E. A., & Parker, J. F. (1962). Factors in the retention and relearning of perceptual-motor skill. *Journal of Experimental Psychology, 64,* 215–226.

Fleishman, E. A., & Rich, S. (1963). Role of kinesthetic and spatial-visual abilities in perceptual-motor learning. *Journal of Experimental Psychology, 66,* 6–11.

Flowers, K. (1976). "Visual closed-loop" and "open-loop" characteristics of voluntary movement in patients with Parkinson's and intention tremor. *Brain, 99,* 260–310.

Formisano, R., Pratesi, L., Modarelli, F., Bonefati, V., & Meco, G. (1992). Rehabilitation and Parkinson's disease. *Scandinavian Journal of Rehabilitation Medicine, 24*(3), 157–160.

Forssberg, H. (1985). Ontogeny of human locomotor control. I. Infant stepping, supported locomotion, and transition to independent locomotion. *Experimental Brain Research, 57,* 480–493.

Forssberg, H., Grillner, S., & Rossignol, S. (1977). Phasic gain control of reflexes from the dorsum of the paw during spinal locomotion. *Brain Research, 132,* 121–139.

Fournier, E., & Pierrot-Deseilligny, E. (1989). Changes in transmission in some reflex pathways during movement in humans. *NIPS 4,* 29–32.

Fowler, C., & Turvey, M. T. (1978). Skill acquisition: An event approach with special reference to searching for the optimum of a function of several variables. In G. Stelmach (Ed.), *Information processing in motor control and learning* (pp. 1–40). New York: Academic Press.

Fox, C. R. (1999). Special senses 3: The visual system. In H. Cohen (Ed.), *Neuroscience for rehabilitation* (pp. 195–206). Philadelphia: Lippincott, Williams & Wilkins.

Franken, R. E. (1982). *Human motivation.* Pacific Grove, CA: Brooks/Cole.

French, K. E., & Thomas, J. R. (1987). The relation of knowledge development to children's basketball performance. *Journal of Sport Psychology, 9,* 15–32.

Fritsch, G., & Hitzig, E. (1870). Uber die elektrische errebarkeit des grosshirns. *Archives of Anatomical Physiologie, 37,* 300–332. (trans. G. von Bonin). In Some papers on the cerebral cortex. (1960) (pp. 73– 96). Springfield, IL: Thomas.

Gabriele, T. E., Hall, C. R., & Buckholz, E. E. (1987). Practice schedule effects on the acquisition and retention of a motor skill. *Human Movement Science, 6,* 1–6.

Gagne, R. M. (1970). *Conditions of learning.* New York: Holt.

Gagne, R. M., Baker, K. E., & Foster, H. (1950). On the relation between similarity and transfer of training in the learning of discriminative motor tasks. *Psychological Review, 57,* 67–79.

Gagne, R. M., Foster, H., & Crowley, M. E. (1948). The measurement of transfer of training. *Psychological Bulletin, 45*, 97–130.

Gallagher, J. D., & Thomas, J. R. (1980). Effects of varying post-KR intervals upon children's motor performance. *Journal of Motor Behavior, 12*, 41–46.

Gallahue, D. L., Werner, P. H., & Luedke, G. C. (1975). *A conceptual approach to moving and learning.* New York: Wiley.

Gandevia, S. (1996). Kinesthesis: Roles for afferent signals and motor commands. In L. B. Rowell & J. T. Shephard (Eds.), *Handbook of physiology. Section 12: Exercise: Regulation and integration of multiple systems* (pp. 128–172). New York: Oxford University Press.

Gandevia, S. C., & McCloskey, D. I. (1977). Changes in motor commands, as shown by changes in perceived heaviness, during partial curarization and peripheral anaesthesia in man. *Journal of Physiology, 272*, 673–689.

Gardlin, G. R., & Sitterly, T. E. (1972). *Degradation of learned skills: A review and annotated bibliography.* Seattle: Boeing Company.

Gardner, E. P., & Kandel, E. R. (2000). Touch. In E. R. Kandel, J. H. Schwartz, & T. M. Jessell (Eds.), *Principles of neural science,* (4th ed.) (pp. 451–471). New York: McGraw-Hill.

Gardner, E. P., & Martin, J. H. (2000). Coding of sensory information. In E. R. Kandel, J. H. Schwartz, & T. M. Jessell (Eds.), *Principles of neural science* (4th ed.) (pp. 411–429). New York: McGraw-Hill.

Gentile, A. M. (1972). A working model of skill acquisition with application to teaching. *Quest* (Monograph XVII), 3–23.

Gentile, A. M. (1987). Skill acquisition: Action, movement, and neuromotor processes. In J. H. Carr, R. B. Shepherd, J. Gordon, A. M. Gentile, & J. M. Held (Eds.), *Movement science: Foundations for physical therapy in rehabilitation* (pp. 93–154). Rockville, MD: Aspen Publications.

Gentile, A. M. (1998). Implicit and explicit processes during acquisition of functional skills. *Scandinavian Journal of Occupational Therapy, 5*, 7–16.

Gentner, D. (1980). *The structure of analogical models in science* (Tech. Rep. 4451). Cambridge, MA: Bolt, Beranek and Newman, Inc.

Gentner, D. (1982). Are scientific analogies metaphors? In D. S. Miall (Ed.), *Metaphor: Problems and perspectives* (pp. 106–118). Brighton, Sussex, UK: Harvester Press, Ltd.

Gentner, D., & Gentner, D. R. (1983). Flowing waters or teeming crowds: Mental models of electricity. In D. Gentner & A. Stevens (Eds.), *Mental models* (pp. 99–127). Hillsdale, NJ: Erlbaum.

Gentner, D., & Stevens, A. L. (1983). *Mental models.* Hillsdale, NJ: Erlbaum.

Georgopoulos, A. P., Kalaska, J. F., Caminiti, R., & Massey, J. T. (1982). On the relations between the direction of two dimensional arm movements and cell discharge in primate motor cortex. *Journal of Neuroscience, 2*, 1527–1537.

Gerst, M. S. (1971). Symbolic coding processes in observational learning. *Journal of Personality and Social Psychology, 19*, 9–17.

Ghatan, P. H., Hsieh, J. C., Wirsen-Muerling, A., Wredling, R., Eriksson, L., Stone-Elander, S., Levander, S., & Ingvar, M. (1995). Brain activation induced by the perceptual maze test: A PET study of cognitive performance. *Neuroimage, 2*(2), 112–124.

Ghez, C., & Krakauer, J. (2000). The organization of movement. In E. R. Kandel, J. H. Schwartz, & T. M. Jessell (Eds.), *Principles of neural science,* (4th ed.) (pp. 653–673). New York: McGraw-Hill.

Ghez, C,. & Thach, W. T. (2000). The cerebellum. In E. R. Kandel, J. H. Schwartz, & T. M. Jessell (Eds.), *Principles of neural science* (4th ed.) (pp. 832–852). New York: McGraw-Hill.

Gibbs, C. B. (1951). Transfer of training and skill assumptions in tracking. *Quarterly Journal of Experimental Psychology, 3*, 99–110.

Gibson, J. J. (1966). *The senses considered as perceptual systems.* Boston: Houghton Mifflin.

Gibson, J. J. (1979). *The ecological approach to visual perception.* Boston: Houghton Mifflin.

Gick, M. L., & Holyoak, K. J. (1987). The cognitive basis of knowledge transfer. In S. M. Cormier & J. D. Hagman (Eds.), *Transfer of learning: Contemporary research and applications* (pp. 9–46). San Diego, CA: Academic Press.

Gilbert, P. F. C., & Thach, W. T. (1977). Purkinje cell activity during motor learning. *Brain Research, 70*, 1–18.

Glanzer, M., & Koppenaal, L. (1977a). The effect of encoding tasks on free recall stages and levels. *Journal of Verbal Learning and Verbal Behavior, 16*, 21–28.

Glanzer, M., & Koppenaal, L. (1977b). Relation between measures of motor educability and learning of specific motor skills. *Research Quarterly for Exercise and Sport, 13*, 43–56.

Glendon, A. I., McKenna, S. P., Blaylock, S. S., & Hunt, K. (1987). Evaluating mass training in cardiopulmonary resuscitation. *British Medical Journal, 294*, 1182–1183.

Glickstein, M., & Yeo, C. (1989). The cerebellum and motor learning. *Journal of Cognitive Neuroscience, 2*(2), 69–79.

Godden, D. R., & Baddeley, A. D. ( 1975). Context-dependent memory in two natural environments: On land and underwater. *British Journal of Psychology, 66*, 325–331.

Goldberg, M. E. (2000). The control of gaze. In E. R. Kandel, J. H. Schwartz, & T. M. Jessell (Eds.), *Principles of neural science* (4th ed.) (pp. 782–800). New York: McGraw-Hill.

Goldberg, M. E., & Hudspeth, A. J. (2000). The vestibular system. In E. R. Kandel, J. H. Schwartz, & T. M. Jessell (Eds.), *Principles of neural science* (4th ed.) (pp. 801–815). New York: McGraw-Hill.

Goode, S. L. (1986). The contextual interference effect in learning an open motor skill. Unpublished doctoral dissertation, Louisiana State University, Baton Rouge, LA.

Goode, S. L., & Magill, R. A. (1986). The contextual interference effect in learning three badminton serves. *Research Quarterly for Exercise and Sport, 57,* 308–314.

Goode, S. L., & Wei, P. (1988). Differential effects of variations of random and blocked practice on novice learning of an open motor skill (Abstract). In D. L. Gill & J. E. Clarke (Eds.), *Abstracts of Research Papers, 1988* (p. 80). American Alliance for Health, Physical Education, Recreation and Dance (AAHPERD) Annual Convention, Kansas City, MO. Reston, VA: AAHPERD.

Goodwin, G. M., McCloskey, D. I., & Matthews, P. B. C. (1972). The contribution of muscle afferents to kinesthesia shown by vibration-induced illusions of movement and by the effects of paralysing joint afferents. *Brain, 95,* 705–748.

Gordon, J. (1987). Assumptions underlying physical therapy intervention: Theoretical and historical perspectives. In J. H. Carr, R. B. Shepherd, J. Gordon, A. M. Gentile, & J. M. Held (Eds.), *Movement Science: Foundations for physical therapy in rehabilitation* (pp. 1–30). Rockville, MD: Aspen Publications.

Gordon, W. C. (1989). *Learning and memory.* Pacific Grove, CA: Brooks/Cole.

Gottlieb, G. L., Corcos, D. M., Agarwal, G. C., & Latash, M. L. (1990). Organizing principles for single-joint movements. I. A speed-insensitive strategy. *Journal of Neurophysiology, 63,* 625–636.

Gould, D. R. (1980). *The influence of motor task types on model effectiveness.* Unpublished doctoral dissertation, University of Illinois, Urbana–Champaign, IL.

Gould, D. R., & Weiss, M. R. (1981). The effects of model similarity and model talk on self-efficacy and muscular endurance. *Journal of Sport Psychology, 3,* 17–29.

Goulet, C., Bard, C., & Fleury, M. (1989). Expertise differences in preparing to return a tennis serve: A visual information processing approach. *Journal of Sport and Exercise Psychology, 11,* 382–398.

Graham G., Holt-Hale, S., & Parker, M. (1993). *Children moving: A reflective approach to teaching physical education.* Mountain View, CA: Mayfield.

Graybiel, A.M. (1998). The basal ganglia and chunking of action repertoires. *Neurobiology of Learning and Memory, 70,* 119.

Grillner, S. (1975). The role of muscle stiffness in meeting the postural and locomotor requirements for force development by the ankle extensors. *Acta Physiologica Scandinavia, 86,* 92–108.

Hagman, J. D. (1978). Specific-cue effects of interpolated movements on distance and location retention in short-term motor memory. *Memory and Cognition, 6,* 432–437.

Hagman, J. D., & Rose, A. M. (1983). Retention of military skills: A review. *Human Factors, 25,* 199–213.

Haken, H. (1977). *Synergetics: An introduction.* Berlin: Springer-Verlag.

Haken, H. (1983). *Advanced synergetics.* Berlin: Springer-Verlag.

Hale, B. D. (1981). *The effects of internal and external imagery on muscular and ocular concomitants.* Unpublished doctoral dissertation, Pennsylvania State University, University Park, PA.

Hale, B. D. (1982). The effects of internal and external imagery on muscular and ocular concomitants. *Journal of Sport Psychology, 4,* 379–387.

Hall, K. G., Domingues, D. A., & Cavazos, R. (1994). Contextual interference effects with skilled baseball players. *Perceptual and Motor Skills, 78,* 835–841.

Hall, K. G., & Magill, R. A. (1995). Variability of practice and contextual interference effects in motor skill learning. *Journal of Motor Behavior, 27,* 299–309.

Hall, S. J. (2003). *Basic biomechanics* (4th ed.). Dubuque, IA: McGraw-Hill.

Hallett, M. (1993). Physiology of basal ganglia disorders: An overview. *Canadian Journal of Neurological Science, 20,* 177.

Hallett, M., Shahani, B. T., & Young, R. R. (1975). EMG analysis of patients with cerebellar deficits. *Journal of Neurology, Neurosurgery, and Psychiatry, 38,* 1163–1169.

Halverson, L., Roberton, M. A., & Langendorfer, S. (1982). Development of the overarm throw: Movement and ball velocity changes by seventh grade. *Research Quarterly for Exercise and Sport, 53,* 198–205.

Hamachek, D. E. (1978). *Encounters with the self* (2nd ed.). New York: Holt, Rinehart & Winston.

Hamill, J., Haddad, J. M., & McDermott, W. J. (2000). Issues in quantifying variability from a dynamical systems perspective. *Journal of Applied Biomechanics, 16,* 407–418.

Hamilton, C. E. (1950). The relationship between length of interval separating two learning tasks and performance on the second task. *Journal of Experimental Psychology, 40,* 613–621.

Hancock, G. R., Butler, M. S., & Fischman, M. G. (1995). On the problem of two-dimensional error scores: Measures and analyses of accuracy, bias, and consistency. *Journal of Motor Behavior, 27,* 241–250.

Hanna, A., Abernethy, B., Neal, R. J., & Burgess-Limerick, R. J. (2000). Triggers for the transition between human walking and running. In W. A. Sparrow (Ed.), *Energetics of human activity* (pp. 124–164). Champaign, IL: Human Kinetics.

Hardy, L., & Nelson, D. (1988). Self-regulation in sport and work. *Ergonomics, 31,* 1573–1583.

Harkema, S. (2001). Neural plasticity after human spinal cord injury: Application of locomotor training to the rehabilitation of walking. *Neuroscientist, 75,* 455–468.

Harlow, H. F. (1949). The formation of learning sets. *Psychological Review, 56,* 51–65.

Harlow, H. F. (1951). Thinking. In H. Helson (Ed.), *Theoretical foundations of psychology* (pp. 452–500). New York: Van Nostrand.

Harlow, H. F. (1959). Learning set and error factor theory. In S. Koch (Ed.), *Psychology: A study of science* (2nd ed.) (pp. 492–537). New York: McGraw-Hill.

Harrison, S. (1958). Problems of piano playing. *Ergonomics, 1,* 273–276.

Hay, J. G. (1988). Approach strategies in the long jump. *International Journal of Sport Biomechanics, 4,* 114–129.

He, S. Q., Dum, R. P., & Strick, P. L. (1993). Topographic organization of corticospinal projections from the frontal lobe: Motor areas on the lateral surface of the hemisphere. *Journal of Neuroscience, 13,* 952–980.

Hebb, D. O. (1949). The organization of behavior. New York: Wiley.

Hebert, E. P., & Landin, D. (1994). Effects of a learning model and augmented feedback on tennis skill acquisition. *Research Quarterly for Exercise and Sport, 65,* 250–257.

Heiderscheit, B. C. (2000). Movement variability as a clinical measure for locomotion. *Journal of Applied Biomechanics, 16,* 419–427.

Helsen, W., & Pauwels, J. M. (1990). Analysis of visual search activity in solving tactical game problems. In D. Brogan (Ed.), *Visual search* (pp. 177–184). London: Taylor & Francis.

Helsen, W. F., Elliott, D., Starkes, J. L., & Ricker, K. L. (1998). Temporal and spatial coupling of point of gaze and hand movements in aiming. *Journal of Motor Behavior, 30,* 249–259.

Helsen, W. F., Elliott, D., Starkes, J. L., & Ricker, K. L. (2000). Coupling of eye, finger, elbow, and shoulder movements during manual aiming. *Journal of Motor Behavior, 32,* 241–248.

Hendrickson, G., & Schroeder, W. H. (1941). Transfer of training in learning to hit a submerged target. *Journal of Educational Psychology, 32,* 205–213.

Henneman, E. (1957). Relation between size of neurons and their susceptibility to discharge. *Science, 126,* 1345–1347.

Henneman, E. (1979). Functional organization of motoneuron pools: The size principle. In H. Asanuma & V. J. Wilson (Eds.), *Integration in the nervous system* (pp. 13–25). Tokyo: Igaku-Shoin.

Henry, F. M. (1958). Specificity vs. generality in learning motor skills. *Annual Proceedings of the College Physical Education Association, 61,* 126–128.

Henry, F. M. (1961). Reaction time-movement time correlations. *Perceptual and Motor Skills, 12,* 63–66.

Henry, F. M. (1974). Variable and constant performance errors with a group of individuals. *Journal of Motor Behavior, 6,* 149–154.

Henry, F. M., & Rogers, D. E. (1960). Increased response latency for complicated movements and a "memory drum" theory of neuromotor reaction. *Research Quarterly for Exercise and Sport, 31,* 448–458.

Herdman, S. (2000). *Vestibular rehabilitation* (2nd ed.). Philadelphia: F. A. Davis.

Heuer, H., & Keele, S. W. (Eds.). (1996). *Handbook of perception and action.* New York: Academic Press.

Hicks, R. E. (1975). Intrahemispheric response competition between vocal and unimanual performance in normal adult human males. *Journal of Comparative and Physiological Psychology, 89,* 50–60.

Hicks, R. E., Gualtieri, T. C., & Schroeder, S. R. (1983). Cognitive and motor components in bilateral transfer. *American Journal of Psychology, 96,* 223–228.

Hinshaw, K. E. (1991). The effects of mental practice on motor skill performance: Critical evaluation and meta-analysis. *Imagination, Cognition and Personality, 11,* 3–35.

Hird, J. S., Landers, D. M., Thomas, J. R., & Horan, J. (1991). Physical practice is superior to mental practice in enhancing cognitive and motor performance. *Journal of Sport and Exercise Psychology, 13,* 281–293.

Ho, L., & Shea, J. B. (1978). Levels of processing and the coding of position cues in motor short-term memory. *Journal of Motor Behavior, 10,* 113–121.

Hoehn, M. M., & Yahr, M. D. (1967). Parkinsonism: Onset, progression and mortality. *Neurology, 17,* 427.

Hogan, J., & Yanowitz, B. (1978). The role of verbal estimates of movement error in ballistic skill acquisition. *Journal of Motor Behavior, 10,* 133–138.

Holding, D. H. (1962). Transfer between difficult and easy tasks. *British Journal of Psychology, 53,* 397–407.

Holding, D. H. (1965). *Principles of training.* Oxford: Pergamon.

Hollerbach, J. M. (1987). *A study of human motor control through analysis and synthesis of handwriting.* Unpublished doctoral dissertation, Massachusetts Institute of Technology, Cambridge, MA.

Holmes, G. (1939). The cerebellum of man. *Brain, 62,* 1–30.

Holyoak, K. J. (1985). The pragmatics of analogical transfer. In G. H. Bower (Ed.), *The psychology of learning and motivation* (Vol. 19, pp. 59–87). New York: Academic Press.

Hornak, J. E. (1971). *The effects of three methods of teaching on the learning of a motor skill.* Unpublished doctoral dissertation, University of Northern Colorado, Greeley, CO.

Housner, L. D., & French, K. E. (1994). Future directions for research on expertise in learning, performance, and instruction in sport and physical activity. *Quest, 46,* 241–246.

Housner, L., & Hoffman, S. J. (1981). Imagery ability in recall of distance and location information. *Journal of Motor Behavior, 13,* 207–223.

Howland, D., & Noble, M. E. (1953). The effect of physical constants of a control on tracking performance. *Journal of Experimental Psychology, 46,* 353–360.

Hubbard, A. W., & Seng, C. N. (1954). Visual movements of batters. *Research Quarterly for Exercise and Sport, 25,* 42–57.

Hurlock, R. E., & Montague, W. E. (1982). *Skill retention and its implications for Navy tasks: An analytical review.* NPRDC SR 82–21, San Diego, CA: Navy Personnel Research and Development Center.

Inglis, J., Campbell, D., & Donald, M. W. (1976). Electromyographic feedback and neuromuscular rehabilitation. *Canadian Journal of Behavioral Science, 8,* 299–323.

Ito, M. O. (1970). Neurophysiological aspects of the cerebellar motor control system. *International Journal of Neurophysiology, 1,* 162.

Ito, M. (1984). *The cerebellum and neural control.* New York: Raven.

Iyer, M. B., Mitz, A. R., & Winstein, C. (1999). Motor 1: Lower centers. In H. Cohen (Ed.), *Neuroscience for rehabilitation* (pp. 209–239). Philadelphia: Lippincott, Williams & Wilkins.

Jackson, J. H. (1932). *Selected writings of John Hughlings Jackson.* (Vol. 2). J. Taylor (Ed.). London: Hodder and Stoughton.

Jacobs, S. E., & Lowe, D. L. (1999). Somatic senses I: The anterolateral system. In H. Cohen (Ed.) *Neuroscience for rehabilitation.* (pp. 77–92.) Philadelphia: Lippincott, Williams & Wilkins.

Janelle, C. M., Barba, D. A., Frehlich, S. G., Tennant, L. K., & Cauraugh, J. H. (1997). Maximizing performance feedback effectiveness through videotape replay and a self-controlled learning environment. *Research Quarterly for Exercise and Sport, 68,* 269–279.

Janelle, C. M., Kim, J., & Singer, R. N. (1995). Participant-controlled performance feedback and learning of a closed motor skill. *Perceptual and Motor Skills, 81,* 627–634.

Jeannerod, M. (1984). The timing of natural prehension movements. *Journal of Motor Behavior, 16*(3), 235–254.

Jeannerod, M. (1994). The representing brain: Neural correlates of motor intention and imagery. *Behavioral and Brain Sciences, 17,* 187–245.

Jelsma, O., & Pieters, J. M. (1989). Practice schedule and cognitive style interaction in learning a maze task. *Applied Cognitive Psychology, 3,* 73–83.

Jelsma, O., & Van Merrienboer, J. J. G. (1989). Contextual interference interactions with reflection-impulsivity. *Perceptual and Motor Skills, 68,* 1055–1064.

Jensen, B. E. (1975). Pretask speed training and movement complexity as factors in rotary-pursuit skill acquisition. *Research Quarterly for Exercise and Sport, 46,* 1–11.

Jobst, E. E., Melnick, M. E., Byl, N. N., Dowling, G. A., & Aminoff, M. J. (1997). Sensory perception in Parkinson disease. *Archives of Neurology, 54*(4), 450–454.

Johansson, G. (1976). Spatio-temporal differentiation and integration in visual motion perception. *Psychological Research, 38,* 379–393.

Johansson, G., von Hofsten, G., & Jansson, G. (1980). Event perception. *Annual Review of Psychology, 31,* 27–63.

Johnson, D. W., & Johnson, R. T. (1975). *Learning together and alone: Cooperation, competition, and individualization.* Englewood Cliffs, NJ: Prentice-Hall.

Johnson, P. (1982). The functional equivalence of imagery and movement. *Quarterly Journal of Experimental Psychology: Human Experimental Psychology, 34A,* 349–365.

Johnson, R. W., Wicks, G., & Ben-Sira, D. (1981). Practice in the absence of knowledge of results: Skill acquisition and retention. In G. C. Roberts & D. M. Landers (Eds.), *Psychology of motor behavior and sport.* Champaign, IL: Human Kinetics.

Jones, L. A. (1995). The senses of effort and force during fatiguing contractions. In S. C. Gandevia, R. M. Enoka, A. J. McComas, et al. (Eds.), *Fatigue: Neural and muscular mechanisms* (pp. 305–313). New York: Plenum Press.

Jones, L. A. (1999). Somatic senses 3: Proprioception. In H. Cohen (Ed.), *Neuroscience for rehabilitation* (pp. 111–130). Philadelphia: Lippincott, Williams & Wilkins.

Jones, L. A., & Hunter, I. W. (1983). Effect of fatigue on force sensation. *Experimental Neurology, 81,* 640–650.

Jones, M. B. (1985). *Nonimposed overpractice and skill retention* (Tech. Rep. No. 86–55). Alexandria, VA: U.S. Army Research Institute for the Behavioral Sciences.

Jonides, J. M., Naveh-Benjamin, M., & Palmer, J. (1985). Assessing automaticity. *Acta Psychologica, 60,* 157–171.

Jordan, T. C. (1972). Characteristics of visual and proprioceptive response times in the learning of a motor skill. *Journal of Experimental Psychology, 24,* 536–543.

Judd, C. H. (1908). The relation of special training to general intelligence. *Educational Review, 36,* 28–42.

Jung, C. (1927). *The theory of psychological type.* Princeton, NJ: Princeton University Press.

Kahn, M. A., Franks, I. M., & Goodman, D. (1998). The effect of practice on the control of rapid aiming movements: Evidence for an interdependency between programming and feedback processing. *The Quarterly Journal of Experimental Psychology, 51,* 425–444.

Kapur, S., Craik, F .I. M., & Jones, C. (1995). Functional role of the prefrontal cortex in retrieval of memories: A PET study. *NeuroReport, 6,* 1880–1884.

Karni, A. (1996). The acquisition of perceptual and motor skills: A memory system in the adult human cortex. *Cognitive Brain Research, 5,* 39–48.

Karni, A., Meyer, G., Jezzard, P., Adams, M. M., Turner, R., & Ungerleider, L. G. (1995). Functional MRI evidence for adult motor cortex plasticity during motor skill learning. *Nature, 377,* 155–158.

Kay, B. A., & Warren, W. H. (1998). Dynamical modeling of the interaction between posture and locomotion. In D. A. Rosenbaum & C. E. Collyer (Eds.), *Timing of behavior: Neural, computational, and psychological perspectives* (pp. 293–322). Cambridge, MA: MIT Press.

Keele, S. W. (1968). Movement control in skilled motor performance. *Psychological Bulletin, 70,* 387–403.

Keele, S. W. (1981). Behavioral analysis of movement. In V. B. Brooks (Ed.), *Handbook of physiology* (Sec. 1, Vol. II, Part 2, pp. 1391–1414). Bethesda: American Physiological Society.

Keele, S. W. & Hawkins, H. L. (1982). Explorations of individual differences relevant to high skill level. *Journal of Motor Behavior, 14,* 3–23.

Keele, S. W., Ivry, R. I., & Pokorny, R. A. (1987). Force control and its relation to timing. *Journal of Motor Behavior, 19,* 96–114.

Keele, S. W., Pokorny, R. A., Corcos, D. M., & Ivry, R. I. (1985). Do perception and motor production share common timing mechanisms? A correlational analysis. *Acta Psychologica, 60,* 173–191.

Keele, S. W., and Posner, M. I. (1968). Processing of visual feedback in rapid movements. *Journal of Experimental Psychology, 77,* 155–158.

Keller, F. S. (1958). The phantom plateau. *Journal of the Experimental Analysis of Behavior, 1,* 1–13.

Kelso, J. A. S. (1977). Motor control mechanisms underlying human movement production. *Journal of Experimental Psychology: Human Perception and Performance, 3,* 529–543.

Kelso, J. A. S. (1981). Contrasting perspectives on order and regulation in movement. In J. Long & A. Bad-deley (Eds.), *Attention and performance IX* (pp. 437–457). Hillsdale, NJ: Erlbaum.

Kelso, J. A. S. (1984). Phase transitions and critical behavior in human bimanual coordination. *American Journal of Physiology: Regulatory, Integrative, and Comparative Physiology, 15,* R1000–R1004.

Kelso, J. A. S. (1995). *Dynamic patterns: The self-organization of brain and behavior.* Cambridge, MA: MIT Press.

Kelso, J. A. S., Buchanan, J. J., & Wallace, S. A. (1991). Order parameters for the neural organization of single, multijoint limb movement patterns. *Experimental Brain Research, 83,* 432–444.

Kelso, J. A. S., & Norman, P. E. (1978). Motor schema formation in children. *Developmental Psychology, 2,* 153–156.

Kelso, J.A.S., & Schoner, G. (1988). Self-organization of coordinative movement patterns. *Human Movement Science, 7,* 27–46.

Kelso, J. A. S., Southard, D. L., & Goodman, D. (1979). On the nature of human interlimb coordination. *Science, 203,* 1029–1031.

Kelso, J. A. S., & Tuller, B. (1984). A dynamical basis for action systems. In M. S. Gazzaniga (Ed.), *Handbook of cognitive neuroscience* (pp. 321–356). New York: Plenum Press.

Kerlinger, F. N. (1973). *Foundations of behavioral research* (2nd ed.). New York: Holt, Rinehart & Winston.

Kernodle, M. W., & Carlton, L. G. (1992). Information feedback and the learning of multiple-degrees-of-freedom activities. *Journal of Motor Behavior, 24*(2), 187–196.

Kerr, R. (1973). Movement time in an underwater environment. *Journal of Motor Behavior, 5,* 175–178.

Kerr, R., & Booth, B. (1977). Skill acquisition in elementary school children and schema theory. In R. W. Christina & D. M. Landers (Eds.), *Psychology of motor behavior and sport—1976* (Vol. 2, pp. 243–247). Champaign, IL: Human Kinetics.

Kieras, D. E., & Boviar, S. (1984). The role of mental models in learning to operate a device. *Cognitive Science, 8,* 255–273.

Kim, G. B. (1989). Relative effectiveness of anxiety reduction techniques on levels of competitive anxiety and shooting performance. In *Commemorative volume dedicated to Professor Hong-Dae Kim, Young-Nam University* (pp. 61–74). Dae-ku, Republic of Korea: Hong-ik Publishing Company.

King, L. A., & Van Sant, A. (1995). The effect of solid ankle-foot orthoses on movement patterns used in a supine-to-stand rising task. *Physical Therapy, 75,* 952–964.

Klapp, S. T. (1975). Feedback versus motor programming in the control of aimed movements. *Journal of Experimental Psychology: Human Perception and Performance, 104,* 147–153.

Knapp, C. G., & Dixon, W. R. (1952). Learning to juggle. II. A study of whole and part methods. *Research Quarterly for Exercise and Sport, 23,* 398–401.

Knapp H. D., Taub, E., & Berman, A. J. (1963). Movements in monkeys with deafferented forelimbs. *Experimental Neurology, 7,* 305–315.

Knutsson, E. (1983). Analysis of gait and isokinetic movements for evaluation of anti-spastic drugs or physical therapies. In J. E. Desmedt (Ed.), *Motor control mechanisms in health and disease* (pp. 1013–1034). New York: Raven Press.

Knutsson, E., & Richards, C. (1979). Different types of distributed motor control in gait of hemiparetic patients. *Brain, 102,* 405–430.

Ko, Y. G., Challis, J. H., & Newell, K. M. (2003). Learning to coordinate redundant degrees of freedom in a dynamic balance task. *Human Movement Science, 22,* 47–66.

Kohl, R. M., & Roenker, D. L. (1980). Bilateral transfer as a function of mental imagery. *Journal of Motor Behavior, 12,* 197–206.

Kolb, D. A. (1985). *Learning-style inventory* (revised). Boston: McBer & Company.

Kowalski, E. M., & Sherrill, C. (1992). Motor sequencing of boys with learning disabilities: Modeling and verbal rehearsal strategies. *Adapted Physical Activity Quarterly, 9,* 261–272.

Krakauer, J., & Ghez, C. (2000). Voluntary movement. In E. R. Kandel, J. H. Schwartz, & T. M. Jessell (Eds.), *Principles of neural science* (4th ed.) (pp. 756–781). New York: McGraw-Hill.

Krampe, R. Th., & Ericsson, K. (1996). Maintaining excellence: Deliberate practice and elite performance in young and older pianists. *Journal of Experimental Psychology: General, 125,* 331–359.

Kugler, P. N., Kelso, J. A. S., & Turvey, M. T. (1980). On the concept of coordinative structures as dissipative structures: I. Theoretical lines of convergence. In G. E. Stelmach & J. Requin (Eds.), *Tutorials in motor behavior* (pp. 3–47). Amsterdam: North-Holland.

Kugler, P. N., Kelso, J. A. S., & Turvey, M. T. (1982). On the control and coordination in naturally developing systems. In J. A. S. Kelso & J. E. Clark (Eds.), *The development of movement control and coordination* (pp. 5–78). New York: Wiley.

Kugler, P. N., & Turvey, M. T. (1987). *Information, natural law and the self-assembly of rhythmic movement.* Hillsdale, NJ: Erlbaum.

Kuhn, T. (1962). *The structure of scientific revolutions.* Chicago: University of Chicago Press.

Kurz, M. J., & Stergiou, N. (2004). Applied dynamic systems theory for the analysis of movement. In N. Stergiou (Ed.), *Innovative analyses of human movement* (pp. 93–120). Champaign, IL: Human Kinetics.

Kuypers, H. G. J. M. (1985). The anatomical and functional organization of the motor system. In M.

Swash & C. Kennard (Eds.), *Scientific basis of clinical neurology* (pp. 3–18). New York: Churchill Livingstone.

Kyllo, L. B., & Landers, D. M. (1995). Goal setting in sport and exercise: A research synthesis to resolve the controversy. *Journal of Sport and Exercise Psychology, 17,* 117–137.

Laabs, G. J. (1973). Retention characteristics of different reproduction cues in motor short-term memory. *Journal of Experimental Psychology, 100,* 168–177.

Landers, D. M., & Landers, D. M. (1973). Teacher versus peer models: Effect of model's presence and performance level on motor behavior. *Journal of Motor Behavior, 5,* 129–139.

Landers, D. M., Wang, M. Q., Daniels, F., & Boutcher, S. (1984, November–December). Unraveling some of the mysteries of archery. *The US Archer,* 260–263.

Landin, D. (1994). The role of verbal cues in skill learning. *Quest, 46,* 299–313.

Lang, C. E., & Bastian, A. J. (1999). Cerebellar subjects show impaired adaptation of anticipatory EMG during catching. *Journal of Neurophysiology, 82*(5), 2108–2119.

Lantz, B. (1945). Some dynamic aspects of success and failure. *Psychological Monographs, 59,* 1–40.

Larish, D. D., & Stelmach, G. E. (1982). Preprogramming, programming, and reprogramming of aimed hand movements as a function of age. *Journal of Motor Behavior, 14,* 322–340.

Lashley, K. S. (1917). The accuracy of movement in the absence of excitation from the moving organ. *The American Journal of Physiology, 43,* 169–194.

Lashley, K. S. (1929). *Brain mechanisms and intelligence.* Chicago: University of Chicago Press.

Lashley, K. S. (1950). In search of the engram. *Symposia of the Society for Experimental Biology, 4,* 454–482.

Laszlo, J. I., & Bairstow, E. J. (1983). Kinesthesia: Its measurement, training and relationship to motor control. *Quarterly Journal of Experimental Psychology, 35A,* 411–422.

Latash, M. L. (1998). *Neurophysiological basis of movement.* Champaign, IL: Human Kinetics.

Laugier, C., & Cadpoli, M. (1996). Representational guidance of dance performance in adult novices: Effect of concrete vs. abstract movement. *International Journal of Sport Psychology, 27,* 91–108.

Lave, J. (1988). *Cognition and practice: Mind, mathematics and culture in everyday life.* Cambridge, UK: Cambridge University Press.

Lave, J., & Wenger, E. (1991). *Situated learning: Legitimate peripheral participation.* Cambridge, UK: Cambridge University Press.

Lavery, J. J. (1962). Retention of simple motor skills as a function of type of knowledge of results. *Canadian Journal of Psychology, 16,* 300–311.

Lee, D. N. (1976). A theory of visual control of braking based on information about time-to-collision. *Perception, 5*, 437–459.

Lee, D. N. (1978). The functions of vision. In H. Pick & E. Salzmann (Eds.), *Modes of perceiving and processing information* (pp. 159–170). Hillsdale, NJ: Erlbaum.

Lee, D. N. (1980). Visuo-motor coordination in space-time. In G. E. Stelmach & J. Requin (Eds.), *Tutorials in motor behavior* (pp. 281–295). Amsterdam: North-Holland.

Lee, D. N., & Aronson, E. (1974). Visual proprioceptive control of standing in human infants. *Perception and Psychophysics, 15*, 527–532.

Lee, D. N., & Lishman, J. R. (1975). Visual proprioceptive control of stance. *Journal of Human Movement Studies, 1*, 87–95.

Lee, D. N., Lishman, J. R., & Thomson, J. A. (1982). Regulation of gait in long-jumping. *Journal of Experimental Psychology: Human Perception and Performance, 8*, 448–459.

Lee, D. N., Lough, F., & Lough, S. (1984). Activating the perceptuo-motor system in hemiparesis. *Journal of Physiology, 349*, 28P.

Lee, D. N., & Young, D. S. (1985). Visual timing of interceptive action. In D. Ingle, M. Jeannerod, & D. N. Lee (Eds.), *Brain mechanisms and spatial vision* (pp. 1–30). Dordrecht, Netherlands: Martinus Nijhoff.

Lee, T. D. (1988). Testing for motor learning: A focus on transfer-appropriate processing. In O. G. Meijer & K. Roth (Eds.), *Complex motor behavior: "The" motor-action controversy* (pp. 201–215). Amsterdam: Elsevier.

Lee, T. D. (1998). On the dynamics of motor behavior research. *Research Quarterly for Exercise and Sport, 69*, 334–337.

Lee, T. D., & Carnahan, H. (1990). Bandwidth knowledge of results and motor learning: More than just a relative frequency effect. *Quarterly Journal of Experimental Psychology, 42A*, 777–789.

Lee, T. D., & Genovese, E. D. (1988). Distribution of practice in motor skill acquisition: Learning and performance effects reconsidered. *Research Quarterly for Exercise and Sport, 59*, 59–67.

Lee, T. D., & Genovese, E. D. (1989). Distribution of practice in motor skill acquisition: Different effects for discrete and continuous tasks. *Research Quarterly for Exercise and Sport, 60*, 297–299.

Lee, T. D., & Magill, R. A. (1983). The locus of contextual interference in motor skill acquisition. *Journal of Experimental Psychology: Learning, Memory, and Cognition, 9*, 730–746.

Lee, T. D., & Magill, R. A. (1985). Can forgetting facilitate skill acquisition? In D. Goodman, R. B. Wilberg, & I. M. Franks (Eds.), *Differing perspectives in motor learning, memory and control* (pp. 3–22). Amsterdam: North-Holland.

Lee, T. D., Magill, R. A., & Weeks, D. J. (1985). Influence of practice schedule on testing schema theory predictions in adults. *Journal of Motor Behavior, 17*, 283–299.

Lee, T. D., Swinnen, S. P., & Serrien, D. J. (1994). Cognitive effort and motor learning. *Quest, 46*, 328–344.

Lee, T. D., Swinnen, S. P., & Verschueren, S. (1995). Relative phase alterations during bimanual skill acquisition. *Quest, 46*, 263–274.

Lee, T. D., & White, M. A. (1990). Influence of an unskilled model's practice schedule on observational motor learning. *Human Movement Science, 9*, 349–367.

Leonard, S. D., Karnes, E. W., Oxendine, J., & Hesson, J. (1970). Effects of task difficulty on transfer performance on rotary pursuit. *Perceptual and Motor Skills, 30*, 731–736.

Lersten, K. C. (1968). Transfer of movement components in a motor learning task. *Research Quarterly for Exercise and Sport, 39*, 575–581.

Lersten, K. C. (1969). Retention of skill on the Rho apparatus after one year. *Research Quarterly for Exercise and Sport, 40*, 418–419.

Lewellen, J. O. (1951). *A comparative study of two methods of teaching swimming*. Unpublished doctoral dissertation, Stanford University, Stanford, CA.

Lewis, D., McAllister, D. E., & Adams, J. A. (1951). Facilitation and interference in performance on the modified Mashburn apparatus: I. The effects of varying the amount of original learning. *Journal of Experimental Psychology, 41*, 247–260.

Liepert, J., Miltner, W. H. R., Bauder, H., Sommer, M., Dettmers, C., Taub, E., & Weiller, C. (2000). Motor cortex plasticity during constraint-induced movement therapy in stroke patients. *Neuroscience Letters, 250*, 5–8.

Lincoln, R. S., & Smith, K. U. (1951). Transfer of training in tracking performance at different target speeds. *Journal of Applied Psychology, 35*, 358–362.

Lindberg, G. A. (1949). A study of the degree of transfer between quickening exercises and other coordinated movements. *Research Quarterly for Exercise and Sport, 20*, 180–195.

Linden, C. A., Uhley, J. E., Smith, D., & Bush, M. A. (1989). The effects of mental practice on walking balance in an elderly population. *Occupational Therapy Journal of Research, 9*, 155–169.

Lirgg, C. D., & Feltz, D. L. (1991). Teacher versus peer models revisited: Effects on motor performance and self-efficacy. *Research Quarterly for Exercise and Sport, 62*(2), 217–224.

Lisberger, S. G. (1988). The neural basis for learning of simple motor skills. *Science, 242*, 728–735.

Liu, J., & Wrisberg, C. A. (1997). The effect of knowledge of results delay and the subjective estimation of movement form on the acquisition and retention of a motor skill. *Research Quarterly for Exercise and Sport, 68,* 145–151.

Livesey, J. P., & Lazlo, J. I. (1979). Effect of task similarity on transfer performance. *Journal of Motor Behavior, 11,* 11–22.

Locke, E. A. (1991). Problems with goal-setting research in sports and their solution. *Journal of Sport and Exercise Psychology, 13,* 311–316.

Locke, E. A., & Latham, G. P. (1985). The application of goal setting to sports. *Sport Psychology Today, 7,* 205–222.

Lockhart, R. S. (1980). Levels of processing and motor memory. In P. Klavora & J. Flowers (Eds.), *Motor learning and biomechanical factors in sport* (pp. 34–40). Toronto, Canada: University of Toronto.

Loeb, G. E., & Ghez, C. (2000). The motor unit and muscle action. In E. R. Kandel, J. H. Schwartz, & T. M. Jessell (Eds.), *Principles of neural science,* (4th ed.) (pp. 674–694). New York: McGraw-Hill.

Loftus, G. R. (1985). Evaluating forgetting curves. *Journal of Experimental Psychology: Learning, Memory, and Cognition, 11,* 397–406.

Lordahl, D. S., & Archer, E. J. (1958). Transfer effects on a rotary-pursuit task as a function of first task difficulty. *Journal of Experimental Psychology, 56,* 421–426.

Lowin, A., & Epstein, G. F. (1965). Does expectancy determine performance? *Journal of Experimental and Social Psychology, 1,* 248–255.

Lutz, R., Landers, D. M., & Linder, D. E. (2002). Procedural variables and skill level influences on preperformance mental practice efficacy. *Journal of Mental Imagery, 25,* 115–134.

Lynch, M. D., Norem-Hebeisen, A. A., & Gergen, K. (Eds.). (1981). *Self-concept: Advances in theory and research.* Cambridge, MA: Ballinger.

Magill, R. A. (1988). Activity during the post-knowledge of results interval can benefit motor skill learning. In O. G. Meijer & K. Roth (Eds.), *Complex motor behavior: "The" motor-action controversy* (pp. 231–246). Amsterdam: Elsevier.

Magill, R. A. (1993a). Modeling and verbal feedback influences on skill learning. *International Journal of Sport Psychology, 24,* 358–369.

Magill, R. A. (1993b). *Motor learning: Concepts and applications* (4th ed.). Dubuque, IA: Wm. C. Brown.

Magill, R. A. (1998). Knowledge is more than we can talk about: Implicit learning in motor skill acquisition. *Research Quarterly for Exercise and Sport, 69,* 104–110.

Magill, R. A. (2001). *Motor learning and control: Concepts and applications* (6th ed.). New York: McGraw-Hill.

Magill, R.A. (2004). *Motor learning and control. Concepts and applications* (7th ed.). Dubuque. IA: McGraw-Hill.

Magill, R. A., & Dowell, M. N. (1977). Serial position effects in motor short-term memory. *Journal of Motor Behavior, 9,* 319–323.

Magill, R. A., & Hall, K. G. (1990). A review of the contextual interference effect in motor skill acquisition. *Human Movement Science, 9,* 241–289.

Magill, R. A., & Schoenfelder-Zohdi, B. (1996). A visual model and knowledge of performance as sources of information for learning a rhythmic gymnastics skill. *International Journal of Sport Psychology, 27,* 7–22.

Magill, R. A., & Wood, C. A. (1986). Knowledge of results precision as a learning variable in motor skill acquisition. *Research Quarterly for Exercise and Sport, 57,* 170–173.

Mahoney, M. J., & Avener, M. (1977). Psychology of the elite athlete: An exploratory study. *Cognitive Therapy and Research, 1,* 135–141.

Maki, B. E., Perry, S. D., Norrie, R. G., & McIlroy, W. E. (1999). Effect of facilitation of sensation from plantar foot-surface boundaries on postural stabilization in young and older adults. *Journal of Gerontology, 54,* M281–M287

Margolis, J. F., & Christina, R. W. (1981). A test of Schmidt's schema theory of discrete motor skill learning. *Research Quarterly for Exercise and Sport, 52,* 474–483.

Marr, D. (1969). A theory for cerebellar cortex. *Journal of Physiology, 202,* 437–470.

Martens, R., Burwitz, L., & Zuckerman, J. (1976). Modeling effects on motor performance. *Research Quarterly for Exercise and Sport, 47(2),* 277–291.

Martin, K. A., Moritz, S. E., & Hall, C. R. (1999). Imagery use in sport: A literature review and applied model. *The Sport Psychologist, 13,* 245–268.

Martin, T. A., Keating, J. G., Goodkin, H. P., Bastian, A. J., & Thach, W. T. (1996). Throwing while looking through prisms. I. Focal olivocerebellar lesions impair adaptation. *Brain, 119,* 1183–1198.

Masdeu, J. C., Sudarsky, L., & Wolfson, L. (Eds.). (1997). *Gait disorders of aging: Falls and therapeutic strategies.* New York: Lippincott-Raven.

Maslow, A. H. (1970). *Motivation and personality* (2nd ed.). New York: Harper & Row.

Masters, R. S. W. (1992). Knowledge, knerves, and know-how: The role of explicit versus implicit knowledge in the breakdown of a complex motor skill under pressure. *British Journal of Psychology, 83,* 343–358.

Matthews, P. B. C. (1981). Proprioceptors and the regulation of movement. In A. L. Towe & E. S. Luschei (Eds.), *Motor coordination. Vol. 5 in Handbook of behavioral neurobiology* (pp. 93–127). New York: Plenum Press.

Mayer, R. E. (1975). Different problem-solving competencies established in learning computer programming with and without meaningful models. *Journal of Educational Psychology, 67,* 725–734.

Mayer, R. E. (1985). Learning in complex domains: A cognitive analysis of computer programming. In

G. H. Bower (Ed.), *The psychology of learning and motivation* (Vol. 19, pp. 89–130). New York: Academic Press.

Mayer, R. E., & Greeno, J. G. (1972). Structural differences between learning outcomes produced by different instructional methods. *Journal of Educational Psychology, 63,* 165–173.

McAllister, D. E. (1953). The effects of various kinds of relevant verbal pretraining on subsequent motor performance. *Journal of Experimental Psychology, 46,* 329–336.

McAuley, E. (1985). Modeling and self-efficacy: A test of Bandura's model. *Journal of Sport Psychology, 7,* 283–295.

McCarthy, B. (1987). *The 4MAT system: Teaching to learning styles with right/left mode techniques.* Barrington, IL: Excel Corporation.

McClelland, D. C. (1965). Toward a theory of motive acquisition. *American Psychologist, 20,* 221–333.

McCloskey, D. I. (1973). Differences between the senses of movement and position shown by the effects of loading and vibration of muscles in man. *Brain Research, 61,* 119–131.

McCloskey, D. I. (1981). Corollary discharges: Motor commands and perception. In V. B. Brooks (Ed.), *Handbook of physiology. Section 1: The nervous system.* (Vol. 2, pp. 1415–1445). Bethesda, MD: American Physiological Society.

McCloskey, D. I., Cross, M. J., Honner, R., & Potter, E. K. (1983). Sensory effects of pulling of vibrating exposed tendons in man. *Brain, 106,* 21–37.

McCloskey, D. I., Ebeling, P., & Goodwin, G. M. (1974). Estimations of weights and tensions and apparent involvement of a "sense of effort." *Experimental Neurology, 42,* 220–232.

McCloy, C. H. (1934). The measurement of general motor capacity and general motor ability. *Research Quarterly for Exercise and Sport, 5* (Suppl. 5), 45–61.

McCracken, H. D., & Stelmach, G. E. (1977). A test of schema theory of discrete motor learning. *Journal of Motor Behavior, 9,* 193–201.

McCrea, D. A. (1992). Can sense be made of spinal interneuron circuits? *Behavioral and Brain Sciences, 15*(4), 633–643.

McCullagh, P. (1986). A model's status as a determinant of attention in observational learning and performance. *Journal of Sport Psychology, 8,* 319–331.

McCullagh, P. (1987). Model similarity effects on motor performance. *Journal of Sport Psychology, 9,* 249–260.

McCullagh, P., & Caird, J. K. (1990). Correct and learning models and the use of model knowledge of results in the acquisition and retention of a motor skill. *Journal of Human Movement Studies, 18,* 107–116.

McCullagh, P., & Meyer, K. N. (1997). Learning versus correct models: Influence of model type on the learning of a free-weight squat lift. *Research Quarterly for Exercise and Sport, 68,* 56–61.

McCullagh, P., Stiehl, J., & Weiss, M. R. (1990). Developmental considerations in modeling: The role of visual and verbal models and verbal rehearsal in skill acquisition. *Research Quarterly for Exercise and Sport, 61,* 344–350.

McCullagh, P., & Weiss, M. R. (2001). Modeling: Considerations for motor skill performance and psychological responses. In R. N. Singer, H. A. Hasenblaus, & C. M. Janelle (Eds.), *Handbook of research on sport psychology* (pp. 205–238). New York: Wiley.

McCullagh, P., & Weiss, M. R. (2002). Observational learning: The forgotten psychological method in sport psychology. In J. L. Van Raalte & B. W. Brewer (Eds.), *Exploring sport and exercise psychology* (2nd ed.) (pp.131–149). Washington, DC: American Psychological Association.

McCullagh, P., Weiss, M. R., & Ross, D. (1989). Modeling considerations in motor skill acquisition and performance: An integrated approach. In K. B. Pandolf (Ed.), *Exercise and sport science reviews* (Vol. 17, pp. 475–513). Baltimore: Williams & Wilkins.

McDonald, P. V., van Emmerik, R. E. A., & Newell, K. M. (1989). The effects of practice on limb kinematics in a throwing task. *Journal of Motor Behavior, 21*(3), 245–264.

McGeoch, J. A., & Irion, A. L. (1952). *The psychology of human learning* (2nd ed.). New York: Longman, Green, and Company.

McGown, C. M., & Schmidt, R. A. (1981). Coordination in two-handed movements. Paper presented at the annual meeting of the North American Society for the Psychology of Sport and Physical Activity, Asilomar, CA.

McIntyre, D. R., & Pfautsch, E. W. (1982). A kinematic analysis of the baseball batting swing involved in opposite-field and same-field hitting. *Research Quarterly for Exercise and Sport, 53,* 206–213.

McKenna, S. P., & Glendon, A. I. (1985). Occupational first aid training. Decay in cardiopulmonary resuscitation (CPR) skills. *Journal of Occupational Psychology, 58,* 109–117.

McPherson, S. (1993). The influence of player experience on problem solving during batting preparation in baseball. *Journal of Sport and Exercise Psychology, 15,* 304–325.

McPherson, S. L., & Thomas, J. R. (1989). Relation of knowledge and performance in boy's tennis: Age and expertise. *Journal of Experimental Child Psychology, 48,* 190–211.

Meany, K. S. (1994). Developmental modeling effects on the acquisition, retention, and transfer of a novel motor task. *Research Quarterly for Exercise & Sport, 65*(1), 31–39.

Meeuwsen, H., & Magill, R. A. (1987). The role of vision in gait control during gymnastics vaulting. In T. B. Hoshizaki, J. Slamela, & B. Petiot (Eds.), *Diagnostics, treatment, and analysis of gymnastic talent* (pp. 137–155). Montreal, Canada: Sport Psyche Editions.

Meichenbaum, D., & Goodman, J. (1971). Training impulsive children to talk to themselves: A means of developing self-control. *Journal of Abnormal Psychology, 77,* 115–126.

Meijer, O. G., & Roth, K. (Eds.) (1988). *Complex motor behavior: "The" motor-action controversy.* Amsterdam: Elsevier.

Melnick, M. (2001). Basal ganglia disorders: Metabolic, hereditary, and genetic disorders in adults. In D. A. Umphred (Ed.), *Neurological rehabilitation* (4th ed.) (pp. 661–695). Philadelphia: Mosby.

Melnick, M. E., & Oremland, B. (2001). Movement dysfunction associated with cerebellar problems. In D. A. Umphred (Ed.), *Neurological rehabilitation* (4th ed.) (pp. 717–740). Philadelphia: Mosby.

Melnick, M. J. (1971). Effects of overlearning on the retention of a gross motor skill. *Research Quarterly for Exercise and Sport, 42,* 60–69.

Melton, A. W., & von Lackum, W. J. (1941). Retroactive and proactive inhibition in retention: Evidence for a two-factor theory of retroactive inhibition. *American Journal of Psychology, 54,* 157–173.

Merton, P. A. (1953). Speculations on the servo control of movement. In G. E. W. Wolstenholme (Ed.), *The spinal cord.* London: Churchill.

Merton, P. A. (1972). How we control the contraction of our muscles. *Scientific American, 226,* 30–37.

Meyer, D. E., Smith, J. E. K., & Wright, C. E. (1982). Models for the speed and accuracy of aimed movements. *Psychological Review, 89,* 449–482.

Meyers, J. L. (1967). Retention of balance coordination learning as influenced by extended layoffs. *Research Quarterly for Exercise and Sport, 38,* 72–78.

Michaels, C. F., & Carello, C. (1981). *Direct perception.* Englewood Cliffs, NJ: Prentice-Hall.

Michaels, J. W. (1977). Classroom reward structures and academic performance. *Review of Educational Research, 47,* 87–98.

Miles, F. A., & Lisberger, S. G. (1981). Plasticity in the vestibulo-ocular reflex: A new hypothesis. *Annual Review of Neuroscience, 4,* 273–299.

Milgram, P. (1987). A spectacle-mounted liquid-crystal tachistoscope. *Behavior, Research Methods, Instruments and Computers, 19,* 449–456.

Miller, G. A. (1956). The magical number seven, plus or minus two: Some limits on our capacity for processing information. *Psychological Review, 63,* 81–97.

Mills, V. M. (1988). Traumatic head injury. In S. B. O'Sullivan & T. J. Schmitz (Eds.), *Physical rehabilitation: Assessment and treatment* (2nd ed.) (pp. 495–514). Philadelphia: F. A. Davis.

Milone, F. (1971). Interference in motor short-term memory. Unpublished master's thesis, Pennsylvania State University, University Park, PA.

Mishkin, M. (1982). A memory system in the monkey. *Philosophical Transactions of the Royal Society of London. 298,* 85–95.

Miyai, I., Fujimoto, Y., Yamamoto, H., Ueda, Y., Saito, T., Nozaki, S., & Kang, J. (2002). Long-term effect of body weight–supported treadmill training in Parkinson's disease: A randomized controlled trial. *Archives of Physical Medicine and Rehabilitation, 83*(10), 1370–1373.

Moberg, E. (1983). The role of cutaneous afferents in position sense, kinesthesia, and motor function of the hand. *Brain, 106,* 1–19.

Mohr, D. R., & Barrett, M. E. (1962). Effect of knowledge of mechanical principles in learning to perform intermediate swimming skills. *Research Quarterly for Exercise and Sport, 33,* 574–580.

Moritani, T., & deVries, H. A. (1979). Neural factors vs. hypertophy in the time course of muscle strength gain. *American Journal of Physical Medicine, 58,* 115–230.

Morris, C. D., Bransford, J. D., & Franks, J. J. (1977). Levels of processing versus transfer-appropriate processing. *Journal of Verbal Learning and Verbal Behavior, 16,* 519–533.

Morris, C. D., Stein, B. S., & Bransford, J. D. (1979). Prerequisites for the utilization of knowledge in recall of prose passages. *Journal of Experimental Psychology: Human Learning and Memory, 5,* 253–261.

Moxley, S. E. (1979). Schema: The variability of practice hypothesis. *Journal of Motor Behavior, 11,* 65–70.

Muir, G. D., & Steeves, J. D. (1997). Sensorimotor stimulation to improve locomotor recovery after spinal cord injury. *Trends in Neuroscience, 20*(2), 72–77.

Müller, G. E., & Pilzecker, A. (1900). Experimentelle beitrage zur lehre vom gedachtniss. *Zeitshrift fur Psychologie und Physiologie der Sinnesorgone. Ergan zungsband, 1,* 1–288.

Munn, N. L. (1932). Bilateral transfer of learning. *Journal of Experimental Psychology, 15,* 342–353.

Murdock, B. B., Jr. (1957). Transfer designs and formulas. *Psychological Bulletin, 54,* 313–326.

Mynark, R. G., & Koceja, D. M. (2001). Effects of age on the spinal stretch reflex. *Journal of Applied Biomechanics, 17,* 188–203.

Nacson, J., & Schmidt, R. A. (1971). The activity-set hypothesis for warm-up decrement. *Journal of Motor Behavior, 3,* 1–15.

Namikas, G., & Archer, E. J. (1960). Motor skill transfer as a function of intertask interval and pretransfer task difficulty. *Journal of Experimental Psychology, 59,* 109–112.

Nashner, L. M. (1976). Adapting reflexes controlling human posture. *Experimental Brain Research, 26,* 59–72.

Nashner, L. M., & Grimm, R. J. (1978). Analysis of multi-loop dyscontrols in standing cerebellar patients. In J. E. Desmedt (Ed.), *Cerebral motor control in man* (pp. 300–319). Basel, Switzerland: Karger.

Naylor, J., & Briggs, G. (1961). Effects of task complexity and task organization on the relative efficiency of part and whole training methods. *Journal of Experimental Psychology, 65,* 217–244.

Neafsey, E. J., Hull, C. D., & Buchwald, N. A. (1978). Preparation for movement in the cat. II. Unit activity in the basal ganglia and thalamus. *Electroencephalography and Clinical Neurophysiology, 44*(6), 714–723.

Nelson, D. O. (1957a). Effect of swimming on the learning of selected gross motor skills. *Research Quarterly for Exercise and Sport, 28,* 374–378.

Nelson, D. O. (1957b). Study of transfer of training in gross motor skills. *Research Quarterly for Exercise and Sport, 28,* 364–373.

Neumann, E., & Ammons, R. B. (1957). Acquisition and long-term retention of a simple serial perceptual-motor skill. *Journal of Experimental Psychology, 53,* 159–161.

Newell, K. M. (1974). Knowledge of results and motor learning. *Journal of Motor Behavior, 6,* 235–244.

Newell, K. M. (1985). Coordination, control and skill. In D. Goodman, R. B. Wilberg, & I. M. Franks (Eds.), *Differing perspectives in motor learning, memory, and control* (pp. 295–317). Amsterdam: North-Holland.

Newell, K. M. (1991). Motor skill acquisition. *Annual Review of Psychology, 42,* 213–237.

Newell, K. M. (1998). Commentary 4: Action and ecological psychology: A Winter's view from Summers. In J. P. Piek (Ed.), *Motor behavior and human skill: A multidisciplinary approach* (pp. 410–411). Champaign, IL: Human Kinetics.

Newell, K. M. (2003). Schema theory (1975): Retrospectives and prospectives. *Research Quarterly for Exercise and Sport, 74,* 383–388.

Newell, K. M., & Carlton, M. J. (1987). Augmented information and the acquisition of isometric tasks. *Journal of Motor Behavior, 19,* 4–12.

Newell, K. M., Carlton, M. J., Fisher, A. T., & Rutter, B. G. (1989). Whole-part training strategies for learning the response dynamics of microprocessor-driven simulators. *Acta Psychologica, 71,* 197–216.

Newell, K. M., Kugler, P. N., van Emmerik, R. E. A., & McDonald, P. V. (1989). Search strategies and the acquisition of coordination. In S. A. Wallace (Ed.), *Perspectives on the coordination of movement* (pp. 85–122). Amsterdam: North-Holland.

Newell, K. M., & McDonald, P. V. (1992). Searching for solutions to the coordination function: Learning as exploratory behavior. In G. E. Stelmach & J. Requin (Eds.), *Tutorials in motor behavior II* (pp. 517–532). Amsterdam: North-Holland.

Newell, K. M., & McGinnis, P. M. (1985). Kinematic information feedback for skilled performance. *Human Learning, 4,* 39–56.

Newell, K. M., Morris, L. R., & Scully, D. M. (1985). Augmented information and the acquisition of skills in physical activity. In R. L. Terjung (Ed.), *Exercise and sport sciences reviews* (pp. 235–261). New York: Macmillan.

Newell, K. M., Quinn, J. T., Sparrow, W. A., & Walter, C. B. (1983). Kinematic information feedback for learning a rapid arm movement. *Human Movement Science, 2,* 255–269.

Newell, K. M., & van Emmerik, R. E. A. (1989). The acquisition of coordination: Preliminary analysis of learning to write. *Human Movement Science, 8,* 17–32.

Newell, K. M., & Walter, C. B. (1981). Kinematic and kinetic parameters as information feedback in motor skill acquisition. *Journal of Human Movement Studies, 7,* 235–254.

Nicholls, J. G. (1979). The role of motivation in education. *American Psychologist, 34,* 1071–1084.

Nicklaus, J. (with Bowden, K.). (1974). *Golf my way.* New York: Simon & Schuster.

Niemeyer, R. K. (1959). Part versus whole methods and massed versus distributed practice in the learning of selected large muscle activities. *Annual Proceedings of the College Physical Education Association, 62,* 122–125.

Nixon, J. E., & Locke, L. F. (1973). Research on teaching physical education. In R. M. W. Travers (Ed.), *Second handbook of research on teaching* (pp. 1210–1242). Chicago: Rand McNally.

Novick, L. (1986). *Analogical transfer in expert and novice problem solvers.* Unpublished doctoral dissertation, Stanford University, Stanford, CA.

O'Sullivan, S. B. (1988). Strategies to improve motor control. In S. B. O'Sullivan & T. J. Schmitz (Eds.), *Physical rehabilitation: Assessment and treatment* (2nd ed.) (pp. 253–280). Philadelphia: F. A. Davis.

O'Sullivan, S. B. (1994). Strategies to improve motor control and motor learning. In S. B. O'Sullivan & T. J. Schmitz (Eds.), *Physical rehabilitation: Assessment and treatment* (3rd ed.) (pp. 225–249). Philadelphia: F. A. Davis.

O'Sullivan, S. B., & Schmitz, T. J., (Eds.). (1994). *Physical rehabilitation: Assessment and treatment.* (3rd ed.). Philadelphia: F. A. Davis.

Okun, M. A., & DiVesta, F. J. (1975). Cooperation and competition in coaching groups. *Journal of Personality and Social Psychology, 31,* 615–620.

Ornstein, P. A., Naus, M. J., & Liberty, C. (1975). Rehearsal and organization processes in children's memory. *Child Development, 26,* 818–830.

Osgood, C. E. (1949). The similarity paradox in human learning: A resolution. *Psychological Review, 56,* 132–143.

Oxendine, J. B. (1984). *Psychology of motor learning* (2nd ed.). Englewood Cliffs, NJ: Prentice-Hall.

Page, S. J. (2000). Imagery improves motor function in chronic stroke patients with hemiplegia: A pilot study. *Occupational Therapy Journal Research, 20*(3), 200–215.

Page, S. J., Levine, P., Sisto, S., Johnston, M. V. (2001). A randomized efficacy and feasibility study of imagery in acute stroke. *Clinical Rehabilitation, 15,* 233–240.

Palmer, S. S., Mortimer, J. A., Webster, D. D., Bistevins, R., & Dickinson, G. L. (1986). Exercise therapy for Parkinson's disease. *Archives of Physical Medicine and Rehabilitation, 67*(10), 741–745.

Papscy, F. E. (1968). The effect of understanding a specific principle upon learning a physical education skill. Unpublished doctoral dissertation, New York University, New York, NY.

Parks, S., Rose, D. J., & Dunn, J. (1989). A comparison of fractionated reaction time between cerebral-palsied and non-handicapped youth. *Adapted Physical Activity Quarterly, 6*(4), 379–388.

Pascuel-Leone, A., Grafman, J., & Hallet, M. (1994). Modulation of cortical motor output maps during development of implicit and explicit knowledge. *Science, 263,* 1287–1289.

Patla, A. E., Prentice, S. D., Robinson, C., & Neufeld, J. (1991). Visual control of locomotion: Strategies for changing direction and for going over obstacles. *Journal of Experimental Psychology: Human Perception and Performance, 17*(3), 603–634.

Patrick, J. (1971). The effect of interpolated motor activities in short-term motor memory. *Journal of Motor Behavior, 3,* 39–48.

Peacock, I. W. (1987). A physical therapy program for Huntington's disease patients. *Clinical Management, 7,* 22.

Pearson, K. G. (2001). Could enhanced reflex function contribute to improving locomotion after spinal cord repair? *Journal of Physiology, 15*(533), 75–81.

Pearson, K., & Gordon, J. (2001). Spinal reflexes. In E. R. Kandel, J. H. Schwartz, & T. M. Jessell (Eds.), *Principles of neural science* (4th ed.) (pp. 713–736). New York: McGraw-Hill.

Penfield, W., & Boldrey, E. (1937). Somatic motor and sensory representation in the cerebral cortex of man as studied by electrical stimulation. *Brain, 60,* 389–443.

Pepper, R. L., & Herman, L. M. (1970). Decay and interference effects in the short-term retention of a discrete motor act. *Journal of Experimental Psychology, 83,* (Monograph Suppl. 2).

Perkins-Ceccato, N., Passmore, S. R., & Lee, T. D. (2003). Effects of focus of attention depend on golfers' skill. *Journal of Sport Sciences, 21,* 593–600.

Pew, R. W. (1974). Levels of analysis in motor control. *Brain Research, 71,* 393–400.

Pew, R. W. (1984). A distributed processing view of human motor control. In W. Prinz & A. F. Sanders (Eds.), *Cognition and motor processes* (pp. 19–27). Berlin: Springer.

Pfurtscheller, G., & Neuper, C. (1997). Motor imagery activates primary sensorimotor area in humans. *Neuroscience Letters, 239,* 65–68.

Piaget, J. (1972). Problems of equilibration. In C. F. Nadine, J. M. Gallagher, & R. D. Humphries (Eds.), *Piaget and Inhelder: On equilibration.* Philadelphia: Jean Piaget Society.

Piek, J. P. (Ed.) (1998). *Motor behavior and human skill.* Champaign, IL: Human Kinetics.

Pigott, R. E., & Shapiro, D. C. (1984). Motor schema: The structure of the variablity session. *Research Quarterly for Exercise and Sport, 55,* 41–54.

Pikler, E. (1968). Some contributions to the study of the gross motor development of children. *The Journal of Genetic Psychology, 113,* 27–39.

Platt, J. R. (1964). Strong inference. *Science, 146,* 347–352.

Pollard, R. (1986). Home advantage in soccer: A retrospective analysis. *Journal of Sport Sciences, 4,* 237–248.

Pollock, B. J., & Lee, T. D. (1992). Effects of the model's skill level on observational motor learning. *Research Quarterly for Exercise and Sport, 63*(1), 25–29.

Popper, K. (1959). *The logic of scientific discovery.* New York: Basic.

Porter, L. A. (1999). Motor 2: Higher centers. In H. Cohen (Ed.), *Neuroscience for rehabilitation* (pp. 243–273). Philadelphia: Lippincott, Williams & Wilkins.

Poto, C. C., French, K. E., & Magill, R. A. (1987). Serial position and asymmetric transfer effects in a contextual interference study. Paper presented at the annual meeting of the North American Society for the Psychology of Sport and Physical Activity, Vancouver, B.C., Canada.

Poulton, E. C. (1956). The precision of choice reactions. *Journal of Experimental Psychology, 51,* 9–17.

Poulton, E. C. (1957). On prediction in skilled movements. *Psychological Bulletin, 54,* 467–478.

Prablanc, C., Echallier, J. F., Komilis, E., & Jeannerod, M. (1979). Optimal response of eye and hand motor systems in pointing at a visual target. I. Spatio-temporal characteristics of eye and hand movements and their relationships when varying the amount of visual information. *Biological Cybernetics, 35,* 113–124.

Priplata, A. A., Niemi J. B., Harry, J. D., Lipsitz, L. A., & Collins, J. J. (2003). Vibrating insoles and balance control in elderly people. *The Lancet, 362,* 1123–1124.

Prophet, W. W. (1976). Long-term retention of flying skills: A review of the literature. (HumRRO Final Report 76–35.) Alexandria, VA: Human Resources Research Organization (ADA036077).

Proske, U., Schaible, H. G., & Schmidt, R. F. (1988). Joint receptors and kinaesthesia. *Experimental Brain Research, 72,* 219–224.

Proteau, L., Marteniuk, R. G., & Levesque, L. (1992). A sensorimotor basis for motor learning: Evidence indicating specificity of practice. *The Quarterly Journal of Experimental Psychology, 44A,* 557–575.

Proteau, L., Marteniuk, R. G., Girouard, Y., & Dugas, C. (1987). On the type of information used to control and learn an aiming movement after moderate and extensive training. *Human Movement Science, 6,* 181–199.

Proteau, L., Tremblay, L., & DeJaeger, D. (1998). Practice does not diminish the role of visual information in on-line control of a precision walking task: Support for the specificity of practice hypothesis. *Journal of Motor Behavior, 30,* 143–150.

Quillian, T. A. (1975). Neuro-cutaneous relationships in fingerprint skin. In H. Kornhuber (Ed.), *The somatosensory system.* Sachs, Germany: Thieme.

Raibert, M. H. (1977). Motor control and learning by the state-space model. Technical Report, Artificial Intelligence Laboratory, Massachusetts Institute of Technology (AI-TR-439), Cambridge, MA.

Raynor, A. J. (1998). Fractionated reflex and reaction times in children with developmental coordination disorder. *Motor Control, 2,* 114–124.

Reeve, T. G., Dornier, L. A., & Weeks, D. J. (1990). Precision of knowledge of results: Consideration of the accuracy requirements imposed by the task. *Research Quarterly for Exercise and Sport, 61,* 284–290.

Reeve, T. G., & Magill, R. A. (1981). Role of components of knowledge of results information in error correction. *Research Quarterly for Exercise and Sport, 52,* 80–85.

Reissman, F. (1977). There is more than one style for learning. In D. E. Hamachek (Ed.), *Human dynamics in psychology and education* (3rd ed.) (pp.14–15). Boston: Allyn & Bacon.

Renshaw, S., & Postle, D. K. (1928). Pursuit learning under three types of instruction. *Journal of General Psychology, 56,* 3–11.

Revien, L., & Gabor, M. (1981). *Sports-Vision.* New York: Workman Publishing Co.

Rhine, R. J. (1957). The effect on problem solving of success or failure as a function of cue specificity. *Journal of Experimental Psychology, 53,* 121–125.

Richardson, A. (1967). Mental practice: A review and discussion. Part I. *Research Quarterly for Exercise and Sport, 38,* 95–107.

Rikli, R., & Smith, G. (1980). Videotape feedback effects on tennis serving form. *Perceptual and Motor Skills, 50,* 895–901.

Roach, N. K., & Burwitz, L. (1986). Observational learning in motor skill acquisition: The effect of verbal directing cues. In J. Watkins & L. Burwitz (Eds.), *Sports science: Proceedings of the VIII Commonwealth and International Conference on Sport, Physical Education, Dance, Recreation and Health* (pp. 349–354). London: E. & F. N. Spoon.

Robertson, S., Tremblay, L., Anson, G., & Elliot, D. (2002). Learning to cross a balance beam: Implications for teachers, coaches, and therapists. In K. Davids, G. Savelsbergh, S. Bennett, & J. van der Kamp (Eds.). *Dynamic interceptive actions in sport: Current research and practical applications* (pp. 109–125). London: E. & F. N. Spoon.

Rogers, C. A. (1974). Feedback precision and post-feedback interval duration. *Journal of Experimental Psychology, 102,* 604–608.

Roland, P. E., Larsen, B., Lassen, N. A., Skinhöf, E. (1980). Supplementary and other cortical areas in organization of voluntary movements in man. *Journal of Neurophysiology, 43,* 118–136.

Rose, D. J. (2003). *Fallproof: A comprehensive balance and mobility program.* Champaign, IL: Human Kinetics.

Rose, D. J., & Clark, S. (1995). Efficacy and transferability of a customized balance training program for "at-risk" older adults. Proceedings of the 5th Asia/Oceania Regional Congress of Gerontology, Hong Kong.

Rose, D. J., & Lucchese, N. (2003). The Fullerton advanced balance scale: Validation of an early identification tool. Paper presented at National Council on Aging—American Society on Aging Joint Conference, Chicago, IL.

Rose, D. J., & Tyry, T. (1994). The relative effectiveness of three model types on the early acquisition of rapid-fire pistol shooting. *Journal of Human Movement Studies, 26,* 87–99.

Rosenbaum, D. A. (1991). *Human motor control.* San Diego, CA: Academic Press.

Rosenbaum, D. A., Inhoff, A. W., & Gordon, A. M. (1984). Choosing between movement sequences: A hierarchical editor model. *Journal of Experimental Psychology: General, 113,* 372–393.

Rosenberg, M. (1979). *Conceiving the self.* New York: Basic Books.

Ross, I. D. (1974). Interference in discrete motor tasks: A test of the theory. Unpublished doctoral dissertation, University of Michigan, Ann Arbor, MI.

Roth, M., Decety, J., Raybaudi, M., Massarelli, R., Delon-Martin, C., Segebarth, C., Morand, S., Germignani, A., Decorps, M., & Jeannerod, M. (1996). Possible involvement of primary motor cortex in mentally simulated movement: A functional magnetic resonance imaging study. *NeuroReports, 7,* 1280–1284.

Rothkopf, E. Z. (1981). A macroscopic model of instruction and purposeful learning. *Instructional Science, 10,* 105–122.

Rothstein, A. L., & Arnold, R. K. (1976). Bridging the gap: Application of research on videotape feedback and bowling. *Motor Skills: Theory into Practice, 1,* 36–61.

Rothwell, J. C. (1994). *Control of human voluntary movement* (2nd ed.). Kent, UK: Croom Helm.

Rothwell, J. C., Taub, M. M., Day, B. L., Obeso, J. A., & Marsden, C. D. (1982). Manual motor performance in a deafferented man. *Brain, 105,* 515–542.

Rouiller, E. M., Yu, X. H., Moret, V., Tempini, A., Wiesendanger, M., & Liang, F. (1998). Dexterity in adult monkeys following early lesion of the motor cortical hand area: The role of cortex adjacent to lesion. *European Journal of Neuroscience, 10,* 729–740.

Ryan, E. D. (1965). Retention of stabilometer performance over extended periods of time. *Research Quarterly for Exercise and Sport, 36,* 46–51.

Ryding, E., Decety, J., Sjoholm, H., Stenberg, G., & Ingvar, D. H. (1993). Motor imagery activates the cerebellum regionally. A SPECT rCBF study with 99mTc-HMPAO. *Cognition and Brain Research 1,* 94–99.

Sage, G. H., & Hornak, J. E. (1978). Progressive speed practice in learning a continuous motor skill. *Research Quarterly for Exercise and Sport, 49,* 190–196.

Salmoni, A. W., Schmidt, R. A., & Walter, C. B. (1984). Knowledge of results and motor learning: A review and reappraisal. *Psychological Bulletin, 95,* 355–386.

Salthouse, T. A. (1991). *Theoretical perspectives on cognitive aging.* Hillsdale, NJ: Erlbaum.

Sanes, J. N., & Donoghue, J. P. (2000). Plasticity and primary motor cortex. *Annual Review of Neuroscience, 23,* 393–415.

Saper, C. B., Iversen, S., & Frackowiak, R. (2000). Integration of sensory and motor function: The association areas of the cerebral cortex and the cognitive capabilities of the brain. In E. R. Kandel, J. H. Schwartz, & T. M. Jessell (Eds.), *Principles of neural science* (4th ed.) (pp. 349–380). New York: McGraw-Hill.

Savelsbergh, G. J. P., Whiting, H. T. A., & Bootsma, R. J. (1991). "Grasping" tau! *Journal of Experimental Psychology: Human Perception and Performance, 17,* 315–322.

Sawle, G. V., & Myers, R. (1993). The role of positron emission tomography in the assessment of neurotransplantation. *Trends in Neuroscience, 16*(5), 172–176.

Scannell, R. J. (1968). Transfer of accuracy training when difficulty is controlled by varying target size. *Research Quarterly for Exercise and Sport, 39,* 341–350.

Schaal, S., Sternad, D., & Atkeson, C. G. (1996). One-handed juggling: A dynamical approach to a rhythmic movement task. *Journal of Motor Behavior, 28*(2), 165–183.

Schendel, J. D., & Hagman, J. D. (1982). On sustaining procedural skills over a prolonged retention interval. *Journal of Applied Psychology, 67,* 605–610.

Schendel, J. D., & Hagman, J. D. (1991). Long-term retention of motor skills. In J. E. Morrison (Ed.), *Training for performance: Principles of applied human learning* (pp. 53–92). New York: Wiley.

Schendel, J. D., Shields, J., & Katz, M. (1978). Retention of motor skills: Review. (Technical Paper 313.) Alexandria, VA: U.S. Army Research Institute for the Behavioral and Social Sciences.

Schieppati, M. (1987). The Hoffman reflex: A means of assessing spinal reflex excitability and its descending control in man. *Progress in Neurobiology, 28,* 345–376.

Schmidt, R. A. (1972). Experimental psychology. In R. N. Singer (Ed.), *The psychomotor domain: Movement behavior* (pp. 18–55). Philadelphia: Lea & Febiger.

Schmidt, R. A. (1975). A schema theory of discrete motor skill learning. *Psychological Review, 82,* 225–260.

Schmidt, R. A. (1976). Control processes in motor skills. *Exercise and Sport Sciences Reviews, 4,* 229–261.

Schmidt, R. A. (1982a). More on motor programs. In J. A. S. Kelso (Ed.), *Human motor behavior. An introduction* (pp. 189–207). Hillsdale, NJ: Erlbaum.

Schmidt, R. A. (1982b). The schema concept. In J. A. S. Kelso (Ed.), *Human motor behavior: An introduction* (pp. 219–235). Hillsdale, NJ: Erlbaum.

Schmidt, R. A. (1988a). Motor and action perspectives on motor behavior. In O. G. Meijer & K. Roth (Eds.), *Complex motor behavior: "The" motor-action controversy* (pp. 3–44). Amsterdam: North Holland.

Schmidt, R. A. (1988b). *Motor control and learning: A behavioral emphasis* (2nd ed.). Champaign, IL: Human Kinetics.

Schmidt, R. A. (1991). Frequent augmented feedback can degrade learning: Evidence and interpretations. In G. E. Stelmach & J. Requin (Eds.), *Tutorials in motor neuroscience* (pp. 59–75). Norwell, MA: Kluwer Academic Publishers.

Schmidt, R. A. (1992). Motor learning principles for physical therapy. In M. Lister (Ed.), *Contemporary management of motor problems. Proceedings of the II STEP Conference* (pp. 65–76). Alexandria, VA: Foundation for Physical Therapy, Inc.

Schmidt, R. A. (2003). Motor schema theory after 27 years: Reflections and implications for a new theory. *Research Quarterly for Exercise and Sport, 74,* 366–375.

Schmidt, R. A., & Bjork, R. A. (1992). New conceptual-izations of practice: Common principles in three paradigms suggest new concepts for training. *Psychological Science, 3*, 207–217.

Schmidt, R. A., Heuer, H., Ghodsian, D., & Young, D. E. (1998). Generalized motor programs and units of action in bimanual coordination. In M. Latash (Ed.), *Bernstein's traditions in motor control* (pp. 329–360). Champaign, IL: Human Kinetics.

Schmidt, R. A., Lange, C. A., & Young, D. E. (1990). Optimizing summary knowledge of results for increased skill learning. *Human Movement Science, 9*, 325–348.

Schmidt, R. A., & Lee, T. D. (1999). *Motor control and learning: A behavioral emphasis* (3rd ed.). Champaign, IL: Human Kinetics.

Schmidt, R. A., & Nacson, J. (1971). Further tests of the activity-set hypothesis for warm-up decrement. *Journal of Experimental Psychology, 90*, 56–64.

Schmidt, R. A., & White, J. L. (1972). Evidence for an error-detection mechanism in motor skills: A test of Adams' closed-loop theory. *Journal of Motor Behavior, 4*, 143–153.

Schmidt, R. A., & Wrisberg, C. A. (1971). The activity-set hypothesis for warm-up decrement in a movement-speed task. *Journal of Motor Behavior, 3*, 318–325.

Schmidt, R. A. & Wrisberg, C. A. (2000). *Motor learning and performance. A problem-based learning approach* (2nd ed.). Champaign, IL: Human Kinetics.

Schmidt, R. A., & Young, D. E. (1987). Transfer of motor control in motor skill learning. In S. M. Cormier & J. D. Hagman (Eds.), *Transfer of learning* (pp. 47–79). Orlando, FL: Academic Press.

Schmidt, R. A., Young, D. E., Swinnen, S., & Shapiro, D. C. (1989). Summary knowledge of results for skill acquisition: Support for the guidance hypothesis. *Journal of Experimental Psychology: Learning, Memory, and Cognition, 15*, 352–359.

Schneider, W., Dumais, S. T., & Shiffrin, R. M. (1984). Automatic and control processing and attention. In R. Parasuraman & D. R. Davies (Eds.), *Varieties of attention*. Orlando, FL: Academic Press.

Schneider, W., & Fisk, A. D. (1983). Attention theory and mechanisms for skilled performance. In R. A. Magill (Ed.), *Memory and control of action* (pp. 119–143). Amsterdam: North-Holland.

Schneider, W., & Shiffrin, R. M. (1977). Controlled and automatic processing: Detection, search, and attention, *Psychological Review, 84*, 1–66.

Schoner, G., & Kelso, J. A. S. (1988). A synergetic theory of environmentally specified and learned patterns of movement coordination. I. Relative phase dynamics. *Biological Cybernetics, 58*, 71–80.

Schunk, D. H. (1987). Peer models and children's behavioral change. *Review of Educational Research, 57*, 149–174.

Schunk, D. H., & Hanson, A. R. (1985). Peer models: Influence on children's self-efficacy and achievement. *Journal of Educational Psychology, 77*, 313–322.

Schunk, D. H., Hanson, A. R., & Cox, C. D. (1987). Peer-model attributes and children's achievement behaviors. *Journal of Educational Psychology, 79*, 54–61.

Schutz, R. W. (1977). Absolute, constant, and variable error: Problems and solutions. In D. Mood (Ed.), Proceedings of the Colorado Measurement Symposium (pp. 82–100). Boulder, CO: University of Colorado.

Scully, D. M. (1986). Visual perception of technical execution and aesthetic quality in biological motion. *Human Movement Science, 5*, 185–206.

Scully, D. M., & Newell, K. M. (1985). Observational learning and the acquisition of motor skills: Toward a visual perception perspective. *Journal of Human Movement Studies, 11*, 169–186.

Seefeldt, V., & Haubenstricker, J. (1982). Patterns, phases, or stages: An analytical model for the study of developmental movement. In J. A. S. Kelso & J. E. Clark (Eds.), *The development of movement control and coordination* (pp. 309–318). New York: Wiley.

Seymore, W. D. (1954). Experiments on the acquisition of industrial skills. *Occupational Psychology, 28*, 77–89.

Shallice, T. (1964). The detection of change and the perceptual-moment hypothesis. *British Journal of Statistical Psychology Record, 17*, 113–135.

Shapiro, D. C. (1977). Bilateral transfer of a motor program. Paper presented at the annual meeting of the AAHPER, Seattle, WA.

Shapiro, D. C. (1978). *The learning of generalized motor programs*. Unpublished doctoral dissertation, University of Southern California, Los Angeles, CA.

Shapiro, D. C., & Schmidt, R. A. (1982). The schema theory: Recent evidence and developmental implications. In J. A. S. Kelso & J. E. Clark (Eds.), *The development of movement control and coordination*, (pp. 113–150). New York: Wiley.

Shapiro, D. C., Zernicke, R. F., Gregor, R. J., & Diestel, J. D. (1981). Evidence for generalized motor programs using gait-pattern analysis. *Journal of Motor Behavior, 13*, 33–47.

Sharon, S. (1980). Cooperative learning in small groups: Recent methods and effects on achievement attitudes and ethnic relations. *Review of Educational Research, 50*, 241–271.

Sharp, R. H., & Whiting, H. T. A. (1974). Information processing and eye movement behavior in a ball-catching skill. *Journal of Human Movement Studies, 1*, 124–131.

Shea, C. H., Lai, Q., Black, C., & Park, J. (2000). Spacing practice sessions across days benefits the learning of motor skills. *Human Movement Science, 19*, 737–760.

Shea, C. H., & Wulf, G. (1999). Enhancing motor learning through external-focus instructions and feedback. *Human Movement Science, 18*, 553–571.

Shea, J. B., & Morgan, R. L. (1979). Contextual interference effects on the acquisition, retention, and transfer of a motor skill. *Journal of Experimental Psychology: Human Learning and Memory, 5*, 179–187.

Shea, J.B., & Zimny, S. T. (1988). Knowledge incorporation in motor representation. In O. G. Meijer and K. Roth (Eds.), *Complex motor behavior: "The" motor-action controversy* (pp. 289–314). Amsterdam: North-Holland.

Shea, J. B., & Zimny, S. T. (1983). Context effects in memory and learning in movement information. In R. A. Magill (Ed.), *Memory and control of action* (pp. 345–366). Amsterdam: North-Holland.

Sheffield, F. D. (1961). Theoretical considerations in the learning of complex sequential tasks from demonstration and practice. In A. A. Lumsdaine (Ed.), *Student response in programmed instruction* (pp. 13– 32). Washington, DC: National Academy of Science–National Research Council.

Sheridan, M. R. (1984). Planning and controlling simple movements. In M. M. Smyth & A. L. Wing (Eds.), *The psychology of movement* (pp. 47–82). London: Academic Press.

Sherrington, C. S. (1906; reprinted 1947). *The integrative action of the nervous system.* New Haven, CT: Yale University Press.

Sherrington, C. S. (1910). Notes on the scratch-reflex of the cat. *Quarterly Journal of Experimental Physiology, 3*, 213–220.

Sherrington, C. S. (1911). *The integrative action of the nervous system.* London: Constable.

Sherwood, D. E. (1988). Effect of bandwidth knowledge of results on movement consistency. *Perceptual and Motor Skills, 66*, 535–542.

Sherwood, D. E., & Lee, T. D. (2003). Schema theory: Critical review and implications for the role of cognition in a new theory of motor learning. *Research Quarterly for Exercise and Sport, 74*, 376–382.

Shiffrin, R. M., & Schneider, W. (1977). Controlled and automatic human information processing: Perceptual learning, automatic attending, and a general theory. *Psychological Review, 84*, 127–190.

Shumway-Cook, A., Anson, D., & Haller, S. (1988). Postural sway biofeedback: Its effect on reestablishing stance stability in hemiplegic patients. *Archives of Physical Medicine and Rehabilitation, 69*, 395–400.

Shumway-Cook, A., Horak, F., & Black, F. O. (1987). A critical examination of vestibular function in motor-impaired learning disabled children. *International Journal of Pediatric Otorhinolaryngology, 14*, 21–30.

Shumway-Cook, A., Woollacott, M., Baldwin, M., & Kerns, K. (1997). The effects of cognitive demands

on postural control in elderly fallers and non-fallers. *Journal of Gerontology, 52*, M232–M240.

Sidaway, B., McNitt-Gray, J., & Davis, G. (1989). Visual timing of muscle preactivation in preparation for landing. *Ecological Psychology, 1*, 253–264.

Siedentop, D. (1991). *Developing teaching skills in physical education.* Mountain View, CA: Mayfield.

Siegel, D., & Davis, C. (1980). Transfer effects of learning at specific speeds on performance over a range of speeds. *Perceptual and Motor Skills, 50*, 83–89.

Siipola, E. M. (1941). The relation of transfer to similarity in habit structure. *Journal of Experimental Psychology, 28*, 233–261.

Silver, H., Strong, R., & Perini, M. (1997). Interpreting learning styles and multiple intelligences. *Educational Leadership, 55*, 22–27.

Singer, R. N. (1966). Transfer effects and ultimate success in archery due to degree of difficulty of the initial learning. *Research Quarterly for Exercise and Sport, 37*, 532–539.

Singer, R. N. (1980). *Motor learning and human performance* (3rd ed.). New York: Macmillan.

Skinner, B. F. (1938). *The behavior of organisms.* New York: Appleton-Century.

Slade, J. M., Landers, D. M., & Martin, P. E. (2000). Muscular activity during real and imagined movements: A test of the inflow hypothesis. *Journal of Sport and Exercise Psychology, 22*, S100.

Slamecka, N. J., & McElree, B. (1983). Normal forgetting of verbal lists as a function of their degree of learning. *Journal of Experimental Psychology: Learning, Memory, and Cognition, 9*, 384–397.

Slavin, R. E. (1980). Cooperative learning. *Review of Educational Research, 50*, 315–342.

Smith J. C., & Feldman, J. L. (1987). In vitro brainstem-spinal cord preparations for study of motor systems for mammalian respiration and locomotion. *Journal of Neuroscience Method, 21*, 321–333.

Smith, J. L. (1969). Fusimotor neuron block and voluntary arm movement in man. Unpublished doctoral dissertation, University of Wisconsin, Madison, WI.

Smoll, F. L. (1972). Effects of precision of information feedback upon acquisition of a motor skill. *Research Quarterly for Exercise and Sport, 43*, 489–493.

Smyth, M. M., & Marriott, A. M. (1982). Vision and proprioception in simple catching. *Journal of Motor Behavior, 14*, 143–152.

Smyth, M. M., & Pendleton, L. R. (1990). Space and movement in working memory. *Quarterly Journal of Experimental Psychology, 42A*, 291–304.

Sotrel, A., Williams R. S., Kaufmann W. E., Myers R. H. (1993). Evidence for neuronal degeneration and dendritic plasticity in cortical pyramidal neurons of Huntington's disease. A quantitative Golgi study. *Neurology, 43*, 2088.

Soucy, M. C., & Proteau, L. (2001). Development of multiple movement representations with practice: Specificity vs. flexibility. *Journal of Motor Behavior, 33*, 243–254.

Sparrow, W. A. (1983). The efficiency of skilled performance. *Journal of Motor Behavior, 15*, 237–261.

Sparrow, W. A., & Irizarry-Lopez, V. M. (1987). Mechanical efficiency and metabolic cost as measures of learning a novel gross motor task. *Journal of Motor Behavior, 19*, 240–264.

Spirduso, W. W., & McCrae, P. G. (1990). Motor performance and aging. In J. E. Birren & K. W. Schaie (Eds.), *Handbook of the psychology of aging* (3rd ed.) (pp. 183–200). Orlando, FL: Academic Press.

Squire, L. R., & Knowlton, B. J. (1994). Memory, hippocampus and brain systems. In M. Gazzaniga (Ed.), *The cognitive neurosciences* (pp. 825–837). Cambridge. MA: MIT Press.

Squire, L. R., & Zola, S. M. (1996). Structure and function of declarative and nondeclarative memory systems. *Proceedings of the National Academy of Sciences, 93*, 13515–13522.

Starkes, J. L., & Deakin, J. M. (1984). Perception in sport: A cognitive approach to skilled performance. In W. F. Straub & J. M. Williams (Eds.), *Cognitive sport psychology* (pp. 115–128). Lansing, NY: Sport Science Associates.

Starkes, J. L., Edwards, P., Dissanayake, P., & Dunn, T. (1995). A new technology and field test of advance cue usage in volleyball. *Research Quarterly for Exercise and Sport, 66*(2), 162–167.

Steigman, M. J., & Stevenson, H. W. (1960). The effect of pre-training reinforcement schedules on children's learning. *Child Development, 31*, 53–58.

Stelmach, G. E. (1969a). Efficiency of motor learning as a function of intertrial rest. *Research Quarterly for Exercise and Sport, 40*, 198–202.

Stelmach, G. E. (1969b). Prior positioning responses as a factor in short-term retention of a simple motor task. *Journal of Experimental Psychology, 81*, 523–526.

Stelmach, G. E. (1974). Retention of motor skills. In J. H. Wilmore (Ed.), *Exercise and sport science reviews* (Vol. 2, pp. 1–31). New York: Academic Press.

Stelmach, G. E., Garcia-Colera, A., & Martin, Z. E. (1989). Force transition control within a movement sequence in Parkinson's disease. *Journal of Neurology, Neurosurgery and Psychiatry, 50*, 296–303.

Stelmach, G. E., Worringham, C. J., & Strand, E. A. (1986). Movement preparation in Parkinson's disease: The use of advance information. *Brain, 109*, 1179–1194.

Stelmach, G. E., Worringham, C. J., & Strand, E. A. (1987). The programming and execution of movement sequences in Parkinson's disease. *International Journal of Neuroscience, 36*, 55–65.

Stergiou, N. (Ed.) (2004). *Innovative analyses of human movement.* Champaign, IL: Human Kinetics.

Stern, G. (1966). The effect of lesions in the substantia nigra. *Brain, 89*, 449.

Sternad, D. (1998). A dynamic systems perspective to perception and action. *Research Quarterly for Exercise and Sport, 69*, 319–325.

Sternberg, S., Monsell, S., Knoll, R. L., & Wright, C. E. (1978). The latency and duration of rapid movement sequences: Comparisons of speech and typewriting. In G. E. Stelmach (Ed.), *Information processing in motor control and learning* (pp. 117–152). New York: Academic Press.

Stevens, J. A., & Stoykov, M. E. P. (2003). Using motor imagery in the rehabilitation of hemiparesis. *Archives of Physical Medicine in Rehabilitation, 84*, 1090–1092.

Stokes, M., & Young, A. (1984). The contribution of reflex inhibition to arthrogenous muscle weakness. *Clinical Science, 67*, 7–14.

Strick, P. L. (1983). The influence of motor preparation on the response of cerebellar neurons to limb displacements. *Journal of Neuroscience, 3*, 2007–2020.

Stroup, F. (1957). Relationship between measurements of fluid motion perception and basketball ability in college men. *Research Quarterly for Exercise and Sport, 28*, 72–76.

Summers, J. (1998). Has ecological psychology delivered what it promised? In J. P. Piek (Ed.), *Motor behavior and human skill* (pp. 385–402). Champaign, IL: Human Kinetics.

Swift, E. J. (1903). Studies in the psychology and physiology of learning. *American Journal of Psychology, 14*, 201–251.

Swinnen, S. P. (1990). Interpolated activities during the knowledge of results delay and post-knowledge of results interval: Effects of performance and learning. *Journal of Experimental Psychology: Learning, Memory, and Cognition, 16*, 692–705.

Swinnen, S. P., Schmidt, R. A., Nicholson, D. E., & Shapiro, D. C. (1990). Information feedback for skill acquisition: Instantaneous knowledge of results degrades learning. *Journal of Experimental Psychology: Learning, Memory, and Cognition, 16*, 706–716.

Swinnen, S. P., Walter, C. B., Lee, T. D., & Serrien, D. J. (1993). Acquiring bimanual skills: Contrasting forms of information feedback for interlimb decoupling. *Journal of Experimental Psychology: Learning, Memory, and Cognition, 19*(6), 1328–1344.

Szafran, J., & Welford, A. T. (1950). On the relation between transfer and difficulty of initial task. *Quarterly Journal of Experimental Psychology, 2*, 88–94.

Szklut, S. E., & Breath, D. M. (2001). Learning disabilities. In D. A. Umphred (Ed.), *Neurological rehabilitation* (4th ed.) (pp. 308–350). St. Louis: Mosby.

Tarver, S., Hallahan, D., Kauffman, J., & Ball, D. (1976). Verbal rehearsal and selective attention in children with learning disabilities: A developmental lag. *Journal of Experimental Child Psychology, 22,* 375–385.

Tatem, J. A. (1973). Personality and physical variables between and among tennis players and other athletes and non-athletes. Unpublished doctoral dissertation, Springfield College.

Taub, E. (1976). Movements in non-human primates deprived of somatosensory feedback. *Exercise and Sport Sciences Reviews, 4,* 335–374.

Taub, E., & Berman, A. J. (1968). Movement and learning in the absence of sensory feedback. In S. J. Freedman (Ed.), *The neuropsychology of spatially oriented behavior* (pp. 173–192). Homewood, IL: Dorsey Press.

Tergerson, R. L. (1964). The relationship of selected measures of wrist strength, vision, and general motor ability to badminton playing ability. Unpublished master's thesis, University of North Carolina.

Terzuolo, C. A., & Viviani, P. (1980). Determinants and characteristics of motor patterns used for typing. *Neuroscience, 5,* 1085–1103.

Tessier-Lavigne, M. (2000). Visual processing by the retina. In E. R. Kandel, J. H. Schwartz, & T. M. Jessell (Eds.), *Principles of neural science* (4th ed.) (pp. 507–522).

Thach, W. T. (1978). Correlation of neural discharge with pattern and force of muscular activity, joint position, and directon of the intended movement in motor cortex and cerebellum. *Journal of Neurophysiology, 41,* 654–676.

Thach, W. T. (1996). On the specific role of the cerebellum in motor learning and cognition: Clues from PET activation and lesion studies in humans. *Behavioral and Brain Sciences, 19,* 411.

Thach, W. T. (1998). A role for the cerebellum in learning movement coordination. *Neurobiology of Learning and Memory, 70,* 177–188.

Thaut, M. H., McIntosh, G. C., Rice, R. R., Miller, R. A., Rathbun, J., & Brault, J. M. (1996). Rhythmic auditory stimulation in gait training for Parkinson's disease patients. *Movement Disorders, 11*(2), 193–200.

Thelen, E., & Fisher, D. M. (1982). Newborn stepping: An explanation for a "disappearing reflex." *Developmental Psychology, 18,* 760–775.

Thelen, E., Kelso, J. A. S., & Fogel, A. (1987). Self-organizing systems and infant motor development. *Developmental Review, 7,* 39–65.

Thomas, J. R. (1980). Acquisition of motor skills: Information processing differences between children and adults. *Research Quarterly for Exercise and Sport, 51,* 158–173.

Thomas, J. R. (1984). Children's motor skill development. In J. R. Thomas (Ed.), *Motor skill development during childhood and adolescence* (pp. 91–104). New York: McGraw-Hill.

Thomas, J. R., French, K. E., & Humphries, C. A. (1985). Knowledge development and sport skill performance: Directions for motor behavior research. *Journal of Sport Psychology, 8,* 259–272.

Thomas, J. R., & Gallagher, G. D. (1986). Memory development and motor skill acquisition. In V. Seefeldt, (Ed.), *Contributions of physical activity to human well-being* (pp. 125–139). Reston, VA: AAHPERD (American Alliance for Health, Physical Education, Recreation and Dance) Publications.

Thomas, J. R., Thomas, K. T., Lee, A. M., Testerman, E., & Ashy, M. (1983). Age differences in the use of strategy for recall of movement in a large scale environment. *Research Quarterly for Exercise and Sport, 54,* 264–272.

Thompson, R. F. (1980). The search for the engram, II. In D. McFadden (Ed.), *Neural mechanisms in behavior: A Texas symposium* (pp. 172–222). New York: Springer-Verlag.

Thomson, D. M., & Tulving, E. (1970). Associative encoding and retrieval: Weak and strong cues. *Journal of Experimental Psychology, 86,* 255–262.

Thorndike, E. L. (1903). *Educational psychology.* New York: Lemcke & Buechner.

Thorndike, E. L. (1914). *Educational psychology: Briefer course.* New York: Columbia University Press.

Thorndike, E. L. (1927). The law of effect. *American Journal of Psychology, 39,* 212–222.

Thorndike, E. L., & Woodworth, R. S. (1901). The influence of improvement in one mental function upon the efficiency of other functions. *Psychological Review, 8,* 247–261.

Thune, L. E. (1950). The effect of different types of preliminary activities on subsequent learning of paired-associate material. *Journal of Experimental Psychology, 40,* 423–438.

Tinetti, M. E. (1994). Prevention of falls among the elderly. *The New England Journal of Medicine, 320,* 1055–1059.

Titzer, R., Smith, L., & Thelen, E. (1995). The effects of infants' experience on the visual cliff and a reaching task. *Journal of Sport and Exercise Psychology, 17* (Suppl.), 103.

Todd, J. T. (1981). Visual information about moving objects. *Journal of Experimental Psychology: Human Perception and Performance, 7,* 795–810.

Toole, T., & Arink, E. A. (1982). Movement education: Its effect on motor skill performance. *Research Quarterly for Exercise and Sport, 53,* 156–162.

Tremblay, L., & Proteau, L. (1998). Specificity of practice: The case of powerlifting. *Research Quarterly for Exercise and Sport, 69,* 284–289.

Tremblay, L., & Proteau, L. (2001). Specificity of practice in a ball interception task. *Canadian Journal of Experimental Psychology, 55,* 207–218.

Trevarthen, C. B. (1968). Two mechanisms of vision in primates. *Psychological Research, 31,* 299–337.

Trumbo, D., Ulrich, L., & Noble, M. E. (1965). Verbal coding and display coding in the acquisition and retention of tracking skill. *Journal of Applied Psychology, 49,* 368–375.

Tubbs, M. E. (1986). Goal setting: A meta-analytic examination of empirical evidence. *Journal of Applied Psychology, 71,* 474–483.

Tulving, E. (1985). How many memory systems are there? *American Psychologist, 40,* 385–398.

Tulving, E., & Pearlstone, Z. (1966). Availability versus accessibility of information in memory for words. *Journal of Verbal Learning and Verbal Behavior, 5,* 381–391.

Tulving, E., & Thomson, D. M. (1973). Encoding specificity and retrieval processes in episodic memory. *Psychological Review, 80,* 352–373.

Turvey, M. T. (1974). Perspectives in vision: Conception or perception. In D. D. Duane & M. B. Rawson (Eds.), *Reading, perception and language* (pp. 131–194). Baltimore: York Press.

Turvey, M. T. (1977). Preliminaries to a theory of action with reference to vision. In R. Shaw & J. Bransford (Eds.), *Perceiving, acting, and knowing* (pp. 211–265). Hillsdale, NJ: Erlbaum.

Turvey, M. T., & Carello, C. (1981). Cognition: The view from ecological realism. *Cognition, 10,* 313–321.

Turvey, M. T., Fitch, H. L., & Tuller, B. (1982). The Bernstein perspective: I. The problems of degrees-of-freedom and context-conditioned variability. In J.A.S. Kelso (Ed.), *Human motor behavior: An introduction* (pp. 239–252). Hillsdale, NJ: Erlbaum.

Ulrich, B., Thelen, E., & Niles, D. (1990). Perceptual determinants of action: Stair climbing choices of infants and toddlers. In J. B. Craik & J. Humphrey (Eds.), *Advances in motor development research* (Vol. 3). New York: AMS Publications.

Ungerleider, L. G. (1995). Functional brain imaging studies of cortical mechanisms for memory. *Science, 270,* 769–775.

Ungerleider, L. G., Doyon, J., & Karni, A. (2002). Imaging brain plasticity during motor skill learning. *Neurobiology of Learning and Memory, 78,* 553–564.

Van Dusen, F., & Schlosberg, H. (1948). Further study of the retention of verbal and motor skills. *Journal of Experimental Psychology, 38,* 526–534.

van Emmerik, R. E. A., den Brinker, B. P. L. M., Vereijken, B., & Whiting, H. T. A. (1989). Preferred tempo in the learning of a gross cyclical action. *The Quarterly Journal of Experimental Psychology, 41,* 251–262.

van Emmerik, R. E. A., & Wagenaar, R. C. (1996). Effect of walking velocity on relative phase dynamics in the trunk in human walking. *Journal of Biomechanics, 29,* 1175–1184.

Van Rossum, J. H. A. (1990). Schmidt's schema theory: The empirical base of the variability of practice hypothesis. *Human Movement Science, 9,* 387–435.

van Wieringen, P. C. W. (1988). Discussion: Self-organization or representation? Let's have both! In A. M. Colley & J. R. Beech (Eds.), *Cognition and action in skilled behaviour* (pp. 247–253). Amsterdam: North-Holland.

van Wieringen, P. C. W., Emmon, H. H., Bootsma, R. J., Hoogesteger, M., & Whiting, H. T. A. (1989). The effect of video-feedback on the learning of the tennis serve by intermediate players. *Journal of Sport Sciences, 7,* 153–162.

Vealey, R., & Greenleaf, C. A. (1998). Seeing is believing: Understanding and using imagery in sport. In J. M Williams (Ed.), *Applied sport psychology: Personal growth to peak performance.* Mountain View, CA: Mayfield.

Vedelli, J. (1986). A study of Revien's sports-vision techniques for improving motor skills (Abstract). Conference of the American Alliance for Health, Physical Education, Recreation and Dance, Cincinnati, OH.

Vereijken, B. (1991). The dynamics of skill acquisition. Unpublished doctoral dissertation, Free University, Amsterdam.

Vereijken, B., van Emmerik, R. E. A., Whiting, H. T. A., & Newell, K. M. (1992). Free(z)ing degrees of freedom in skill acquisition. *Journal of Motor Behavior, 24*(1), 133–142.

Vereijken, B., & Whiting, H. T. A. (1988). A comparison of echokinetic and synkinetic paradigms in the learning of a complex cyclical action. *Pre-proceedings of the Second Workshop on Imagery and Cognition.*

Vickers, J. N. (1988). Knowledge structure of expert-novice gymnasts. *Human Movement Science, 7,* 47–72.

Wadman, W. J., Denier van der Gon, J. J., Geuze, R. H., & Mol, C. R. (1979). Control of fast goal-directed arm movements. *Journal of Human Movement Studies, 5,* 3–17.

Wallace, S. A., & Weeks, D. L. (1988). Temporal constraints in the control of prehensive movements. *Journal of Motor Behavior, 20,* 81–105.

Walter, C. B. (1998). An alternative view of dynamical systems concepts in motor control and learning. *Research Quarterly for Exercise and Sport, 69,* 326–333.

Ward, L. B. (1937). Reminiscence and rote learning. *Psychological Monographs, 49,* No. 220.

Warren, W. H. (1984). Perceiving affordances: Visual guidance of stairclimbing. *Journal of Experimental Psychology: Human Perception and Performance, 10,* 683–703.

Warren, W. H., & Whang, S. (1987). Visual guidance of walking through apertures: Body-scaled information for affordances. *Journal of Experimental Psychology: Human Perception and Performance, 12,* 259–266.

Warren, W. H., Jr., Young, D. S., & Lee, D. N. (1986). Visual control of step length during running over irregular terrain. *Journal of Experimental Psychology: Human Perception and Performance, 12,* 259–266.

Waters, R. H. (1928). The influence of tuition upon ideational learning. *Journal of General Psychology, 1,* 534–549.

Weeks, D. L., & Sherwood, D. E. (1994). A comparison of knowledge of results scheduling methods for promoting motor skill acquisition and retention. *Research Quarterly for Exercise and Sport, 65*(2), 136–142.

Wehner, T., Vogt, S., & Stadler, M. (1984). Task-specific EMG characteristics during mental training. *Psychological Research, 46,* 389–401.

Weinberg, D. R., Guy, D. E., & Tupper, R. W. (1964). Variations of post-feedback interval in simple motor learning. *Journal of Experimental Psychology, 67,* 98–99.

Weinberg, R. S. (1994). Goal setting and performance in sport and exercise settings: A synthesis and critique. *Medicine and Science in Sports and Exercise, 26,* 469–477.

Weinberg, R. S., Hankes, D., & Jackson, A. (1991). Effect of the length and temporal location of the mental preparation interval on basketball shooting performance. *International Journal of Sport Psychology, 22,* 3–14.

Weiner, B. (1972). *Theories of motivation: From mechanism to cognition.* Chicago: Markham.

Weiskrantz, L., Warrington, E. K., Sanders, M. D., & Marshall, J. (1974). Visual capacity in the hemianopic field following a restricted cortical ablation. *Brain, 97,* 709–728.

Weiss, M. R. (1983). Modeling and motor performance: A developmental perspective. *Research Quarterly for Exercise and Sport, 54,* 190–197.

Weiss, M. R., Ebbeck, V., & Rose, D. J. (1992). "Show and tell" in the gymnasium revisited: Developmental differences in modeling and verbal rehearsal effects on motor skill learning. *Research Quarterly for Exercise and Sport, 63,* 292–301.

Weiss, M. R., & Klint, K. A. (1987). "Show and tell" in the gymnasium: An investigation of developmental differences in modeling and verbal rehearsal of motor skills. *Research Quarterly for Exercise and Sport, 58,* 234–241.

Weiss, M. R., McCullagh, P., Smith, A. L., & Berlant, A. R. (1998). Observational learning and the fearful child: Influence of peer models on the swimming skill performance and psychological responses. *Research Quarterly for Exercise and Sport, 69,* 380–394.

Werner, P. (1972). Integration of physical education skills with the concept of levers at intermediate grade levels. *Research Quarterly for Exercise and Sport, 43,* 423–428.

Wernig, A., Muller, S., Nanassy, A., & Cagol, E. (1995). Short communication: Laufband therapy based on "rules of spinal locomotion" is effective in spinal cord injured persons. *European Journal of Neuroscience, 7,* 823–829.

Wernig, A., Nanassy, A., & Muller, S. (1998). Maintenance of locomotor abilities following Laufband (treadmill) therapy in para- and tetraplegic persons: Follow-up studies. *Spinal Cord, 36,* 744–749.

West, K. L., & Bresson, E. S. (1996). The effects of a general versus specific visual skills training program on accuracy in judging length-of-ball in cricket. *International Journal of Sports Vision, 3,* 41–45.

Whitall, J. (1996). On the interaction of concurrent verbal and manual tasks: Which initial task conditions produce interference? *Research Quarterly for Exercise and Sport, 67*(3), 349–354.

Whiting, H. T. A. (1970). An operational analysis of a continuous ball-throwing and catching task. *Ergonomics, 13,* 445–454.

Whiting, H. T. A., Bijlard, M. J., & den Brinker, B. P. L. M. (1987). The effect of the availability of a dynamic model on the acquisition of a complex cyclical action. *The Quarterly Journal of Experimental Psychology, 39,* 43–59.

Whiting, H. T. A., Gill, E. B., & Stephenson, J.M. (1970). Critical time intervals for taking in flight information in a ball-catching task. *Ergonomics, 13,* 265–272.

Wieg, E. L. (1932). Bilateral transfer in the motor learning of young children and adults. *Child Development, 3,* 247–267.

Wightman, D. C., & Lintern, G. (1985). Part-task training strategies for tracking and manual control. *Human Factors, 27,* 267–283.

Williams, A. M., Davids, K., Burwitz, L., & Williams, J. G. (1994). Visual search strategies in experienced and inexperienced soccer players. *Research Quarterly for Exercise and Sport, 65,* 127–135.

Wilson, D. M. (1961). The central nervous control of flight in a locust. *Journal of Experimental Biology, 38,* 471–490.

Winstein, C. J., Christensen, S., & Fitch, N. (1993). Effects of summary knowledge of results on the acquisition and retention of partial weight bearing during gait. *Physical Therapy Practice, 2*(4), 40–51.

Winstein, C. J., & Garfinkel, A. (1985). Qualitative dynamics of disordered human locomotion: A preliminary investigation. *Journal of Motor Behavior, 21*(4), 373–391.

Winstein, C. J., & Schmidt, R. A. (1990). Reduced frequency of knowledge of results enhances motor skill learning. *Journal of Experimental Psychology: Learning, Memory, and Cognition 16,* 677–691.

Winther, K. T., & Thomas, J. R. (1981). Developmental differences in children's labeling of movement. *Journal of Motor Behavior, 13,* 77–90.

Wolf, S. L. (1983). Electromyographic feedback for spinal cord injured patients: A realistic perspective. In J. V. Basmaijian (Ed.), *Biofeedback: Principles and practice for clinicians* (3rd ed.) (pp. 130–134). Baltimore: Williams & Wilkins.

Wolpaw, J. R., & Carp, J. S. (1990). Memory traces in the spinal cord. *Trends in Neuroscience, 13*(4), 137–142.

Wolfson, L. (1997). Balance decrements in older persons: Effects of age and disease. In J. C. Masdeu, L. Sudarsky, & L. Wolfson (Eds.). *Gait disorders of aging: Falls and therapeutic strategies* (pp. 79–92). New York: Lippencott-Raven.

Wood, C. A., Gallagher, J. D., Martino, P. V., & Ross, M. (1992). Alternate forms of knowledge of results: Interaction of augmented feedback modality on learning. *Journal of Human Movement Studies, 22,* 213–230.

Wood, J. M., & Abernethy, B. (1997). An assessment of the efficacy of sports vision training programs. *Optometry and Vision Science, 74,* 646–659.

Woods, J. B. (1967). The effect of varied instructional emphasis upon the development of a motor skill. *Research Quarterly for Exercise and Sport, 38,* 132–142.

Woodworth, R. S. (1899). The accuracy of voluntary movement. *Psychological Review Monographs, 3* (Whole No. 302).

Wright, D. L., & Shea, C. H. (1991). Contextual dependencies in motor skills. *Memory and Cognition, 19,* 361–370.

Wright, D. L., & Shea, C. H. (1994). Cognition and motor skill acquisition: Contextual dependencies. In C. R. Reynolds (Ed.), *Cognitive assessment: A multidisciplinary perspective* (pp. 89–106). New York: Plenum.

Wrisberg, C. A. (1975). Serial-position effect in short-term motor memory. *Journal of Motor Behavior, 7,* 289–295.

Wrisberg, C. A., & Anshel, M. H. (1993). A field test of the activity-set hypothesis for warm-up decrement in an open skill. *Research Quarterly for Exercise and Sport, 64,* 39–45.

Wrisberg, C. A., & Gerard, N. C. (1977). A further investigation into the serial position curve for short-term motor memory. *Proceedings of the IX Canadian Psychomotor Learning and Sport Psychology Symposium* (pp. 241–248).

Wulf, G., Höss, M., & Prinz, W. (1998). Instructions for motor learning: Differential effects of internal versus external focus of attention. *Journal of Motor Behavior, 30,* 169–179.

Wulf, G., Lauterbach, B., & Toole, T. (1999). The learning advantages of an external focus of attention in golf. *Research Quarterly for Exercise and Sport, 70,* 120–126.

Wulf, G., McNevin, N. H., & Shea, C. H. (2002). The automaticity of complex motor skill learning as a function of attentional focus. *Quarterly Journal of Experimental Psychology, 34,* 171–182.

Wulf, G., & Schmidt, R. A. (1988). Variability of practice: Facilitation in retention and transfer through schema formation or context effects? *Journal of Motor Behavior, 20,* 133–149.

Wulf, G., Shea, C. H., & Park, J-H. (2001). Attention and motor performance: Preferences for and advantages of an external focus. *Research Quarterly for Exercise and Sport, 72,* 335–344.

Wulf, G., & Weigelt, C. (1997). Instructions about physical principles in learning a complex skill: To tell or not to tell. *Research Quarterly for Exercise and Sport, 68,* 362–367.

Young, A., Stokes, M., & Iles, J. F. (1987). Effects of joint pathology on muscle. *Clinical Orthopaedics and Related Research, 219,* 21–27.

Young, D. E., & Schmidt, R. A. (1990). Units of motor behavior: Modifications with practice and feedback. In M. Jeannerod (Ed.), *Attention and performance XIII* (pp. 763–795). Hillsdale, NJ: Erlbaum.

Young, D. E., & Schmidt, R. A. (1992). Augmented kinematic feedback and motor learning. *Journal of Motor Behavior, 24,* 261–273.

Zelaznik, H. N., Schmidt, R. A., Gielen, S. C., & Milich, M. (1983). Kinematic properties of rapid aimed hand movements. *Journal of Motor Behavior, 15,* 217–236.

Zimmerman, B. J. (1989). Models of self-regulated learning and academic achievement. In B. J. Zimmerman & D. H. Schunk (Eds.), *Self-regulated learning and academic achievement theory, research, and practice: Progress in cognitive development research* (pp. 1–26). New York: Springer-Verlag.

# CREDITS

## Photo Credits

**p. 4**    (left) Dimitri Lundt/Corbis; (right) Corbis
**p. 8**    Elsa/Getty Images
**p. 21**   Kathleen Olson
**p. 22**   Reuter's/Corbis Bettmann
**p. 23**   Farjana K. Godhuly/AFP/Getty Images
**p. 27**   Tom Stillo
**p. 28**   Bob Daemmrich/Stock Boston
**p. 33**   (left) Michael Wong/Corbis;
            (right) Jamie Squire/Getty Images
**p. 36**   Wally McNamee/Corbis
**p. 54**   Dr. Risto Ilmoniemi/Nexstim Ltd.
**p. 82**   Allsport/Getty Images
**p. 85**   J. Sutton/Duomo
**p. 87**   Don Mason/Corbis
**p. 100**  Kent Warwick/Photolibrary.com
**p. 102**  John Gress/Reuters/Corbis
**p. 106**  Pete Saloutos/Corbis
**p. 110**  Geert Savelsbergh
**p. 118**  NASA/John F. Kennedy Space Center
**p. 122**  Jed Jacobsohn/Allsport USA/Getty Images
**p. 147**  Dan Porges/Peter Arnold, Inc
**p. 285**  Frank Siteman/Rainbow
**p. 363**  Kathleen Olson
**p. 364**  NASA Headquarters

## Art Credits

**p. 44, Figure 2.3** *Source:* Enoka, R. M., Miller, D. I., & Burgess, E. M., Below-knee amputee running gait. *American Journal of Physical Medicine and Rehabilitation,* 1982. Reprinted with permission.

**p. 46, Figure 2.4** *Source:* McIntyre, D. R., & Pfautsh, E. W., A kinematic analysis of the baseball batting swing involved in opposite-field and same-field hitting. *Research Quarterly for Exercise and Sport, 53,* 206–213, 1982. Reprinted with permission.

**p. 47, Figure 2.5** *Source:* Winstein, C. J., and Garfinkel, A. Qualitative dynamics of disordered human locomotion: A preliminary investigation. *Journal of Motor Behavior, 21,* 4, 373–391, 1985. Reprinted with permission of the Helen Dwight Reid Educational Foundation. Published by Heldref Publications, 1319 Eighteenth Street., N.W., Washington D.C. 20036. Copyright 1985.

**p. 50, Figure 2.7** *Source:* Horak, F. B., & Nashner, L. M., Central programming of postural movements: Adaptation to altered support surface of configurations. *Journal of Experimental Psychology: Human Perception and Performance, 17,* 315–322, 1991. Copyright 1991 by the American Psychological Association. Reprinted with permission.

**p. 64, Figure 3.2** *Source:* Germann, William and Stanfield, Cindy, *Principles of Human Physiology,* 2nd ed., Benjamin Cummings Publishing. San Francisco: CA. 2004.

**p.66, Figure 3.3** *Source:* Germann, William and Stanfield, Cindy, *Principles of Human Physiology,* 2nd ed., Benjamin Cummings Publishing. San Francisco: CA. 2004.

**p. 95, Figure 4.1** *Source:* Germann, William and Stanfield, Cindy, *Principles of Human Physiology,* 2nd ed., Benjamin Cummings Publishing. San Francisco: CA. 2004.

**p. 110, Highlight** *Source:* Savelsbergh, G. J. P., Whiting, H. T. A., and Bootsma, R. J. Grasping tau! *Journal of Experimental Psychology: Human Perception and Performance, 17,* 315–322, 1991. Copyright 1991 by the American Psychological Association. Reprinted with permission.

**p. 115, Figure 4.3** *Source:* Germann, William and Stanfield, Cindy, *Principles of Human Physiology,* 2nd ed., Benjamin Cummings Publishing. San Francisco: CA. 2004.

**p. 116, Figure 4.4** *Source:* Germann, William and Stanfield, Cindy, *Principles of Human Physiology,* 2nd ed., Benjamin Cummings Publishing. San Francisco: CA. 2004.

**p. 117, Figure 4.5** *Source:* Germann, William and Stanfield, Cindy, *Principles of Human Physiology,* 2nd ed., Benjamin Cummings Publishing. San Francisco: CA. 2004.

**p. 132, Figure 5.3** *Source:* Johnson, Michael. *Human Biology: Concepts and Current Issues,* 2nd edition. Benjamin Cummings Publishing: San Francisco, CA. 2003.

**p. 141, 143 Figure 5.5a-b** *Source:* Germann, William and Stanfield, Cindy, *Principles of Human Physiology,* 2nd ed., Benjamin Cummings Publishing. San Francisco: CA. 2004.

**p. 153, Figure 5.6** *Source:* Germann, William and Stanfield, Cindy, *Principles of Human Physiology,* 2nd ed., Benjamin Cummings Publishing. San Francisco: CA. 2004.

**p. 156, Figure 5.7** *Source:* Merton, P. A., How we control the contraction of our muscles. *Scientific American,* May 1972. All rights reserved. Reprinted with permission of author.

**p. 180, Figure 6.2:** *Source:* Reprinted from *The Coordination and Regulation of Movements,* Bernstein, N. Copyright 1967, with permission from Elsevier.

**p. 188, Figure 6.4** *Source:* Learning Style Inventory, Copyright 1976, revised 1985. Experience Based Learning Systems Inc. Developed by David A Kolb. Printed with permission from the Hay Group. Tel: (617) 425-4500.

**p.201, Figure 7.2** *Source:* Stelmach, G. E., Efficiency of motor learning as a function of inter-trial rest. *Research Quarterly for Exercise and Sport, 40,* 198–202, 1969.

**p. 213,** *Source:* Williams, A. M., Davids, K., Burwitz, L., and Williams, J. G. Visual search strategies in experiences and inexperienced soccer players. *Research Quarterly for Exercise and Sport, 65,* 127–135, 1994.

**p. 226, Figure 8.1** *Source:* Boyce, B. A., Effects of assigned versus participating set goals on skill acquisition and retention of a selected shooting task. *Journal of Teaching in Physical Education, 11*(3): 227, 1992.

**p. 235, Figure 8.2** *Source:* McCullagh, P., Weiss, M. R., and Ross, D. Modeling considerations in motor skill acquisition and performance. In Pandolf, K. B., *Exercise and Sport Science Reviews, 17,* 475–513, 1989. Baltimore, MD: Lippincott, Williams & Wilkins.

**p. 238, Figure 8.3** *Source:* McCullagh, P., and Caird, J. A comparison of exemplary and learning sequence models and the use of model knowledge of results to increase learning and performance. *Journal of Human Movement Studies, 18,* 107–116, 1990.

**p. 243, Figure 8.4** *Source:* Weiss, M. R., Ebbeck, V., and Rose, D. J., "Show and tell" in the gymnasium revisited: Developmental differences. *Research Quarterly for Exercise and Sport, 63,* 292–301, 1992.

**p. 246, Figure 8.5** *Source:* Vereijken, B., van Emmerik, R. E. A., Whiting, H. T. A., and Newell, K. M. Freezing degrees of freedom in skill acquisition. *Journal of Motor Behavior, 24*(1), 133–142. Washington D.C.: Heldref Publications, 1992.

**p. 273, Figure 9.4** *Source:* Stelmach, G. E., Efficiency of motor learning as a function of inter-trial rest. *Research Quarterly for Exercise and Sport, 40,* 198–202, 1969.

**p. 299, Figure 10.2** *Source:* Swinnen, S. P., Walter, C. B., Lee, T. D., & Serrien, D. J. (1993). Acquiring bimanual skills: Contrasting forms of information feedback for interlimb decoupling. *Journal of Experimental Psychology: Learning, Memory, and Cognition, 19,* 1328–1344.

**p. 301, Figure 10.3** *Source:* Kernodle, M. W., & Carlton, L. G. (1992). Information feedback and the learning of multiple-degree-of-freedom activities. *Journal of Motor Behavior, 24,*187–196. Washington D.C.: Heldref Publications. Reprinted by permission.

**p. 306, Figure, 10.5** *Source:* Winstein, C. J., & Schmidt, R. A. (1990). Reduced frequency of knowledge of results enhances motor skill learning. *Journal of Experimental Psychology: Learning, Memory, and Cognition, 16,* 677–691.

**p. 308, Figure, 10.6** *Source:* Lavery, J. J. (1962). Retention of simple motor skills as a function of type of knowledge of results. *Canadian Journal of Psychology, 16,* 300–311.

**p. 315, Figure, 10.7** *Source:* Swinnen, S. P., Schmidt, R. A., Nicholoson, D. E., & Shapiro, D. C. (1990). Information feedback for skill acquisition: Instantaneous knowledge of results degrades learning. *Journal of Experimental Psychology: Learning, Memory, and Cognition, 16,* 706–716.

# AUTHOR INDEX

# SUBJECT INDEX

Page references followed by *fig* indicate an illustrated figure; followed by *t* indicate a table; *p* indicate a photo.